STUTTERING

Second Edition

Edward G. Conture

Syracuse University

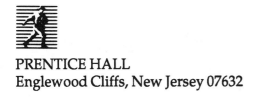

PRENTICE HALL
Englewood Cliffs, New Jersey 07632

Library of Congress Cataloging-in-Publication Data

Conture, Edward G.
  Stuttering / Edward G. Conture. — 2nd ed.
    p.   cm.
  Includes bibliographical references.
  ISBN 0-13-853631-7
  1. Stuttering. I. Title
    RC424.C575   1990
    616.85'54—dc20   89-23179
                                          CIP

REMEDIATION OF COMMUNICATION DISORDERS SERIES

Series Editor, Frederick N. Martin

To My Past and Present Students

Editorial/production supervision: Cyndy Lyle Rymer
Cover design: Diane Saxe
Manufacturing buyer: Ed O'Dougherty

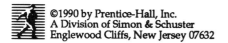©1990 by Prentice-Hall, Inc.
A Division of Simon & Schuster
Englewood Cliffs, New Jersey 07632

Printed in the United States of America
10 9 8 7 6 5 4 3 2 1

0-13-853631-7

Prentice-Hall International (UK) Limited, *London*
Prentice-Hall of Australia Pty. Limited, *Sydney*
Prentice-Hall Canada, Inc., *Toronto*
Prentice-Hall Hispanoamericana, S.A., *Mexico*
Prentice-Hall of India Private Limited, *New Delhi*
Prentice-Hall of Japan, Inc., *Tokyo*
Simon & Schuster Asia Pte. Ltd., *Singapore*
Editora Prentice-Hall do Brasil, Ltda., *Rio de Janeiro*

CONTENTS

SIX CONCLUSIONS *256*

APPENDIX A   INTERVIEW QUESTIONS FOR THE PARENT(S) OF A DISFLUENT CHILD   *293*

APPENDIX B   ONSET OF STUTTERING: A CASE STUDY   *297*

APPENDIX C   NOTE TO A BEGINNING SPEECH-LANGUAGE PATHOLOGIST   *304*

PREFACE

Stuttering has neither been "cured" nor its cause(s) discovered since the first edition of this book was published. As the second edition will reveal, however, a variety of substantive issues have emerged in the past seven to ten years of research and clinical practice, issues which are extremely relevant to the assessment, evaluation, treatment, and understanding of stuttering. Although it would be nice to see the treatment and understanding of stuttering rapidly advance through a quantum leap in knowledge based on a once-in-a-lifetime discovery, the plain truth is that most disciplines advance through the systematic, albeit rather slow, accretion of relatively small bits of information.

So too has our theoretical understanding, as well as therapeutic management of stuttering steadily but slowly advanced through the accumulation of small bits of information resulting from a myriad of research studies as well as clinical practices. Making sense of as well as describing these various "bits of information," particularly in a text having an applied, clinical orientation, is not always easy, but wherever possible we've tried to touch all bases—not just the good ones but the bad and the ugly as well. It is especially challenging to make abstract theoretical and therapeutic issues more concrete and applicable to everyday clinical practice, but we hope that the reader will feel we met this challenge in a readable as well as beneficial fashion. Most of all we have tried not to give the second edition the appearance of a simplistic, unidimensional solution to the complex, multidimensional problem of stuttering.

This clinically oriented book is intended for graduate-level clinicians as well as beginning clinicians in speech-language pathology who are assessing, evaluating, remediating, and trying to further understand stuttering. More experienced clinicians should also find that the second edition covers a variety of issues that they may want to know more about or review in light of current information. I have tried to strike a balance between formal, scholarly documentation, and less formal, clinical or practical experiences as a basis for discussing the evaluation and remediation of stuttering. I have also tried to balance a presentation between the stutterer as a stutterer and the stutterer as a human being. An attempt has been made to view stutterers within the totality of their experiences and existence: a child, teenager, or adult who is a human first and a stutterer second. Hopefully, I have been relatively successful in striking such balances.

ACKNOWLEDGMENTS

A book ultimately requires *one* person to put pen to paper or, in this day and age, fingers to keyboard. No one writes alone, however, since the author, while writing, constantly considers conversations, lectures, and experiences shared with teachers, students, colleagues, friends, and family. While I accept full responsibility for the text and attribute whatever mistakes it may contain, totally to myself, I owe a great deal to others. In the preface to the first edition I acknowledged the many contributions to my personal and professional life made by my parents, family, and professors at Emerson College, Northwestern University, and the University of Iowa, particularly my mentor, Dr. Dean E. Williams; however, the influences of past and present students on my development of the second edition deserves special recognition.

Many consider the influence of teaching to be unidirectional, that is, the teacher influences the student; however, many times this influence is bidirectional, that is, the teacher influences the student and the student influences the teacher. In my experience, such bidirectionality of influence is particularly apparent with doctoral students, and I have been fortunate to have solely or jointly directed the doctoral studies of a series of individuals at Syracuse University. These past and present doctoral students—E. Brayton, A. Caruso, E. Kelly, L. LaSalle, L. Louko, J. Mahshie, D. Metz, H. Schwartz, L. Wolk, and P. Zebrowski—have helped clarify, refine, and shape my theoretical as well as therapeutic approaches to stuttering. These individuals' diverse and manifold influence on my thinking is reflected throughout the second edition. Indeed, it is doubtful whether this book could or would have been written without the influence and help of these doctoral students. Certainly their clinical and classroom interactions and instructions of bachelors' and masters' level students at Syracuse University, either with or without my assistance, have helped me disseminate and test out various ways of expressing my ideas in a manner I could have never accomplished by myself. Thank you all and may you be as fortunate as I and have students as good as you are.

We would also like to acknowledge the manuscript preparation assistance of Pat Grimsley and Donna-Jean Marsula, as well as Linda Cohen's assistance with the development and illustration of figures and tables. I would also like to thank the following for their reviews of the manuscript: Cindy S. Spillers, University of Minnesota–Duluth; Howard D. Schwartz, Northern Illinois University; and Patricia M. Zebrowski, University of Iowa. We were also fortunate to have the administrative support and encouragement of colleagues in Syracuse University's Department of Communication Sciences and Disorders and Division of Special Education and Rehabilitation. Special thanks to the many stutterers, their parents and families, and friends whom we have evaluated, remediated, and interacted with over the years and for whom we have gained so many insights into the problem of stuttering, the world around us and, most certainly, ourself. Preparation of this book was supported in part by a NINCDS contract (N01-NS-0-2331) and OSEP research grants (G000850252 and H023C80008) to Syracuse University.

Bidirectional influences not only occur between students and teachers but between writers and readers. As I wrote, I continually thought about you, the reader, and your varied backgrounds, needs, and interests and this heavily influenced the content and nature of my writing. Now, however, it is my turn to influence you through your reading of my writings. May my influence on you be as positive as I felt yours was on me.

Edward G. Conture

ONE
INTRODUCTION

SOMETHING OF WHAT THIS BOOK IS ABOUT

Stuttering is a complex, multidimensional problem that has defied a variety of simple, unidimensional explanations. Indeed, some explanations have become part of rather than solution for the problem. While some explanations deal nicely with one facet of the problem, they seemingly overlook many others. To paraphrase Sinclair Lewis (1920), the reality of our clinical days has all too often failed to live up to the dreams of our theoretical nights.

And yet, despite these concerns, more and more is known about stuttering and the treatment for this problem slowly but steadily improves. Clearly, stutterers and those who work with them and study their problem have every reason to be optimistic. If asked, however, why one should feel so hopeful, we would reply in one word: honesty. Increasingly, both clinicians and researchers seem more willing to say the magical phrase: I don't know.

For example, I don't know what causes stuttering. I also don't know the best way to treat it. I don't even know if there is *one* way. I'm not sure if anyone else does either. Of one thing I am sure, however: The history of stuttering reflects a multidimensional problem that has repeatedly and successfully defied unidimensional solutions. So, if readers of this book hope that I'm going to reveal *the* cause of stuttering or the silver bullet for "curing" it, they are probably going to be disappointed.

Instead, my purpose in writing this book is to share with the reader approaches to the evaluation and remediation of stuttering that I have found useful and the rationale behind them. I will also discuss problems encountered in their application. Problems? Yes, problems because I think we can learn as much by exploring the darkness of our failures as we can by basking in the light of our successes. This approach is, of course, contrary to the modern tendency toward claiming incredible success rates for this or that therapy.

Indeed, the hype surrounding certain therapies has contributed to feelings of inadequacy by clinicians who are less successful than the famous Dr. X, even though in reality the famous Dr. X also has clinical failures with stutterers. Instead, we need to stop ignoring or downplaying our clinical failures and begin to realize that systematic study of our failures can lead to powerful new insights into the problem. For example, such study may help us identify, prior to beginning therapy, clients most apt to take longer to recover and/or relapse and thus help us to make the necessary adjustments. To paraphrase a popular song, our mistakes are one of the few things we can truly call our own, and if we can't learn from them, who can?

This book, therefore, should not be considered a "how-to" book; rather, it might more appropriately be called a "this is what needs to be considered" book. We will present concepts, ideas, notions, procedures, and strategies that we have found pertinent to consider in the evaluation and management of stuttering. Reading this material will not make the reader an instant expert nor will he or she gain instant expertise or success in the management of stuttering. Rather, we hope to provide both the student-clinician and the practicing speech-language pathologist with meaningful insights into some of the more central, relevant aspects that need to be considered when evaluating or remediating stuttering in children, teenagers, and adults.

GENERAL ORIENTATION

The Common Cold and Stuttering

Discussing the remediation of stuttering is a bit like discussing the remediation of the common cold. Many "remedies" exist for both stuttering and the common cold, with each remedy backed by various forms of evidence. Some professionals advocate one form of remediation while others support different forms with equal enthusiasm. Each approach has its enthusiasts and its skeptics. The enthusiasts claim tremendous success with their approach while the skeptics, hoping to land a knockout punch, continually jab away at the rationale and method.

Possibly, the reason that so many different approaches work is that the terms *common cold* and *stuttering* represent catchalls for a number of related but different problems with different causes. Conversely, others support the notion that common colds or stuttering have unitary symptoms and causes. It is our hunch, however, based on our work as well as others' (for example, Daly, 1981; Preus, 1981; Prins and Lohr, 1972; Schwartz and Conture, 1988) that not only are the speech and related behaviors of stutterers subtly and not so subtly different, but that the reasons for their problems also differ. Just like bananas, oranges, and apples are all called fruit, they all come from different seeds and have somewhat different functions; likewise, some of the things we label and react to as stuttering may have different etiologies and courses of development and may in turn be more or less responsive to different therapeutic approaches. While folk wisdom suggests that chicken soup helps people with colds, similar wisdom suggests that stutterers may be helped by instructing them to "slow down, take a deep breath, and think about what you're saying." Of course, by chance alone, such unidimensional solutions might "cure," at least in some instances, a multidimensional problem. Does this mean that chicken soup "cures" the common cold or that the aforementioned instructions "cure" stuttering? We think not.

Cures Are for Hams and Other Edibles

Anyone who has clinically managed the common cold or the problem of stuttering recognizes one reality: We are not yet at the point where we can meaningfully discuss *curing* most people's common colds or stutterers' stuttering. Cures, outside those applied to hams and other edibles, suggest total, complete, and for all time recovery—something a bit short of miraculous, but nevertheless a remarkable event. While we cannot categorically deny the present existence of a cure for stuttering, it seems far more appropriate at this point in time to discuss our abilities, as speech-language pathologists, to facilitate positive change in the speech and related aspects of individuals who stutter. No, my purpose in writing this book is not to discuss or tout a cure for stuttering. Instead, I would like to keep as close as I can to the facts of the matter and ground my approach in the agony as well as the ecstasy of reality.

Certainly, therapeutic success of a particular method is important; however, success, because of its highly elusive nature, is extremely difficult to determine. For example, how does one define *success*? How long and how many times *after* formal therapy ended was stuttering behavior sampled and under what conditions? What was the nature of the problems exhibited by the clients who received the method? What was their behavior like *before* therapy began? We think these and other questions quickly put into perspective the many claims that this or that therapy procedure results in 80 percent to 90 percent success (cf. Van Riper, 1973, for a more complete overview of therapeutic success with stutterers).

Stuttering, Like a Pendulum, Never Stops in the Middle

One of the first realities about stuttering is that it is first and foremost a behavior that characteristically varies with time and place of communication. It is not static; it is ever changing, particularly in the speech of young children. To ignore such change is to overlook one of the fundamental aspects of this problem: variability.

Researchers are not the only ones who must concern themselves with ranges, variances, standard deviations, and the like. Clinicians, too, must understand that their stuttering client's stuttering varies. Clinicians must try, as best they possibly can, to capture variations in stuttering so that they will not be fooled into thinking that their client's change during therapy is due to their therapy when in actuality it is nothing more than a "natural" variation in the problem. Although it is nice to know about the central tendency (average, median, or mode) of a stutterer's stuttering, if the clinician doesn't also know something about the dispersion of values around that central tendency (for example, the range, variance, standard deviation, or semi-interquartile range), it is very difficult to interpret the representativeness of the central tendency. Stuttering is a fluctuating, dynamically varying behavior. No matter how static or fixed our terms are for describing it, we cannot change its highly variable nature.

To expect that a stutterer's average stuttering frequency reflects what would be observed from minute to minute or day to day would be like expecting to find the next ten people you meet to have an IQ of 100 just because that is the mean for the population. To work with stuttering is to work with a behavior that has a highly variable frequency of occurrence. We are talking plastic here, not concrete.

Nature Interacts with Nurture

In an ideal world things would be clean, simple, and straightforward; unfortunately, this is an imperfect world where things are often dirty, complex, and intertwined with one another. It might be nice, in some ways, if stuttering had a straightforward genetic (cf. Kidd, 1983) or environmental (cf. Johnson et al., 1959) origin; however, neither "pure" nature nor nurture models have been able to adequately explain stuttering (cf. Cox, 1988, for a more recent description of genetic aspects of stuttering and how environmental variables may interact with these aspects). While each nicely describes a piece of the action, neither completely circumscribes the event.

At present, therefore, I take what I believe to be a reasonable, middle-of-the-road approach that considers both nature *and* nurture. This type of approach has been described as an interactionist approach (cf. Purser, 1987, pp. 258–59). In essence, I believe that stuttering relates to a complex *interaction* between the stutterer's environment and the skills and abilities the stutterer brings to that environment. We will elaborate on this notion in the latter part of this chapter, but for now let us make our point by paraphrasing a colloquialism: For most stutterers, it takes two to tango. That is, we believe it takes a unique child in a unique environment for stuttering to have its highest likelihood of occurring and continuing.

Although it is possible that a unique environment (for example, one containing overly critical, perfectionistic, nonsupportive parents) can, by itself, cause stuttering in an otherwise typical youngster, we believe such situations are relatively rare. Likewise, it is possible that a unique child (for example, a child with a delayed and/or deviantly developing neuromotor system) can, by him- or herself, develop stuttering in the presence of an otherwise typical environment; such situations are, we believe, relatively rare. Indeed, we would venture to guess that remediating a young stutterer whose problem relates to an interaction between the child's unique abilities and his/her environment should, in an ideal world, be different from those therapy processes employed for a unique child in a typical environment or for a typical child in a unique environment. Unfortunately, we are still not at a point where we can easily and readily discriminate among young stutterers relative to their etiologies; however, we must continually strive to do so if we are ever to improve the long-term results of our therapy programs for young stutterers.

"Label Jars, Not People"*

Now that I've got your attention, what am I talking about? Simply this: It is not particularly helpful for you to talk to yourself (and you do have to do this many times), fellow professionals, your clients, or their families employing the same terms that your clients use. Rather, you should make every attempt to ensure that your description of your client's concerns, problems, and so forth is as *descriptive, objective,* and *nonjudgmental* as possible. Yes, such terms as stuttering, stutterer, and blocks have their place in our oral and written discussions but not to the exclusion of other far more behavioral, descriptive, and objective terms that actually *describe* what the client is *doing.*

For example, let us say you want to help a friend who has a drinking problem. You might want to begin by telling the friend that he seems to have a drinking problem. To do this, you would have to confront him verbally with the fact of his inappropriate imbibing. You could do this in a variety of ways, but in terms of the types of words you would use you have two choices: (1) Subjective labels carrying judgmental qualities and negative connotations, for example, drunk, souse, alkie, wino versus (2) objective behavioral descriptions, such as, frequently drink too much in too many situations. Likewise, we can label someone as a stutterer or we can say that he is an individual or person who stutters (cf. Conture 1987c). Similarly, we can say

*Poster, Center on Human Policy, Syracuse University

that a person blocked or that the person pressed his lips together for too long and with too much physical tension. Granted, using subjective labels is a convenient and generally shorter means of talking about people and their behavior; however, it is also a means of perpetuating negative stereotypes (cf. Woods and Williams, 1976, for discussion of traits typically assigned to stutterers by speech-language pathologists [SLPs]). What needs to be made clear, however, is that these terms generally don't describe or tell the listener what he or she is actually *doing*. Objective descriptions, on the other hand, while sometimes more verbose, are far less apt to carry negative connotations, be pejorative in nature, and they clearly tell the listener the nature of the behavior being discussed (that is, what the behavior actually sounds, looks, and maybe even feels like).

All of this may sound like a semantic shell game, but a moment's reflection says otherwise. For example, would anyone of sensitivity, social conscience, and tolerance question whether the word "black" is a more appropriate adjective than "colored" for a male or female member of a nonwhite minority group. Similarly, can there be any doubt that the term "Down's Syndrome" is preferable to "mongoloid" or that "not working hard enough" is more descriptive and less pejorative than calling someone "lazy"? The list can go on and on, but the point is that words can hurt you as well as the people you are describing (as the old saying goes, "our words should be soft because we never know when we'll have to eat them"). Words can be used to communicate or they can be used to inappropriately ostracize or segregate. Words used by a professional should be, as much as possible, descriptive in nature, as objective as possible, and carry as many positive or at least neutral connotations as possible. Our words should contribute to a solution for the problem rather than become part of the problem itself.

Psyche as Well as the Soma

Our behavior influences our thinking and our thinking influences our behavior. My orientation to stuttering is based on the belief that the stutterer's psychosocial processes are complexly related to his or her speech production behavior. In my opinion, to understand the psychosocial aspects of stuttering without understanding the physiological aspects (or vice versa) means that one doesn't really understand the problem at all.

It seems inappropriate for a clinician to attempt modifying the disturbed speech production associated with stuttering (for example, Adams, Freeman and Conture, 1984) without considering the psychosocial or emotional components of stuttering and vice versa. It just seems to make common sense that we consider both the psyche (see Sheehan 1970b for overview) and the soma (see Perkins, 1970; Adams, 1974; Freeman, 1979; Adams, Freeman and Conture, 1984; Starkweather, 1982 for overview) of stuttering if we are to adequately diagnose and manage it. Our concern for the psychosocial adjustment problems of the young as well as older stutterer must not, of course, preclude our concern with these clients' speech behavior.

We realize that after all is said and done, our index of clinical success with stutterers will be related to the amount of positive change we have brought about in their speech behavior. Unlike an individual afraid of snakes, who has successfully managed to avoid snakes for years without anyone's noticing, our client's speech behavior is there for the whole world to hear. Unless the stutterer essentially avoids all speaking or happens to be a cave-dwelling hermit, sooner or later he or she will have to speak. And if that stutterer has just gone through your therapy program, every person he or she comes in contact with will shortly know (or at least think they know) the relative success or failure of such therapy. Thus, our consideration of stutterers' psychosocial concerns must take place in the context of our simultaneous consideration of their speech behavior.

Stutterers as People

One of our biggest mistakes is to forget to consider the person who stutters as a person first and a stutterer second. All too often in our sincere, but sometimes overly eager rush to help, we tend to ignore the context of the person's life in our clinical dealings with that person. And, when we do so, we begin to attribute problems and concerns to the fact that the person stutters rather than consider the fact that these issues might just as well be related to other variables in the person's life.

People who stutter have likes and dislikes, highs and lows, brothers and sisters, in-laws and bills to pay, dreams and schemes, just like everyone else. They share in the same human condition that we all experience. To diagnose and remediate people who stutter as if they are isolates, living in a hermetically sealed environment free from concerns of family, society, and life is not only inappropriate, but also poor therapy. Speech-language pathologists need to consider the context of the stutterer's life. This will help them see the individual who stutters as a person, as a functioning individual interacting on a number of levels with a number of people, and as a person, like you and me, unique and without duplicate. This sort of approach helps us put the client's behavior into perspective as we go about evaluating and remediating that client.

As an example, let me describe one of our younger clients with a severe stuttering problem, who opted to join Cub Scouts rather than continue to receive therapy from us. This young client was, right from the beginning, struggling for success in one of our weekly parent-child (P/C) fluency groups (to be discussed in Chapter 3). He was developmentally behind (communicatively and physically) other children of his chronological age and thus he found it quite difficult to compete in the P/C group that contained "older children" of about his same age. Conversely, when placed in another P/C group with younger children, he reacted strongly: He felt these young children were "babies" and he didn't like "the baby games" used with this younger group (not an uncommon reaction, we might add). Stymied, we shared the above information with his mother, who had also observed the same situation, and seemed as perplexed as we were on how to proceed. During our discussion with the mother, it became clear that this boy had really wanted to join a local Cub Scout group ("all his classmates are") but the P/C group was scheduled at the same time as the weekly Cub Scout meeting. A scheduled break from therapy ensued and when we next contacted the mother to resume therapy with her son she informed us that she had enrolled her son in Cub Scouts rather than our P/C group. Our first reaction, naturally enough, was, "How could you?" (or words to that effect). We explained the seriousness of her son's problem and his needs for continued therapy. However, after cooling down a bit and listening to the mother, it became clear that at this point in time Cub Scouts, its attendant socialization, and sense of being similar to one's peers were far more important for this child than our therapy. We told the mother to continue with the Cub Scouts, but to tell her son that sometime in the future he would need to resume therapy and that once he got established with his Cub Scout group that perhaps he could be late once in a while for the beginning of the meetings. After a four-month break, the boy resumed with our "younger" P/C group, and continued attending his weekly Cub Scouts meetings. He is making excellent, if slow progress. Whatever he has gotten from participating in Cub Scouts seems to have given him the security necessary to handle the approaches we use with the younger children and benefit from the experience.

What is the point? Well, by assuming that the child's needs for our therapy outweighed his needs for the socialization associated with Cub Scouts, we would have been making a big mistake. As hard as it was at the time, we were luckily able to realize that there might be more to this client's life than just becoming more fluent (like being one of the guys) and we were able to resolve a clinical dilemma. We wish that all our clinical problems were so easily solved. Keeping the perspective that the person who stutters is a person first, and a stutterer second, helps us to understand, if not resolve, many such issues.

Individuals Stutter but They Are Still Individuals

Similarly, when considering stutterers as people, we should also consider each stutterer's individuality (Van Riper, 1973). While there may be important commonalities among our clients, what may be appropriate in Sally's situation may not work with John. Of course, gearing therapy procedures to the individual needs and abilities of various clients is not always easy or possible. Nevertheless, we should at least recognize each client's individuality and not generalize.

Procedures that make good sense to Mr. and Mrs. Brown for their little Joey may totally baffle and confuse Mr. and Mrs. Peterson in their dealings with their daughter Jane. Likewise, some clients need explicit rationale and reason for each and every step of our clinical attempts to change their stuttering whereas others simply want the procedure and not the explanation. What may take one client a couple of sessions to learn or understand may take another individual who stutters many sessions of intensive remediation. Reasons for these individual differences are not necessarily related to intelligence; such differences may relate to a stutterer's relative willingness to work at change, different levels of motivation, and high degrees of emotionality surrounding the stuttering problem that make it difficult for the client to deal objectively with the problem.

In other words, while we must strive to recognize certain commonalities among our clients who stutter, we must also recognize the range of individuals who surround, on both sides, such typicalness. Just as the fact that the average IQ is 100 does not mean that the "average" individual has an IQ equal to 100, so do we find that all stutterers' problems and related concerns are not identical. Stuttering is a behavior that varies around some central tendency. To overgeneralize and expect every individual who stutters to be the same, just because they stutter, is to oversimplify. Remember, stutterers don't enter your clinical doors in a group—they walk in as individuals.

Tolerating Individual Differences

My clinical experience indicates that speech fluency is one area of human behavior in which we have little tolerance for individual differences. We appear to accept the fact that some people can run, jump, climb, and calculate farther, faster, higher, and more accurately and at earlier ages than other people. We are somewhat tolerant of height and weight differences among people. We are not quite as tolerant, however, of differences among people in terms of speech fluency and speech and language behavior.

Many individuals implicitly or explicitly express their unwillingness to accept the fact that some children go through periods of disfluency for longer durations than other children or that some children go through these periods of disfluency at later or earlier periods than their peers do. For example, my son, when nearing his ninth birthday, went through a period of about two weeks in which he produced a fair number of whole-word repetitions and more than his normal amount of part-word repetitions. Up to that time, his speech (dis)fluency had never been something we or anyone else had ever thought particularly different from that of other children his age. Other parents have reported similar increments in speech disfluency in the communication of their eight- to ten-year-old children.

Are these instances of disfluency peculiar to this age group? Are they indicative of particular pressures we parents or the schools or society place on this age child? Are these disfluencies related to sudden spurts in vocabulary growth or language or cognitive development? Do these disfluencies represent a discoordination in the timing and spatial movements of speech structures that may be related to some as yet unknown neuromotor or similar developmental change peculiar to this age child? (See, for example, Perkins and others, 1976; Perkins, 1978; Caruso, Conture and Colton, 1988; Conture, Colton and Gleason, 1988). The answers to these questions are still vague, but we believe that the speech fluency of *all* speakers, particularly children, is highly variable within as well as between speakers and that these differences are complexly related to a myriad of nature as well as nurture factors.

So, who cares? Of what earthly good is making such an apparent, as-plain-as-the-nose-on-your-face observation? Well, too often, the apparent and the familiar are overlooked in our attempts to be creative and novel. At the least, continually recognizing that not everybody is as fluent and articulate as Walter Cronkite, at least most of the time, helps us recognize that the individual we are evaluating may be developing, no matter how slowly or unevenly, in a "normal" fashion. We will shortly discuss our belief that as many as 40 percent to 50 percent of children frequently exhibiting within-word disfluencies will probably eventually become fluent with or without therapeutic intervention. Our job, of course, is to decide which children should and which should not receive our services. Conversely, if we fail to make these decisions and merely include *everybody* on our clinical caseloads, it then becomes rather problematic how we can claim high degrees of success when perhaps as many as 50 percent of our cases would have improved on their own. Speech disfluency, whether of the within- or between-word kind, is first and foremost a behavior, and simply put, a behavior that varies within and among people.

While a sizable proportion of the lay public may remain relatively intolerant of such differences, we as speech-language pathologists, while recognizing the importance of fluent, articulate speech to a full and productive life, must demonstrate our tolerance in word and deed for individual differences and stop trying to fix what may not be broken but merely different. As Starkweather (1987) so aptly said, "The goal of therapy is not total fluency but normal disfluency." Here he recognizes that people, no matter how apparently "normally fluent," are also sometimes normally disfluent and that to try to make our clients who stutter *totally* fluent is about as realistic a goal as to make everybody perfect. Individuals are and will continue to differ in their speech fluency and such differences don't mean that they are bad people, just people.

Categorizing Noncategorical Behavior

We are inclined to view fluency and stuttering along a continuum rather than as discrete categories. For example, on one occasion listeners would problably accept as "marginally fluent" a young stutterer's /p/ in the production of the word popcorn that contained a slightly longer than normal stop phase (an *alpha* behavior to be discussed shortly). Or on another occasion, if the young stutterer maintains the stop phase for a bit longer, for example, 100 ms to 200 ms, listeners might judge it as a silent sound prolongation, block, hesitation, or stuttering.

First, we can consider categorizing on the basis of *frequency* of disfluency. Table 1–1, based on data reported by Johnson and others (1959), mirrors our clinical experience. This table shows that very few, if any, children who produce an average of 3 or more *within-word* disfluencies per 100 words are *apt* to be called stutterers. However, as Table 1–1 also shows, the populations—stutterers and normally fluent speakers—overlap in terms of the number of exhibited *within-word* speech disfluencies, and thus there will always be some "stutterers" who produce 1 to 2 within-word disfluencies per 100 words as well as some "normally fluent" speakers who produce 1 or 2 within-word disfluencies per 100 words.

Thus, try as we might, categorizing stutterers and normally fluent speakers by frequency of stuttering or within-word disfluencies will always mean that a small percentage of normally fluent speakers will produce a frequency of within-word disfluencies similar to that of stutterers and vice versa. In essence, our decision rules for demarking or placing categorical boundaries onto a process based on a continuum means that some constant error will be produced. Therefore, the only debate can be the size and nature of the error because such an error (false positive/false negative) will always

TABLE 1–1. Decile distribution of frequency of *within-word* disfluencies (sound/syllable repetitions+broken words+sound prolongations) per 100 words spoken by 68 young male stutterers, 68 young male normally fluent speakers, 21 young female stutterers, and 21 young female normally fluent speakers.

DECILE DISTRIBUTION OF FREQUENCY OF WITHIN-WORD DISFLUENCY	YOUNG MALE STUTT (N = 68)	YOUNG MALE NF (N = 68)	YOUNG FEMALE STUTT (N = 21)	YOUNG FEMALE NF (N = 21)
1	0.43	0.00	0.50	0.00
2	0.93	0.00	0.64	0.25
3	1.68	0.22	1.53	0.26
4	2.84	0.40	2.38	0.29
5	3.77	0.55	2.80	0.53
6	5.04	0.60	4.47	0.55
7	7.06	0.95	6.01	0.95
8	10.07	1.22	7.29	1.60
9	17.47	2.16	11.95	2.37

STUTT = Stutterer and NF = Normally Fluent.

Diagnosis

"Reality"	Positive (Stutterer)	Negative (Normally Fluent)
True	(Hit) Call a child a Stutterer who actually is	(Correct Rejection) Call a child a normally fluent speaker who actually is
False	(False Positive) Call a child a stutterer who is actually normally fluent	(Miss) Call a child a normally fluent speaker who actually is a stutterer

FIGURE 1–1. Four possible relations between the diagnostic decision that (a) an individual is or is not a stutterer and (b) the "reality" of whether the person actually is or is not a stutterer. While many clinicians seem concerned about committing false positives relative to stuttering, it is the writer's experience that a "miss" or false negative is just as likely if not more likely to occur (adapted from Thorner and Remein, 1982).

take place (cf. Thorner and Remein, 1982, for excellent discussion of this issue). Figure 1–1 shows the various types of diagnostic decisions and errors that can be made when evaluating stuttering; however, there are no published data, to my knowledge, specifying the number or percentage of times the average clinician makes each of these decisions/errors.

Second, we might try to categorize or dichotomize stuttering and fluency into two separate categories on the basis of the *type* of speech disfluency exhibited; however, even this approach has some difficulties. One typical way of making such dichotomies is to consider within-word disfluencies (for example, sound/syllable repetitions) as *stuttered* and between-word disfluencies (for example revisions) as *normal* disfluencies (cf. Conture, 1982). However, sometimes even within-word disfluencies will be judged as "normal" or fluent. Let us return to our previous example. If the stop phase of a young stutterers's /p/ in the word popcorn is held a bit longer than typical, for example, 100 ms to 200 ms, some might judge it as a silent sound prolongation or stuttering, whereas if the same stutterer holds the stop phase on a /p/ in another production of popcorn for a shorter duration, say, 50 ms to 75 ms, some might judge this to be fluent or at least marginally fluent. That is, in this case, the judgment of stuttered versus fluent merely has to do with the duration of the stop phase and not the fact that the two speech events represent two different kinds or types of speech production. Indeed, differences in the duration of speech behavior are just as apt to result in a judgment of stuttering as are differences in the actual nature of speech production. It is as if the duration of a certain speech disfluency has to cross over some as yet unknown *threshold of acceptability* and once having done so, the disfluency becomes labeled as "stuttered."

The point in all this is that even such within-word disfluencies as sound/syllable repetitions and sound prolongations, which are most apt to be considered stuttered, are sometimes produced in such a way as to be judged fluent (Boehmler, 1958; Williams and Kent, 1958; Schiavetti, 1975). In essence, try as we might, our definition of what is and what is not stuttered will have to remain relative and not absolute. Guidelines can be put forth in terms of the type and frequency of disfluency that may be considered stuttered or that might warrant an individual speaker being considered a stutterer, but these guidelines are just that—guidelines—and major exceptions to the rule can and will be observed.

Rationales versus Recipes

We believe that clinicians should try to understand, as best they can, the reasons behind a method as well as the method itself. We, as clinicians, should try to understand why an advocated method is believed to work (I am not referring to simple recipes for clinical success that must be dutifully followed step by step).

If a clinician does not know why a method is advocated, why it is thought to work, and how it might be modified or adapted to suit the needs of each individual case, the clinician may blindly follow one set of instructions in all therapy situations. Granted, it is important to know how to follow the instructions *quickly and correctly* in order to make the method work. However, if all we know is the method itself, then we become like poorly trained auto mechanics who wonder why their standard tools don't work with a "new" car that has metric fittings. Eventually, the day comes when the procedure does not work with this or that client. Without knowing why the procedure was supposed to work in the first place and its basic rationale, the clinician will find it difficult to adjust the procedure to meet the client's individual needs.

Tightly structured programs for the remediation of stuttering may give clinicians the impression that they know what they are about, what they need to do, and how to do it. Such programs are many times suitable for certain stutterers or for certain aspects of certain stutterers; however, difficulties arise when exceptions to the rule or new information occur that cast doubts on the prescribed program. One should not confuse the confident manner of the cookbook-oriented clinician who works with stutterers with that clinician's expertise and ability to handle *all* clinical problems relative to stuttering. Such clinicians, in my experience, may reject or vigorously disagree with information or approaches that fall outside the realm of their rigidly prescribed approach. Clinicians who seek and want to learn only *the program* often find it difficult to adjust to the clinical exception and to be flexible enough to deal with new information and changing approaches. The *recipe* or *cookbook* approach, particularly in view of the present state of our clinical art in stuttering, appears to hamper future growth in a clinician's ability to evaluate and remediate stuttering. With stuttering, change is apt to be constant.

WHAT IS STUTTERING?

Types of Disfluency Labeled Stuttering

Table 1–2 lists a variety of disfluency types and the probability that each will be considered by listeners to be a "stuttered" versus "normal" disfluency. As this table shows, listeners are most *apt* to perceive a speech disfluency as stuttering when a speaker produces a word that contains any one or combination of the following: (1) a sound or syllable repetition, (2) a sound prolongation, (3) an unusual pause between the sounds or syllables of a word, and (4) (in some instances) a repetition of a monosyllabic whole word. Of course, other types of speech disfluency and behavior can and are associated with listener perceptions of stuttering (cf. Young, 1984), but these other disfluency types, while not unimportant, are not the *usual* or typical associates of listeners' perceptions of stuttering.

Notice the phrase "listeners' perceptions of stuttering"; we need to be clear that perceptions of stuttering involve listener evaluations. At present there are no machines—analog, digital, or otherwise—into which we can input audio- or videotapes of speech and related behavior of suspected stutterers that can readily tell us (1) which sounds, syllables, words, phrases, or sentences are *stuttered* or contain instances of *stuttering*, and (2) whether the speaker who produces these speech events is a *stutterer*. We, the trained listener, must decide, after careful and (hopefully) objective assessment, whether we consider a particular speech behavior indicative of stuttering as well as whether the person who produced that behavior is or is not a stutterer.

Listeners' Judgments Differ as Much as the Behavior They Judge

Herein lies the problem: Judgments of stuttering involve perceptual evaluations. When two or more people observe and report an event such as an auto crash, their judgments and evaluations are subjective, variable, and difficult to make. These differences in listener judgments, if given a moment's thought, should not surprise us. If a speaker's speech fluency is a behavior that differs among and between speakers, why wouldn't listener perceptions

TABLE 1–2. Examples of various types of within-word ("stuttered") and between-word ("normal") speech disfluencies.

DISFLUENCY TYPE	CATEGORY WITHIN-WORD*	BETWEEN-WORD	EXAMPLES
Sound/syllable repetitions	X		"He is run-ruh-running." "It is abou-about time." "See the ba-ba-baby." "You t-t-take it."
Sound prolongation	X		"Mmmmmmore cake please." "T-(silence while person holds articulatory posture for 't')-oday is Monday."
Broken word	X		"I was g-(pause)-oing." Distinguishing broken words from sound prolongations is not always possible or easy.
Monosyllabic whole-word repetitions	X	X	"I-I-I can't do that." "He-he-he is a big boy."
Multisyllabic whole-word repetitions		X	"She really-really is here."
Phrase repetition		X	"I was - I was there."
Interjection		X	"I will, uhm, you know, be late."
Revision		X	"She is - she was here"

*Within-word disfluencies are most apt to be considered "stuttered" and between-word disfluencies most likely to be perceived as "normal" (cf. Bloodstein, 1987). One exception is monosyllabic whole-word repetitions which are sometimes judged stuttered and other times as nonstuttered. This judgment seems to be dependent on associated physical tension, rate of repetition, and other, as yet unknown, factors (cf. Conture, 1982a). For the present discussion, monosyllabic whole-word repetitions will be considered to be within-word or stuttered disfluencies.

Source: After Conture, 1982a, p. 164.

of these events differ among and between listeners? Recognizing the variability and difficulty of making such perceptual evaluations need not discourage us from developing a reasonably complete index of those events that are most apt to be perceived as stuttered, but it should alert us to the fact that this is not a simple undertaking.

Relative versus Absolute Definitions of Stuttering

It is very difficult, if not impossible, as we will discuss later in this chapter, to develop *absolute* definitions of what is and what is not a stuttering and who is and who is not a stutterer (Bloodstein, 1987). However, it is possible to develop *relative* definitions that capture the essentials of what is stuttering and who is a stutterer (Wingate, 1964). We use the word *apt* purposely to highlight the fact that this definition involves a statement of probability rather than one of certainty. For example, it is a statement of certainty that the sun will come up tomorrow, but a statement of probability that this or that horse will win the Kentucky Derby. Comics who attempt to imitate stutterers as part of their act are *apt* or *most likely* to select within-word rather than between-word disfluencies. Once again, the phrase *most likely* denotes an event that is relatively (probably) rather than absolutely (certainly) likely to occur. It is, of course, possible that a listener may perceive a particular between-word disfluency (for example, a revision) as stuttered and a particular within-word disfluency (for example, a sound prolongation) as normally disfluent. Possible but not as probable.

Nonspeech Behaviors Associated with Instances of Stuttering

Besides those speech events that are most probably associated with listener perceptions of stuttering, listeners may also see and hear at least two other events associated with stuttering: (1) (non)verbal reports of bodily movement and tension and (2) (non)verbal reports of psychosocial discomfort and concern (Bloodstein, 1987). These two events, along with the speech behavior itself, make up a behavioral composite that many SLPs have difficulty describing clearly and adequately. Indeed, the beginning SLP or student SLP may be so challenged by trying to describe and understand these (non)verbal behaviors and reports of bodily movement, tension, and psychosocial discomfort and/or concern that he or she totally misses the client's actual speaking behavior.

In our opinion, SLPs who remediate stuttering should be able to do what we term *parallel-process* (with all due apologies to my colleagues in speech science): simultaneously process or handle different types of information coming from different sources or modalities. In our opinion, remediating stuttering should not be undertaken by an SLP who cannot or will not simultaneously process different events, each perhaps related to one another, but with its own seriated time course and meaning to the overall problem.

As early as 1940, Barr suggested that nonspeech behavior should be considered when evaluating stutterers' speech. While we think many clinicians would agree with this observation, it is interesting that to our knowledge there have been very few empirical studies of nonverbal behavior associated with stuttering (Prins and Lohr, 1972; Krause, 1982; Schwartz and Conture, 1988; Conture and Kelly, 1988a). Thus, although tests like the Iowa Scale Stuttering Severity (Johnson, Darley and Spriestersbach, 1963) or the Stuttering Severity Instrument (Riley, 1980) attempt to assess nonverbal associates of stuttering, and (non)verbal movements and tension are commonly observed to be associated with stuttering (Brutten and Shoemaker, 1967), the fact remains that we have little objective information regarding the average range, number, and nature of nonverbal behaviors during stuttering, particularly during typical parent-child communicative interaction.

In attempts to rectify this paucity of information, we (Conture and Kelly, 1988a) have undertaken and nearly completed a study of 30 young (3 to 7 year old) stutterers' and their mothers' nonverbal behavior during stuttering in comparison to that of their normally fluent peers and their mothers during comparable fluent utterances. As part of this study, we assessed more than 50 different nonverbal "gestures" and found that the young stutterers produced more nonverbal behaviors during their stutterings than their normally fluent peers did during comparable fluent production. Furthermore, while there was similarity between the two talker groups in terms of nonverbal behavior, there were also differences. That is, the young stutterers were much more likely to move their eyeballs to the left or right or to partially or completely obscure their view of the listener by blinking eyelids and/or raising their lower lip in apparent reactions of disgust (and as Atkins [1989] shows, "poor" eye contact adversely affects a listener's perceptions of a speaker's personality). Although space does not permit an in-depth evaluation of the meaning of these behaviors, the following conclusions can be stated at this point: (1) Children who stutter, at or near the onset of their problem, exhibit a relatively large number and variety of nonverbal behaviors in association with their stutterings, and (2) most of these nonverbal behaviors seem to minimize young stutterers' visual information about their listening partners' reactions to their speech behavior and/or themselves (this would be an example of disruption in "oculesics," cf. Egolf and Chester, 1973).

In essence, facial gestures, bodily movements, and tensing may suggest that the stutterer is trying to cope with the stuttering itself. (In a slightly different vein, Sheehan, 1958, speculated that the nature of these nonverbal behaviors is projective of the individual "behind" the stuttering; that is, "active" or "aggressive" individuals who stutter might produce a greater number and variety of associated behaviors than a more "passive" individual who stutters.)

Perhaps, a head turn to the right, neatly time-locked with the initiation of the articulatory contact of a feared sound or syllable, may indicate the stutterer's belief that this head turning will "get the sound out." And as others have previously discussed (Williams, 1971), if a little bit of movement and tensing helps, in this case head movement and probably neck/shoulder muscle contraction, then a great deal more should really help.

Unfortunately, these associated nonverbal behaviors occasionally "work!" That is, by seemingly chance association with successful forward movement through a sound, syllable, or word, these associated behaviors appear to become reinforced in much the same way that the green shirt the pitcher wore on the day he pitched a no-hitter takes on special properties (see Skinner, 1953; Lefrancois, 1972; Hill, 1985, for discussion of superstitious behavior). Both the green shirt and the head turning are respectively viewed by the pitcher and stutterer as helping or being essential to successful completion of the task at hand. Unfortunately for the person who stutters, behavior cannot be discarded as easily as a shirt and all too often stutterers' associated behavior becomes once again, part of, rather than solution for, the problem.

Along with these nonverbal behaviors and verbal reports of bodily movement and/or tension in (non)speech structures and musculature, we may see and hear, from individuals who stutter, events indicative of psychological discomfort and concern. These reports (and they are generally, though not exclusively, verbal) may indicate that the stutterer is feeling fearful, frustrated, embarassed, nervous, anxious, angry, uncomfortable, or some other affective state. Basically, these reports indicate that during and/or in anticipation of moments of stuttering and during speech in general, the stutterer is in a state of emotional discomfort. In fact, the very act of stuttering (the repeating and prolonging of sounds) is taken by many to mean that the individual who produced them is "tense," or "nervous," or "anxious." Disregarding for the time being speech behaviors like sound/syllable repetitions, we are specifically referring to such things as consistent aversion of eye contact with listeners that may indicate fear, anxiety, or awareness of a problem. Sometimes observers note that even the body posture of the individual who stutters may appear different. For example, we have noticed, particularly with adults who have been stuttering for some time, that their general body posture seems to become increasingly rigid or nonmovable when they speak, especially when they are about to stutter or are in the middle of an instance of stuttering.

These observations, I hasten to add, are in need of empirical testing. Frequent breaks in listener eye contact by means of turning the eyeballs, closing the eyelids, turning the head, or any combination of these behaviors, particularly with young children, may be a sign that all is not right regarding the children's feelings about themselves, their speaking ability, and speaking in general (cf. Schwartz and Conture, 1988). In later sections we discuss the apparent feelings associated with some of the more common nonverbal and verbal reports of psychosocial discomfort. It is our opinion that if we do not deal with these feelings, they may stand in the way of long-term successful remediation.

Parental Reaction to Child Stuttering and Associated Behavior

Interestingly, certain aspects of both the nonverbal behaviors themselves and self-reports of psychosocial concerns are of particular concern to the parents of the young stutterer. For example, parents often seem to show considerable concern about their child's facial grimacing, head jerking, and verbal reports of fear or embarrassment. However, these same parents, as well as other listeners and the stutterers themselves, may be apt to show less concern about sound prolongations than they are about sound/syllable repetitions. There appear to be different responses, on the part of the listener, to various aspects of a speaker's disfluent speech production and associated behavior (for example, Williams and Kent, 1958; Huffman and Perkins, 1974; Zebrowski and Conture, 1989). Not all speech and nonspeech behaviors associated with stuttering are judged equally noxious; an individual listener may be particularly intolerant of a specific aspect of disfluent speaking behavior. We have seen more than one parent who could listen to their child prolong sounds all day and not seem to care very much; however, let that same child repeat the same sounds and the parent would respond with, "You know better than that," or "Stop that this instant."

Listeners are most apt to judge, as an instance of stuttering, those speech events in which a word contains a sound/syllable repetition, a sound prolongation, an inappropriate pause between sounds or syllables, or (on some occasions) repetitions of monosyllabic whole words. Other events, as we have said, may also on occasion be considered as stuttering (for example, repetition of between-word interjections like "uh-uh-uh"). However, as mentioned above, most speech behavior that listeners label as stuttering may be associated with one or both of the following: (1) nonverbal and verbal reports of bodily movement and tension in (non)speech structures and musculature, and/or (2) (non)verbal reports of psychosocial discomfort and concern. And, as we mentioned, within-word disfluencies are most apt to be perceived by listeners as stuttered (for example, Boehmler, 1958; Williams and Kent, 1958; Zebrowski and Conture, 1989); however, this is a statement of relative rather than absolute certainty. We are still far from clearly knowing why listeners react in this way, but in later sections we present some speculation about listener reactions.

At this point, however, we shift our attention to considerations of the onset and development of stuttering, with particular reference to the speech production aspects of this development. We hope that the following discussion is not taken as the *truth*, but rather as one possible means by which we can view the development of stuttered speech behavior. Although much has been learned in recent years regarding disturbances in speech production associated with stuttering, we are not in a position, at this time, to pour such knowledge into concrete. Instead, we believe that we must be tolerant about the evolving state of the art and science of stuttering in this area and that we should be most willing to consider *likely* rather than *certain* explanations. Furthermore, the more sources of input we get from as many different perspectives as possible the greater the possibility that no relevant issue will be overlooked.

We can appreciate the sentiments of some (Smith and Weber, 1988) that we may be suffering from a cornucopia of perspectives relative to stuttering. The too-many-cooks-spoil-the-broth status of stuttering theory and therapy is quite confusing, particularly for students in training. Disagreement for disagreement's sake is, to put it mildly, ludicrous. However, it is only through this apparent heterogeneity of opinion and the resulting tension of divergent perspectives that the truth, if it is ever to be found, will emerge. Disagreements, not agreements, foster and encourage new insights into old problems and are the stuff from which progress is made. However, while we may agree to disagree, we should be able to do this without becoming disagreeable.

ONSET AND DEVELOPMENT OF STUTTERING

Stuttering has been called a disorder of childhood (for example, Bloodstein, 1987). Indeed, it is probably safe to assume that the rather long duration sound prolongations of an adult with a severe stuttering problem did not develop overnight. Surely, when this adult stutterer was a child, his or her instances of stuttering were somewhat shorter in duration, probably less frequently exhibited, and possessed less audible manifestations of physiological tension than the adult form of the problem.

What We Know about Young Stutterers' Speech Production

What do we actually know about the beginning nature of stutterers' stuttering, particularly on the level of speech production? In the early to mid-1980s, when I first posed this rhetorical question, I answered by saying that there was very little information about young stutterers' speech production, despite the plethora of investigations of adult stutterers' speech production during stuttering and fluency available at that time (for example, Conture, McCall, and Brewer, 1977; Conture, Schwartz and Brewer, 1985; Freeman and Ushijima, 1978; Zimmerman, 1980a, 1980b; Shapiro, 1980; Stromsta and Fibiger, 1980). Now, in the late 1980s, several studies of young stutterers' speech production during stuttering and fluency have been reported (for example, Adams, 1987; Pindzola, 1986; Caruso, Conture and Colton, 1988; Conture, Colton and Gleason, 1988; Conture, Rothenberg and Molitor, 1986; McMillan and Pindzola, 1986; McNight and Cullinan, 1987; Schwartz, 1987; Zebrowski, Conture and Cudahy, 1985). These studies now provide us with much more freedom to speculate regarding the ways children who stutter may or may not use their speech production mechanism.

Let us try to ground this discussion in known fact. Caruso, Conture and Colton (1988) reported that the "integrity of young stutterers' speech production mechanism remains intact during stuttering. That is, even during stuttering, the relative sequence of movement and muscle activity onsets is generally similar (for approximately 85 percent of all stutterings analyzed in this study) to that of normally fluent youngsters' fluent utterances" (p. 75). Similarly, Conture, Colton and Gleason (1988) report that "there were no apparent differences during perceptually fluent speech between young stutterers and their normally fluent peers in terms of the selected temporal measures of speech production. . . .that, at least for perceptually fluent speech production, youngsters who stutter are similar to normally fluent children in terms of temporal onsets, offsets and durations of speech production events" (p. 24).

Thus, relatively "gross" indexes of temporal aspects of speech production indicate that young stutterers are not appreciably different from their normally fluent peers; however, other studies indicate that young stutterers may produce brief, subtle disruptions in speech production more often than their normally fluent peers (for example, Conture, Rothenberg, and Molitor, 1986). Finding brief, subtle disruptions in speech production is consistent with Conture's (1982) speculation of "alpha" behavior (pp. 11–14) that will be discussed below.

Children Are Not Adults, Just Smaller

Prior to such discussion, a word or two must be said about research into the speech production abilities of adults versus children who stutter (cf. Conture, 1987, for review of this area). First, it is not clear how much one can readily apply findings about adults who stutter to children who stutter and vice versa. This apparent inability to extrapolate from adult to child and vice versa seems to come from two sources:

1. *History*—It is possible that the aberrant speech behaviors of adult stutterers could be the result of a well-established, long-term history of dealing with and/or reacting to stuttering.
2. *Probability*—Figure 1–2 shows two different models. One model suggests that not every child who stutters has an equal probability of becoming an adult who stutters. That is, an adult who stutters was different as a child from the average child who stutters. Figure 1–2 also shows that the converse model may be true: All young stutterers may have an equal probability of becoming an adult who stutters. That is, an adult who stutters was no different as a child from the average child who stutters.

It is unclear which of these two models—*unequal* or *equal* probability—best explains the relation between adults and children who stutter, but we are betting that the "unequal" model, or something like it, will eventually be shown to be the truth.

Second, procedures used to study the speech production of adults cannot be readily applied to children unless significant modifications are made (cf. Conture, 1987), and as findings are not always based on similar

EQUAL PROBABILITY

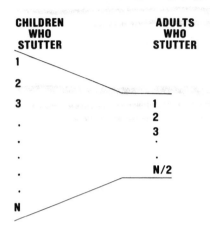

UNEQUAL PROBABILITY

FIGURE 1-2. Two models—"equal" versus "unequal" probability—describing the relation between the number of children and the number of adults who stutter. The total number of children (N) is conservatively estimated to decrease approximately 50% (N/2) by adulthood. With the *equal probability* model all children who stutter are equally likely to become an adult who stutters, while the *unequal probability* model suggests that only a certain strata level or subgroup of children who stutter are likely to become adults who stutter.

methodologies, comparison is difficult. Third, children are still developing their speech production abilities, whether they are stutterers are not, and thus comparing these still-developing abilities to those of supposed established adult speakers would appear to be problematic.

In summary, although aberrancies in the speech production of adults who stutter may tell us little about the speech production abilities of the typical child who stutters, they may still have a great deal of salience for understanding what adult stutterers do when they talk (for example, Conture, Schwartz and Brewer, 1985; Guitar, Guitar, Neilson, O'Dwyer and Andrews, 1988).

Alpha-Delta Hypothesis Revisited

Given the above caveats, we speculate that children who stutter, particularly those who will require some period of therapy, are exhibiting brief, subtle inefficiencies during the entirety of their speech production, the fluent as well as disfluent aspects. Such inefficient, atypical behavior is also exhibited by normally fluent children but children who stutter more frequently exhibit these atypical behaviors (for example, Conture, Rothenberg and Molitor, 1986). It should be stressed that in all my studies of young stutterers I have never found one behavior exhibited by them that was not also exhibited, at least on occasion, by their normally fluent peers or vice versa. It is as if the child who stutters is producing speech by using one of several different means but the means used may be less resistant to internal and external stressors, for example, cognitive or psychosocial demands.

We might draw an analogy to walking. Many different gaits and steps are used by different people to walk, but as long as they get the person from point A to point B, no one is concerned. However, it is possible that some of these gaits and steps are more resistant to stress than other gaits (for example, "stressors" like having to walk faster to catch a bus, walking on crowded sidewalks where one is jostled or hurried along, or walking on slippery pavements where one could fall). Since some forms of walking are less likely to result in halting, tripping, stumbling, or shuffling during stress, their continued use during stress will ensure a minimum of disruption in rate, effort, and smoothness of stride.

Likewise, some forms of speech production might be more resistant to stress than others and continue to perform with a minimum disruption in such things as fluency, rate, and efficiency. These resistant to stress (RTS) speech productions are to be contrasted with those speech productions that are relatively sensitive to stress (STS). This notion is somewhat similar to previous speculation by Brutten and Shoemaker (1967) that certain "fine" motor acts may be more susceptible to disruption through internal/external stressors (termed "negative emotion" by Brutten and Shoemaker) that can become associated with and thus "conditioned" to occur in the presence of various stimuli.

We speculate, therefore, that the speech of children who stutter more frequently contains alpha behaviors (speech that is more STS and less RTS) and that the relatively high frequency of these alpha behaviors puts the young stutterer at risk for disruptions in fluency. This is in contrast to his or her normally fluent peers whose speech contains far fewer alpha behaviors (speech that is less STS and more RTS). In essence, the young stutterer's ratio

TABLE 1–3.   Possible developmental stages of speech production and related behavior associated with stuttering.

	DEVELOP-MENTAL STAGE	BEHAVIORAL DESCRIPTION	COMMENTS
Early	(1) *Alpha*	(1) Brief, nonperceptible (to listener) *inefficiencies* or *aberrancies* in speech production, for example, brief within-word pauses, laryngeal catches, or articulatory arrests at beginning of utterance or at transition between sounds and syllables	(1) *Alpha* resulting from one of three combinations of child and environment (i) Typical child speaking in unique environment or (ii) unique child speaking in typical environment or (iii) unique child speaking in unique environment
	(2) *Beta*	(2) Brief to lengthy *repetitive* or *oscillatory* speech productions used as compensatory and/or coping reactions to *Alpha*, for example, laryngeal adduction (inspiratory gesture and nostril flaring) alternating with adduction	(2) *Beta* results in sound-syllable repetitions; child "uses" *Beta* to adjust to, override, or release from *Alpha*
Listed in order of occurrence	(3) *Gamma*	(3) Brief to lengthy *stabilized* or *fixed*, relatively tense, speech production used as compensation or coping reactions to *Beta*, for example, fixed laryngeal adductory posture, labial contact, or lingual posturing	(3) *Gamma* results in audible or inaudible sound prolongation or cessation in speech productions; child uses this to minimize the highly variable, repetitive behavior of *Beta* but still atypical end product
Later	(4) *Delta*	(4) Brief to lengthy *adjustive* or *reactive* speech or nonspeech behavior used as coping reactions to *Gamma*, sometimes *Beta* and, possibly in some instances, to *Alpha*; for example, pharyngeal muscle constriction, vocal fold lengthening (pitch rises), vocal fold shortening, where arytenoids approximate base of epiglottis (bearing down), blinking of eyelids, eyeball movements used to break listener eye contact	(4) *Delta* adjustive or reactive behavior may or may not have acoustic correlate, but probably does; one of more noticeable aspects of an instance of stuttering

TABLE 1–4. Three possible developmental sequences of Alpha-Delta behavior associated with stuttering and speculations regarding chronicity/recovery with and without therapy. Arrows pointing toward right indicate direction of Alpha-Delta development; arrows pointing down and/or to the left indicate interactions shown between Alpha-Delta behavior.

Developmental Sequence & Nature of Recovery (Approx. % of all young stutts.)	**ALPHA** (Brief, subtle inefficiencies in speech production)	**BETA** (Repetitive speech productions)	**GAMMA** (Relatively tense stabilized/fixed speech productions)	**DELTA** (Nonverbal/verbal reactions to Beta & Gamma)
Most apt to Recover with or without therapy (40 - 50%)	**ALPHA → BETA** (ALPHA behavior generally completely resolves itself)		(Minimal Occurrence)	(Minimal Occurrence)
Most apt to Recover only if they receive therapy (40 - 50%)	**ALPHA → BETA → GAMMA → DELTA** (ALPHA slowly and, in some cases, minimally resolves itself)			
Most apt to need psycho-social eval. and counsl. for effective Recovery (5 - 10%)	**?** (Amount and nature of ALPHA behavior unknown/unclear)	(Minimal Occurrence)	**GAMMA → DELTA**	

of STS to RTS speech behaviors places him or her at greater risk for fluency disruption than normally fluent children.

Although the data are limited, we believe that they support our notion that young stutterers produce more alpha behaviors than do their normally fluent peers. We speculate that these alpha behaviors are more STS. It is also possible, although we don't know for certain, that young stutterers' "degree" (duration, amount of associated muscular tension, and difference from the norm) of alpha differs from that of their normally fluent peers, but this must await further research.

Table 1–3 presents our previous speculation (Conture, 1982) regarding four interdependent stages, from beginning to end, of speech production associated with (dis)fluent speech. The first phase (*alpha*) is characterized by brief, subtle *atypical* speech productions. The second phase (*beta*) is characterized by *oscillatory* or *reiterative* speech production. The third phase (*gamma*) is typified by relatively *fixed* or *stabilized* speech production. The fourth stage, (*delta*) is characterized by *adjustive* or *reactive* speech and nonspeech behavior.

Table 1–3 is similar to our previous theorizing (Conture, 1982); however, as Table 1–4 indicates, we have somewhat revised our previous thinking in this area and are now positing three subgroups of stutterers for whom these developmental sequences may differ:

1. Children most apt to recover from stuttering with or without therapeutic intervention. We speculate that this represents between 40 percent to 50 percent of the population.
2. Children most apt to recover from stuttering only if they receive some form of therapeutic intervention. We speculate that this represents between 40 percent to 50 percent of the population.
3. Children with a sudden, generally traumatic and dramatic onset and/or whose family or themselves may need psychosocial evaluation and counseling. We speculate that this represents between 5 percent to 10 percent of the population.

In essence, we still believe in the existence of these four interdependent stages but believe that not all stutterers (1) start at the same stage, (2) progress through all or similar stages, and/or (3) proceed through these stages at the same rate of development.

Children Apt to Recover Without Therapy

In the children apt to recover without therapy (as seen in the top row of Table 1–4), the first stage (*alpha*) of development is characterized by brief, generally nonperceptible (to listeners) atypical speech productions; for example, increasing vocal fold adduction at a point in time when it should be abducting or slightly longer than typical articulatory contact time. As we said before (Conture, 1982), it is unclear whether such alpha behavior results from environmental or inherited factors (or some complex mix of both), but recent findings by Conture, Rothenberg and Molitor (1986) strongly suggest the presence of these behaviors in the speech of young stutterers. Zebrowski, Conture and Cudahy (1985) also showed that young stutterers are less likely than their normally fluent peers to exhibit "trading relations" between laryngeal and supralaryngeal behaviors during fluent speech, a finding confirmed by Borden, Kim and Spiegler (1987) with adult stutterers. Thus, there is mounting evidence for the existence of alpha behavior, that we speculate is STS and when produced with sufficient frequency places young stutterers "at risk" for continuing to stutter.

For most of these children, alpha behavior is followed by beta behavior that involves the reiterative posturing of speech production gestures. Beta behaviors would, in most cases, be apparent to most listeners and might be, in many children, one of the essential elements of what Johnson and associates (1959) termed *normal* nonfluency. We speculate that beta comes about as a compensatory/coping reaction to alpha behavior; for example, when a brief, within-word articulatory arrest is reacted to by relatively rapid opening and closing of supraglottal and glottal structures in apparent attempts to restart or "free up" or change the perceived stricture within the vocal tract.

The good news is that most of these children never go much beyond the beta stage; that is, most of these children don't start to exhibit the relatively tense, fixed, or stabilized speech production gestures we term gamma. Instead, for a variety of reasons, their beta behavior waxes and wanes, but like ripples further and further out from the center of a disturbance in the water, the cycles of increments followed by decrements in beta behavior exhibit less and less amplitude until finally they disappear from view.

While some of these children may also exhibit gamma (stabilized) speech productions in reaction to beta (repetitive) behaviors as well as delta (adjustive) behavior in reaction to both the inappropriate repetitive and stabilized speech productions, most of them will exhibit only beta for a varying period of time before they will no longer stutter. It is entirely possible that these children may infrequently exhibit alpha behavior and/or their alpha behavior may essentially "drop out" as they mature leaving them with less and less reason for exhibiting beta reactions. Whatever the case, we would expect these children to have essentially normal articulation, language, and neuromotor development or, at the most, slight delays in their development. Using data reported by Schwartz and Conture (1988, figure 1, p. 66), we would speculate that these children are members of clusters 1 and 2: children exhibiting mainly sound/syllable repetitions and a small number and variety of (non)verbal behaviors associated with their stutterings.

Children Apt to Recover Only with Therapy

As shown in the second row of Table 1–4, alpha behavior is followed by beta behavior and for many children it leads to gamma behavior. Ironically, as we have previously mentioned (Conture, 1982) and will discuss later, both our young clients and their parents demonstrate much more concern about beta behavior than they do gamma behavior even though we and others believe that the stabilized, fixed or prolonged pauses, contacts, and transitions of this third stage are a definite step toward a worsening of the child's stuttering (for example, Ainsworth and Fraser, 1988). It is our speculation that these children are members of clusters 3 and 4 (Schwartz and Conture, 1988, figure 1, p. 66): children with frequent sound prolongations and whose stutterings are associated with relatively more as well as greater varieties of associated (non)speech behavior.

Why these children are more apt to "move into" gamma behavior and then delta is, of course, unclear. It is possible that the frequency and type of their alpha behavior leads them, right from the beginning, to a higher frequency of beta which, in turn, increases the chances that they will react with the fixed or stabilizing, albeit inappropriate, gamma speech productions. It is also possible that these children's alpha may take longer to drop out with development; in fact, alpha behavior for these children may never entirely fade away. We further speculate that these children have the highest likelihood of exhibiting delayed and/or deviant speech sound articulation/phonlogical difficulties (for example, Louko, Edwards and Conture, 1988) as well as other concomitant difficulties, such as language delays, voice problems (for example, St. Louis and Hinzman, 1988).

One of the unfortunate aspects in all of this, in our experience, is the increasing number and variety of delta behaviors that these children produce. We say unfortunate because these delta behaviors give the child's parents a great deal of concern (and are many times the reason these children are finally referred to the SLP). These youngsters' delta behaviors are also unfortunate because some individuals, with all good intentions, try to change these rather obvious, noticeable (non)speech behaviors because (a) they are easily identifiable and as such are viewed as objectionable; (b) they are relatively easy to change; and (3) once changed, give at least the visual appearance of an improvement in the problem.

However, it is our contention that these delta or adjustive behaviors are reactions on the part of the young stutterer to other, more central behaviors such as beta and gamma and until these more central behaviors are modified, delta behaviors will continue, albeit in some other form.

Children Exhibiting Sudden, Often Traumatic Onset

Children exhibiting sudden, often traumatic onset make up a very small percentage of children who stutter, but they do exist. It is our experience, apparently shared by Van Riper (1971), that these children begin with fixed articulatory ("blocking" or pronounced gamma) behavior. Although it is possible that these children also exhibit alpha behavior, it is our speculation that the origins and course of their problem are quite different from those of the other 85 percent to 95 percent of young stutterers. Quickly, probably within a matter of hours or days after the reported onset, these children are exhibiting gamma behavior of long duration with much apparent associated physical tension; they also quickly start exhibiting a great number and variety of delta behaviors during their stutterings. Once again, examining data (Schwartz and Conture, 1988; figure 1, p. 66), we would believe that children in cluster 5 are good representatives of this group: They exhibit frequent sound prolongations and a wide number and variety of associated (non)speech behaviors. It is our clinical hunch that these children and their families should receive, at the very least and prior to speech therapy, a psychosocial evaluation because we suspect that this group of children stutters for reasons related more to psychosocial adjustment than anything else.

We end this section with a cautionary note. Knowing the objective detail of young stutterers' speech production should not cloud our view of these youngsters (and their families) as feeling, socially interacting individuals; however, neither should our consideration of these childrens' psychosocial activities obfuscate our detailed knowledge of their speech production. We can and should consider both the soma (speech production) and psyche (feelings, attitudes, and beliefs) of our clients during our evaluation and remediation of these individuals' stuttering problem.

WHO IS A STUTTERER?

From the previous discussion, it can be seen that we would not automatically label an individual as a stutterer if he or she produces a within-word disfluency or two. Someone who has just experienced one bout of alcoholic intoxification does not immediately seek out the local AA chapter; neither should a temporary period of within-word disfluencies mean that a person would or should immediately seek out therapy for stuttering. Just as the *frequency* and *predictability* of alcoholic consumption and intoxification, not just drinking itself, give cause for concern, we only start to become really concerned about a person's speech when his or her exhibited within-word speech disfluency becomes *persistent, predictable,* and *consistent,* and not just occasional.

Those at High Risk

We begin considering the fact that individuals may be stuttering when their exhibited within-word disfluencies become *predictable* parts of their speech, when these disfluencies *persist* over sufficiently long periods of time (no matter how cyclical their appearance may be), and when these disfluencies are *consistently* associated with certain sound-syllables, words, or speaking situations. People may be considered to be stutterers or at high risk for becoming stutterers when we know, with a relatively high degree of certainty, that they will stutter when they talk (*predictable*), when they continue to do so for some some time (*persistent*), and when their disfluencies regularly occur in association with observable events (*consistent*).

We must remember, however, that the terms *persistent, predictable* and *consistent* (PPC), despite sounding definitive and absolute, are still terms whose meanings are relative to the person who has stated them. We know that we can go to extremes in stating that this or that is relative to its surrounds and that there are no absolutes regarding stuttering; however, we have had too many experiences with stuttering where one person's *persistent* is another person's *occasional*. Even in the presence of reports, particularly verbal ones based on second-hand information, that a particular person is consistently stuttering, we should proceed with caution and avoid making a rush to judgment. I am not going to advocate a see-no-evil-hear-no-evil stance, but blasting onto the scene with plans for remediating stuttering on the basis of one person's report of chronic or seemingly chronic stuttering is not particularly appropriate.

Those at Moderate to High Risk

Where the PPC criteria fall down, however, is with the person "at risk" for stuttering, a person who is usually, although not exclusively, a child under ten years of age. With a child who may appear "at risk" for stuttering, we cannot nor should we wait until his or her stutterings become *consistently* associated with stimuli. Likewise, we may also want to begin therapeutic intervention before the child's stuttering becomes *predictable* every time the child speaks.

Instead, with a person "at risk" for stuttering, we must generally rely on the observation that the *frequency of within-word disfluencies* has been *persistent* over a sufficiently long enough period of time to warrant our attention. For most children, this period of time will be between three to six months; however, for some, particularly those whose outset was associated with relatively long, fixed articulatory posturing (that is, audible and inaudible sound prolongations of relatively long duration), this period of time may be days or weeks. Surely, we want to know, as soon as possible, if an individual's problem is or is not going to fade away with or without therapy, but at present we are still developing our abilities to determine these facts.

Those at Low to No Risk

A person is probably at little or no risk for becoming a stutterer if her or his frequency and type of within-word disfluency have been highly variable over a three- to six-month period of time or longer, if she or he exhibits little predictability of speech fluency (may or may not be disfluent when talking), and if her or his disfluencies appear unrelated to other events or stimuli. Of course, any person who, at one point, appears at no or low risk for stuttering can become at moderate to high risk, but the probability is low for such a change to take place.

Other variables, for example, concomitant speech/language problems, attention deficit disorders (cf. Riley and Riley, 1988), can also be factors in determining whether or not a person is highly likely to be or become a stutterer. It takes much, much more than the mere presence of within-word disfluencies in the speech of an individual to determine that he or she has or will have a problem with stuttering.

These decisions, while not easy, are nevertheless important if we are to improve our chances of delivering services to those people who would benefit the most from receiving them. It would seem that judgments of persistency, predictability, and consistency of speech disfluency and related events involve a person-by-person decision.

Although we might like to use group norms (for example, more than 10 speech disfluencies per 100 words = stuttering) to assist us in establishing who is and who is not a stutterer, the data do not appear sufficient to provide us with good group norms. Tests like the Stuttering Severity Instrument (Riley, 1980) and the Stuttering Prediction Instrument (Riley, 1981) are excellent beginning points, but what is needed is more information, on a year-by-year or month-by-month basis, regarding the mean (plus range) number and type of speech disfluencies produced by children from say two to six years of age.

Previous research in this area is commendable (for example, Davis, 1939, 1940; Johnson and associates, 1959; Winitz, 1961; Williams, Silverman and Kools, 1969; Yairi and Clifton, 1972; Yairi and Jennings, 1974; Yairi and Lewis, 1984; Yairi, 1981, 1982). However, the continued massive exposure to and influence of television, computers, and the other media on our children's language and cognitive development, as well as changes in the traditional family structure where both parents now work outside the home, strongly suggest that such research needs further updating and expanding. Furthermore, if at all possible, such information should be based on longitudinal (several samples sequentially spaced out over time) versus cross-sectional (a sample taken at only one point in time) studies. For further general discussion of longitudinal versus cross-sectional studies, see Ventry and Schiavetti, 1986, pp. 55–57, 284–90).

Those Who Appear to Stutter in Their Heads, Not Their Mouths

Clinicians who have worked with children, teenagers, and adults who stutter will recognize that some individuals consider themselves to be stutterers despite objective evidence to the contrary. These individuals are typically adults, and anyone who has clinically served these people knows the difficulties of dealing with people who are objectively fluent but who subjectively feel they stutter and should be considered as stutterers (Douglass and Quarrington, 1952; Prins, 1974). These clients point out the fact that besides what we can hear and see (speech disfluencies, bodily movement, tension, and psychosocial discomfort and/or concerns), we must also consider aspects of the individual's self-concept (for lack of a better phrase) that are not as easily viewed and heard.

If an individual considers him- or herself to be a stutterer, despite what the person sounds or looks like when talking, this should not be ignored by the speech-language pathologist. In a way, these clients are like those clients Daly (1988) describes who, after a period of therapy, are "fluent in the mouth but not the head." Many times, careful observation of the so-called "fluent" stutterer by the SLP will reveal a wide variety of subtle behavior that the person is producing to get the sound or word out, to avoid saying the word, to get the listener to fill-in or complete his utterance or to circumlocute the situation, sound, or word. When asked, these people, like their more obviously disfluent peers, seem to complain universally that speech is a chore, that it is not automatic ("like everyone else"), and that they have to spend too much time thinking about *how* they are going to say something rather than *what* they are going to say (we discuss these concerns in some detail in Chapter 5). Sometimes, if brought into a group of other stutterers, they will express feelings of uneasiness or guilt that they "don't stutter as much as the rest of group" and that they are wasting or taking up the group's time with their problem that is real to them but nearly invisible to external observers. Although some of these people also have other concerns, suffice it to say at this point that the SLP should be able to assess the nonobservable as well as the observable (particularly the *subtly* observable) in order to determine who is and who is not a stutterer.

SOME PARTING THOUGHTS

Stuttering is a multidimensional problem that has and will continue to defy any unidimensional solution. Ideally, our approaches to stuttering, both theoretical as well as therapeutic, should contribute to a solution rather than become part of the problem. Recognizing that there is some overlap between the two populations—stutterers and nonstutterers—in terms of the frequency and nature of exhibited disfluent behavior (cf. Johnson and associates, 1959), our definitions of what is stuttering and who is a stutterer must be *relative* rather than *absolute*. Otherwise, the use of *absolute* criteria will mean that some people who are and will become normally fluent will be considered stutterers and vice versa.

The better approaches, we believe, are those that recognize, at the outset, that (1) no one currently knows what causes stuttering, (2) no one knows with certainty whether differences among stutterers are greater and/or as significant as those between stutterers and nonstutterers, (3) no one has developed a program that eradicates stuttering in all clients for all time despite all claims to the contrary, and (4) there may not be any *one* treatment approach that can effectively deal with the myriad of concerns one encounters with people who stutter.

We are definitely not trying to suggest that we will never know the answers to (1) through (4) above or that we should stop trying to resolve these issues or find the answers. However, at present we don't have these answers, in any definitive, absolute sense, and possibly, if we can recognize this truth, it will eventually set us free to find the answers rather than let us think they have already been found.

Individuals who *persistently*, *predictably*, and *consistently* produce within-word disfluencies during verbal communication are likely candidates for being considered as stutterers. Their candidacy becomes even more likely if we observe, associated with these speech disfluencies, verbal and nonverbal indicators of bodily movement, tension, and psychosocial discomfort and concerns. The SLP should recognize that the PPC criteria are relative to both the observer and the observed. The mental, physiological, and chronological age of the client, in particular, needs to be considered in making judgments regarding the PPC of the person's stuttering. Furthermore, an individual's belief that he or she stutters and should be considered a stutterer may not always square with the objective information available to the clinician. To ascertain who is and who is not a stutterer is a complex decision based on many different considerations and, to some degree, must be determined relative to the particular clients, their developmental and chronological age, and their internal feelings, attitudes, and beliefs.

In later sections of this book, we deal in more detail with the making of this decision and the basis for making it. For now, we should recognize the challenge inherent in making such decisions while at the same time realizing that such decisions can, and in many instances must, be made for the benefit of the client and his or her relations. Although we can harm by making rushes to judgment and remediating in situations where, given enough time, and relatively simple changes in the client's environment, a problem might disappear, we also harm by not wanting to hurt the client and inappropriately delay the delivery of needed clinical services. What we must all strive to develop is the ability to discern the difference between (1) those individuals who truly stutter and who need our services, and (2) those individuals who are truly not stuttering and are not in need of our services. We also need to develop the ability to recognize the presence of individual differences among our clients and to realize that related concerns, although perhaps present, may be neither sufficient nor of a kind to warrant our services.

SUMMARY

Stuttering most likely results from a complex *interaction* between the stutterer's environment (for example, parental standards for child behavior) *and* the skills/abilities the stutterer brings to that environment (for example, gross and fine motor coordination). Listeners are most apt to perceive an instance of stuttering when they hear a within-word disfluency, particularly a sound/syllable repetition, monosyllabic whole-word repetition, sound prolongation, or within-word pause. While there are no absolute criteria for who is a stutterer, one characteristic of children who are at high risk for stuttering is that they typically produce a greater frequency of within-word disfluencies than their normally fluent peers; however, even for children who are quite at risk for stuttering, the nature and frequency of stuttering is highly variable across time and from one speaking situation to another. Stuttering typically begins during childhood, and if the problem does not change by itself or through remediation, it continues to progressively develop with time through a series of stages which are still unclearly understood but often speculated about.

Remediation of stuttering is helpful to many, particularly the younger client, and in this author's opinion should involve modification of two factors: (1) selected aspects of the stutterer's environment, for example, by means of parent counseling and information sharing, help the parents to more often adopt a slower, less physically tense manner of speaking, and (2) selected aspects of speech-language behavior, for example, by changing stutterers' overly rapid, physically tense strategies for initiating or continuing speech production. While therapy regimens need to be developed for a class of individuals, the author views individuals who stutter as people first and stutterers second, and individual needs and differences must be accounted for in any successful treatment program. Within this viewpoint, the problem of stuttering has been defined and in subsequent chapters will be dealt with initially in terms of assessment and evaluation, and then remediation.

Stuttering is a multidimensional problem that has and will continue to defy any unidimensional solution. Thus, this book was not written to be taken as the definitive word regarding the cause or treatment of stuttering; neither was it written to be a cookbook for selecting this or that recipe to cure, eradicate, or eliminate this or that aspect of stuttering. Instead, this book was written in an attempt to describe and discuss the various things that need to be considered when trying to understand, evaluate, and remediate stuttering. Our orientation throughout is toward a problem solving approach to stuttering that permits the speech-language pathologist to independently problem solve and deal with the individual client who stutters according to the client's individualistic needs and concerns.

TWO
ASSESSMENT
AND EVALUATION

Speech and language pathologists who remediate stuttering should have sufficient training and experience with the assessment and evaluation of stuttering in children and adults. While this training and experience are similar to those for dealing with other communicative problems, for example, phonological disorders and expressive language difficulties, it also has its unique aspects that are best learned and appreciated through experience. It is entirely appropriate before discussing the remediation of stuttering that we devote some time to considering its evaluation. Fortunately, there are now a number of sources that interested readers can use to find out something about the assessment and evaluation of stuttering and we will try not to duplicate previous efforts in this chapter (Johnson et al., 1963; Williams, 1974, 1978; Hayhow, 1983; Pindzola, 1986; Ham, 1986; Conture and Caruso, 1987).

SOME BASIC BELIEFS THAT GUIDE
OUR ASSESSMENT PROCEDURES

In this chapter, we present assessment and evaluation procedures that we have found useful as well as those procedures we haven't found as useful.

However, we have three beliefs about stuttering that heavily influence our assessment and evaluation procedures: (1) Stuttering relates to a complex interaction between the stutterer's environment and the skill and abilities the stutterer brings to that environment; (2) stuttering rarely operates in a vacuum, but many times relates to subtle and not-so-subtle difficulties in other areas; and (3) individuals who stutter are individuals first and stutterers second—there is more to their lives than stuttering (cf. Conture, 1987c).

With regard to the first belief—stuttering relates to a complex interaction between the stutterer and his/her environment—we discuss ways to assess the stutterer as well as the stutterer's environment. Regarding the second belief—stuttering rarely operates in a vacuum—we discuss assessment and evaluation of related behaviors such as speech articulation, expressive/receptive language, voice, neuromotor speech and nonspeech skills, nonverbal associates, reading, and so forth. In terms of the third belief—individuals who stutter are individuals first and stutterers second—we discuss ways and means by which we can gain perspective on their individual lives by understanding the client's achievements and aspirations in school and work, parental standards for child raising and behavior, and so forth.

GAINING PERSPECTIVE ON CLIENT'S UNIQUE CIRCUMSTANCES

All of these considerations should help the SLP gain perspective regarding the particular circumstances that surround each client's stuttering and related problems. For example, we gain this perspective when we consider that one stutterer may have *limited* intellectual and employment capabilities while another may have *unlimited* intellectual and employment capabilities. During assessment, as in remediation, the examiner should try to keep in mind that stuttering, in and of itself, does not encompass all of the client as a person or the client's problems. Stuttering is but one of many components that make up an individual; some of these other components may play just as big a role as stuttering itself in terms of recovery from the problem.

EXAMINING THE EXAMINER

During the initial diagnostic, no matter how obvious it seems, it is nonetheless true that the client and his or her associates will be evaluating the clinician. And, as the saying goes, first impressions are lasting (as a current ad states, "one never gets a second chance to make a first impression"). It is therefore desirable that the clinician behave in such a way that the client regards him or her as (1) a person concerned not only with the client's problems but also with the client as an individual; (2) a person who is nonjudgmental regarding both the client as a person and the client's problem; (3) a person who demonstrates a belief in the client's capacity for self-help; and (4) a person who demonstrates professional understanding and knowledge regarding the client's stuttering and related issues. Obviously, the SLP can't be all things to all people but at the very least we should realize that our clients and their associates are also assessing us and that many times what they perceive, be it right or wrong, has a powerful influence on whether they will listen to our advice and benefit from our therapy.

In general, the SLP's evaluation of stutterers involves demonstrating to the client an understanding of stuttering while employing appropriate clinical affect and interpersonal skills. Shriberg and associates (1975) have detailed these professional, technical, and interpersonal skills, and Van Riper (1975) has discussed some of the clinical affects thought to be of relevance to successful clinical intervention (see Schum, 1986, for further discussion of the client-clinician relationship). In our opinion, these professional and personal qualities of the clinician warrant consideration and study by any speech and language pathologist involved in the evaluation and remediation of stuttering and other communicative problems. (Beginning SLPs or student-clinicians might want to read, at this point, Appendix A, which discusses some of the professional/personal qualities and concerns SLPs must consider in their daily work.)

FACILITIES

If first impressions are lasting, probably nothing is more influential on the client and associates than the setting for the diagnostic. While the busy SLP may see only the client and his/her needs, the client is scanning the total environment trying to get a handle on who and what the SLP is all about. Some attention to detail on the part of the SLP is warranted and will help everybody focus on the client and his/her needs.

First, the ideal environment for evaluating stuttering (or any other communicative disorder for that matter) should not possess auditory and visual stimuli that call *undue* attention to themselves. Distracting sights and sounds from outside as well as inside the evaluation room should be reasonably attenuated. A compromise is needed. While the evaluation room should not be overly cluttered, neither should it necessarily convey the sterility of a medical operating suite.

Second, remember that for both you and your client the evaluation will take mental effort, concentration, and attention to detail, and the client may find it difficult to recall some of this detail from the backroads of his or her mind. We can assist the client with this task and reduce, as much as possible, distractions in the environment so that both the client and we can concentrate on the business at hand.

Third, as obvious as it might seem, try to ensure that the chairs, tables, and nature of objects used in various tests are age-appropriate. The client doesn't know, in advance, the purposes of your procedures and can only assume on the basis of that which is familiar to him or her, for example, "play" versus "real" objects, what you might be thinking. Be as sensitive as you can to the older client's needs and try not to be patronizing through the use of seemingly "juvenile" procedures. Also consider the young client's feelings of intimidation when faced with seemingly "grown-up" chairs, tables, and objects.

EQUIPMENT

It is my clinical experience that SLPs need to be more aware of the single most important piece of equipment they use: the audio or video tape recorder and its associated microphones. Far too often, we observe professionals who seem insensitive to the fact that high-quality acoustic and/or video tape recordings are crucial in the establishment of adequate behavioral indexes (baseline, before- or pretreatment measures) of stuttering and related behavior. The quality of these recordings will become even more important in years to come as computer-assisted acoustic analysis packages move from the research labs into the clinics (for example, see Mann's 1987 review of DSPS acoustic-analysis software or Friedman's 1989 review of Speech Viewer Software).

Audio Recordings

Most poor quality audio tape recordings of stutterings result from inappropriate microphone placement. Ideally, the recording surface of the the microphone should be (1) placed perpendicular to the path or plane of the acoustic speech signal (for example, if the client is talking to a clinician across a table, the recording surface of the microphone should be pointed toward the ceiling or toward the wall to the client's immediate left or right), and (2) placed at a relatively constant distance from the client's lips and mouth. The *biggest* mistake most clinicians make, especially with children, is to place the microphone too far away from the child's mouth. In our experience, the microphone should be kept six inches or less from the child's mouth; a variety of small tie-tack or lapel or lavalier microphones (for example, Sony Models ECM–50 or ECM–55, Realistic, Model 33-1063) are available for this purpose and can be easily clipped on or fastened to the child's shirt or shirt collar, as we've done with hundreds of young children.

Whatever the brand of microphone, however, we have found that even the most expensive, sensitive microphone can't make up for one basic mistake: having too great a distance between the client's mouth and the microphone. Sometimes, a young client will resist the wearing of a tie-tack or lapel microphone and/or seems to be unable to forget about the microphone and continues to handle or touch it. One relatively easy way we've found to deal with this problem is for the clinician to fasten a similar microphone on the child's mother or even on the clinician herself (this works, we suppose, on the premise that misery loves company). The microphone on the mother or clinician doesn't even have to be connected to a recorder, just as long as it is visible to the child on the parent or clinician. This procedure seems to help the child forget about the microphone and get on with the business at hand.

If both of the above requirements for microphone placement are met, the clinician should next ensure that the record gain of the tape recorder be set or regulated so that the recorded level of the client's speech is neither too low (soft) nor high (loud); that is, the level of the VU meter is centering, during the recording, around the 0 mark. If we seriously desire to achieve consistent, high quality audio recordings of stutterers' speech behavior, we should *not* employ tape recorders that have glow tubes for VU meters, that lack VU meters, or that have built-in (nondetectable) microphones. Speech-language pathologists who desire audio tape recordings for the purposes of molecular and microscopic analysis of speech behavior (for example, narrow phonetic transcriptions, vocalized versus nonvocalized pauses, voice quality associated with stuttering) are well advised to take the minimal time necessary to learn how to set up and implement proper audio recordings. It takes very little extra time and money to do it right and, with modest amounts of practice, these recording procedures become second nature and the resulting recordings are far and away superior (and are much easier for the clinician to listen to and analyze *after* the client leaves).

Video Recordings

Most poor quality video tape recordings come from two sources: (1) low or inappropriate lighting of the subject, and (2) relatively insensitive cameras or poor camera-to-subject position. Unfortunately, both lighting and cameras involve spending money, money that is frequently not part of clinicians' budgets. At the very least, however, the clinician can, without spending any extra money, do the following: (1) Ensure that the room used for recording has reasonably decent overhead room lighting, and (2) ensure that the background behind the client is neutral in color and without a lot of distracting material, for example, toys, books, desks. Spending a little money, the clinician can purchase a camera tripod (to maximize camera stability) with a smooth or fluid-filled pan tilt head (the head is the part at the top of the tripod that the camera rests on and permits side-to-side swiveling as well as up/down camera movement) so that the camera can be easily, smoothly, and quickly adjusted to follow the ever-moving, ever-squirming child.

Spending even more money, the clinician can purchase a low-priced light kit for illumination of the subject (we have used such a lighting schema to videotape conversations of over 100 children—between two and seven years of age—and their mothers, and with very few exceptions, these lights were tolerated by these young children and their mothers). Finally, if interest and budget permit, the clinician can purchase cameras that either operate in low-light situations (20 or less candlewatts of illumination) or have far greater sensitivity than the typical consumer grade camera. Just as with acoustic recordings, a little attention to detail *prior* to recording will make all the difference in terms of the brightness, contrast, and resolution of videotape recordings.

INFORMED CONSENT, OR THE CLIENT'S RIGHT-TO-KNOW

A word or two is in order regarding clients' and their associates' right-to-know, or informed consent, regarding all of your clinical procedures and practices. Particularly if the client and associates are to be observed, taped (either audio or audiovideo), or otherwise scrutinized by yourself, your colleagues, or students-in-training, the client and associates should be so informed in as matter-of-fact a manner and tone as possible. Right from the beginning of the evaluation, it is important to provide the client an atmosphere of openness and honesty because the atmosphere we send out to clients will often be reflected in the atmosphere clients send back to us.

Telling a client that such observational procedures are routine and essential to help you help him is not only an honest but also a wise policy. Surely, such openness may make some clients more visibly concerned when they know they are being observed and taped. They may ask many lengthy questions about the observational procedure and the use to which the observed information will be put as well as who is doing the observing, but the client clearly has the right to ask such questions. Later in this chapter, we discuss our belief that clients and whoever they designate should get copies of our full-scale diagnostic reports. After all, it is more than likely that this is the way you would want to be dealt with if you were in your client's shoes.

COMPONENTS OF THE STUTTERING EVALUATION

If we disregard, for the moment, the age of the client you will assess and evaluate, the *ideal* evaluation of stuttering should include the following components: (1) an intake form, filled out in advance of the evaluation by the client and/or parents, teacher, doctor, and so forth, providing identification plus basic information regarding history of the problem and related matters; (2) an interview with the client and, if available, associates, regarding history, current and possible future status of the problem plus motivation, need, and desire for clinical services; (3) standardized and nonstandardized assessment and evaluation of communicative and related skills; and (4) preparation and dissemination of a written documentation of findings and interpretations based on assessment. While none of these four components is any more important than the other, it is my experience that those aspects of the evaluation that involve the clinician's interviewing and writing skills are those parts which seem the most difficult to master.

The Intake Form

The first component, an intake form, should ideally be completed *in advance* of the evaluation, and should, at the very least, include information identifying the client and associates, a general history of the problem and related matters, and *full* addresses of all parties to whom the client and associates want the written report sent. It is really important to obtain complete and accurate identification information: addresses, zip codes, telephone numbers (home and office), birthdates and date of evaluation (day, month, and year), present occupation, education, and so forth. It is our experience that this type of information is all too often missing or inaccurate; however, it often serves as the basis for the clinician's first remarks to the client.

Don't hesitate, during the diagnostic itself, to ask the client to provide information on your intake form that appears missing, unclear, or seemingly inaccurate. Even more important than the use of this information in the opening remarks to the client is its later use in the writing up of the diagnostic report, in making referrals, planning remediation, follow-up contacts, and the like. Furthermore, the client's or the client's parents, in the case of the child, taking the time in advance to complete such forms suggests that the client or associates are at least willing to expend some effort in self-help. Conversely, when an evaluation begins *without* the client's having completed or only partially completing the form, we ask ourselves: If this client is not willing and able to find the time and energy to fill out such forms, how willing and able will he or she be to put the necessary time and effort into speech therapy? (This, of course, would not be true of a client who has real difficulties reading and writing because of illiteracy, speaking English as a second language, or similar problems).

The Interview Procedure

The second, and perhaps most important, component of the stuttering assessment is the interview. The interview involves a structured conversation between the clinician and client (and associates) for the purpose of facilitating the clinician's ability to help the client. Generally, the interview consists of the clinician's questioning the client and associates regarding past, present, and future events that directly or indirectly relate to the client's concerns. No aspect of the evaluation requires more training, attention, listening, or observational skills than the interview. It is, therefore, understandable that many clinicians find this a challenging aspect of assessment and evaluation. Let us next consider the number and variety of questions typically used in a diagnostic interview.

Questions: Their general nature Flynn (1978, pp. 268–69) describes a number of specific types of questions or "elicitors" that may be used during the diagnostic (Flynn reportedly adapted these from Goyer et al., 1968).

1. *Direct questions*—Ask for a reply on a specific topic
   Example: "What did you do last summer?"
   a. *Closed questions*—Direct, but with greatly narrowed response field
      Example: "What did you do with Jim on the Fourth of July?"
   b. *Yes-No*—The most restrictive direct questions
      Example: "Did you go to the parade?"
2. *Open-ended questions*—Specify only the topic and leave great latitude in replying
   Example: "Tell me about yourself."
            "Make up your own story about it."
3. *Leading questions*—Imply a specific kind of answer
   Example: "You are a happy person, aren't you?"
   a. *Loaded questions*—Leading questions with emotional connotation
      Example: To a loyal Republican: "Don't you agree that Ronald Reagan was a poor president?"
   b. *Yes-response questions*—Leading questions expressed in such a way as to encourage respondent to agree with statement
      Example: "Of course you'll be the new group leader of the adult stuttering group, won't you?"
4. *Nondirective questions and statements*—Provide encouragement to the respondent to say more
   Example: "I really like to watch hockey. You said you play hockey on the high school team?"
   a. *Mirror question*—Intended to get added comment on previous response
      Example: "I feel real sad...You say that you are sad?"
   b. *Verbal probes*—"I see." "Tell me more." "Umhum." "Interesting." "I'm not sure I understand." These "probes" generally get the client to talk more but the content of the client's conversation can take a variety of directions, some more beneficial than others to the purposes of the diagnostic.

In our experience, the beginning clinician feels most comfortable with direct, closed, and yes-no questions while the more experienced clinician more frequently employs nondirective questions. Ideally, the interview should be a constant blending and switching among these various types of questions: a direct question here, followed by an open-end question, back to a yes-no question, followed by a mirror question, and a verbal probe or two. It is our experience that all these types of questions have a place in the diagnostic and that the clinician should work on learning when each type of question is and is not appropriate to use. For example, when interviewing an older stutterer who is, at the beginning of the diagnostic, having a great deal of trouble talking, you may find that a series of direct, closed, or yes-no questions, interspersed with a verbal probe or two, may be preferable to asking a group of open-ended and/or loaded questions.

Questions: General issues that need to be addressed The previously mentioned questions can be related to three interdependent issues the examining clinician will want to consider:

1. *Questions leading to testing:* These are questions clinicians ask themselves about the client that lead them to test the client to find the answer(s); for example, "Is this client more or less fluent when he reads than when he speaks?"
2. *Questions directly asked of the client and associates:* These are questions clinicians directly ask the client, his or her parents, or associates; for example, "Why do you want, at this point, to receive speech therapy?"
3. *Questions answered by inference and guesstimation:* These are questions clinicians ask themselves about the client that require inferences in order to try to find the answer(s); for example, "What is the source of this person's desire to receive speech therapy (parental, peer, spouse, or employment pressure)?"

Questions that lead to testing are quite familiar to most clinicians: Is the client more fluent when reading than when speaking? On the average, how many of the client's words or syllables per 100 words or syllables are stuttered? What is the client's most frequently produced disfluency type? Are the client's hearing, articulation, and language skills within normal limits? Can we get perceptual clues from the client's voice quality during instances of stuttering that indicate how he or she is using the larynx during stuttering? Are the client's intellectual and reading skills on a level that permit this person to derive sufficient benefit from remediation at this point in his or her life? These and other questions like them form the essence of what a speech-language pathologist will need to know about a client who is suspected or known to stutter.

Such questions as the following are asked directly of the client and associate during the interview: How would you describe to me your or your child's stuttering speech behavior? Would you please show or demonstrate for me how you or your child stutter? What is the theory of why you or your child stutter? Did your stuttering (or your child's stuttering) begin with a sound prolongation or repeating of sounds and syllables? What types of therapy have you or your child previously received? Tell me more about why such therapies did or did not help you or your child? What are your or your child's general strengths or weaknesses?

We will later present a serial listing of questions that we use in the assessment and evaluation of stuttering that may serve as a guide to you in the development and implementation of your own interview procedure. By no means, however, should such a listing preclude or restrict you from developing different and additional questions to be used for your own interview procedure.

Questions that are answered by inference and guesstimation are also important to the diagnosis of stuttering. These types of questions require the SLP to develop the ability to judge, but not be judgmental of, people and their actions. Interestingly, clinicians frequently do not seem to realize that they are asking or need to ask such questions.

One important issue, relative to these types of questions, is the clinician's ability to judge whether the client has sufficient skills or potential for developing skills to make the necessary changes in speech and related behavior. To arrive at such judgments, clinicians will find themselves asking themselves the following types of questions: Is this person capable of expending the necessary mental and physical effort and time to change behavior? What seem to be the sources of motivation and desire for therapy (Prins, 1974; Starbuck, 1974)? Why is this person seeking services? How reliable, honest, and straightforward is this client in his or her responses to me? Does this person really appear to understand what I am saying and asking? Does this client appear to be assuming a *cure me* (passive consumer) or is he or she assuming a *self-effort with guidance* role (active producer)? Are these parents setting reasonable standards for child behavior and child raising?

Of course, all of these questions are not asked independently of one another; they obviously dovetail and are at times redundant in terms of the information they provide. Redundancy, however, is not necessarily a vice; it may indeed be a virtue during the diagnostic because it provides a means for checking on the consistency and stability of the client's and associate's statements and behaviors. It should be clear, therefore, that the types of question the SLP asks are not restricted to this or that section of the evaluation. In fact, the answer to one type of question may partly or completely answer another type of question.

LISTENING TO AND FOLLOWING UP ON ANSWERS

Perhaps even more challenging than structuring the number and nature of your questions is knowing how to listen to and follow up on your client's responses. Sometimes, as Flynn (1978) suggests, "an interested, attentive, relaxed silence" may be an appropriate way to respond to your client. We would agree with Flynn, however, that frequent and prolonged use of such silence gives the client a less than positive image of you and/or may make the client somewhat uncomfortable. Most of the time, though, your follow up to your client's responses will be verbal. Knowing when and how to follow up is a complex skill that needs to be mastered if one is to become a successful interviewer.

COMMON LISTENING PROBLEMS

In the beginning, clinicians often have trouble listening to their clients because they are too busy listening to themselves. That is, instead of listening to their client's responses they are too busy thinking of the next question they are going to ask (media interviewers are frequently guilty of this). As clinicians gain a bit more experience, they sometimes think they hear things or read things into their client's response that are probably best left unsaid. For example, a mother tells about her son's pet garter snake to which the SLP responds by asking the mother, "Has Johnny had any sexual adjustment problems that you know of?" Conversely, clinicians sometime hear the content of the question but not its attendant emotion (and vice versa). For example, when a mother softly cries as she relates a story of a near drowning of one of her children that occurred shortly before her other child began to stutter, the clinician responds, "I bet you now know how to perform CPR, right?"

Sometimes the best response is no response, particularly if you start to feel that you are talking too much or asking too many questions. Silence is particularly golden when the client becomes upset, uncomfortable, or in other ways emotionally concerned. A simple gesture like handing the client a packet or box of tissues makes it clear that you have nonjudgmentally recognized the person's feelings *and* her or his right to self-expression. On the other hand, as Flynn (1978) mentions, there is really no reason to remain silent when a client who has rambled on and on about interesting but ancillary issues finally decides to take a breath. In short, clinicians who interview must be as adept at listening to the client's answers to their questions as they are at asking the questions in the first place. The skill of knowing when and how to switch from speaker to listener and back to speaker during the diagnostic interview presents a challenging, but very interesting part of the entire diagnostic.

FOLLOWING UP ON QUESTIONS

A clinician's ability to follow up the client's responses to questions is based on his or her ability to listen and observe. Like a human form of an artificial intelligence program, the clinician narrows down the possibilities with follow up questions. For example, the clinician asks, "Did Johnny start stuttering before or after the birth of your second child?" and the mother says "After." The clinician then asks, "Did you notice Johnny's stuttering before or after the second child began to speak" and the mother says, "Shortly after the second child began to talk." The clinician next asks, "Was the second child talking more or less than Johnny at that time?" and the mother says, "More. My second child has been a talkative, motor mouth right from the beginning." And so forth. As we can see, the clinician rapidly, and hopefully fluidly, switches back and forth between listening and speaking: She listens to a client's responses to her questions and then asks a question or makes a comment based on that response.

For an actual example of follow up, consider the situation where we suspected a father of having unreasonably high standards for his daughter's verbal communication. The father said, in an extremely fluent, articulate fashion, that he had always had to sell himself through verbal communication. Following up on this comment, we asked the father about his boyhood and that of his relatives (an open-ended question), and he said that both he and his father had been champion debaters in school and had won many individual as well as team honors. We followed up on this by asking him to tell us more about his debating experience (a verbal probe), and the father stated that he had hoped the family tradition of debating would be carried on by his daughter and that he had been helping her learn to develop the necessary communication skills. Unfortunately, his daughter was not only eight years old, but it was also our observation she was not exactly what we would consider an oral-laryngeal athlete. This information, developed from our follow up, together with other observations, led us to strongly suspect that the father had somewhat unreasonable standards for his daughter's verbal communication.

It was not that the father was unwilling, unable, or reluctant to tell us about his debating days (although sometimes this is the case); rather, he just did not think it too relevant. And, perhaps, such information might not be relevant for certain clients; however, we cannot consider the relevance of any information unless we know about it in the first place. Follow up to clients' responses, we have found, often provides this sort of information. We are not advocating, we hasten to add, that clinicians use follow up as free license or carte blanche to snoop and poke through their stuttering client's and associates' private affairs. However, if the clinician believes the information is necessary to gain perspective or better understanding of the client's history, then the information is worthy of the clinician's attempts to retrieve it.

Questions: Some specific ones to ask Appendix C shows a series of questions that may be asked of the parents or associates of young children. (They may be, as the wording in some of these questions suggests, adapted to use with older children, teenagers, and adults.) As noted previously, these questions should be viewed as a *guide* and in no way should they preclude or restrict the reader from developing his own set of questions or variations of those presented. Tanner and Cannon (1978) developed a commercially available series of diagnostic questions that the clinician may ask the mother and/or father of a child who is (or who is suspected of being) a stutterer. Likewise, Zwitman (1978) has presented a similar series of questions and Thompson has developed similar questions that may be asked of a child's classroom teacher. Rather than go through each and every question, we will cover the groupings of questions and give an example of each and the rationale behind it.

INTRODUCTION

You've got to start somewhere and an open-ended question (for example, "What can we do to help you?") helps clarify the purpose and set an appropriate "tone" to the interview. While some (Flynn, 1978) suggest avoiding the use of the word "problem" in the beginning of the interview, we have found that a few open-ended questions (like those given in Appendix C), stated in a matter-of-fact way, start the interview in a positive direction and easily lead into subsequent questioning.

GENERAL DEVELOPMENT

We next like to cover past history to the extent that the person can and will remember such events and detail. Starting with the past does two things: (1) It provides you with perspective on the person, the person's associates and/or the person's life, and (2) it helps the person begin by thinking and talking about things that may not have the same degree of emotionality attached to them as present events (that is, time heals all wounds). With parents, in particular, questions like, "How does his general development from birth to present compare with his brother or sister or other children his age?" provides you perspective on their observational powers as well as their understanding of general childhood development.

FAMILY HISTORY

The family history questions are the first ones that directly deal with stuttering and/or speech-language-hearing problems. We have found that the general question, "Are there any speech, hearing, or language problems in any other family members (living or deceased)?" is far more apt to uncover stuttering in the family than the simple question, "Does anyone else (alive or deceased) stutter?" You can always follow up the general question with the stuttering question, and sometimes you will be surprised at the responses; for example, a response of "no" to the general question, but "yes" to the question about stuttering and vice versa.

Perhaps all this says is that the client wasn't listening, but we are inclined to think that it means that the client and associates attach different meaning to the words "speech problem" and "stuttering" and that some clients may even be trying *not* to reveal information about the past that they think may unduly influence your opinion about them or their child. Whatever the case, as we learn more about the genetics of stuttering, it may turn out to be very important diagnostically to know whether immediate family members or another relative (alive or deceased) ever stuttered (cf. Cox, 1988; Kidd, 1983; Howie, 1981).

SPEECH/LANGUAGE DEVELOPMENT AND HISTORY

The rationale behind these types of questions, we believe, is fairly straightforward. However, responses to these types of questions are generally going to be more unclear when reported by teenagers and adults than when reported by, say, the parents of a four-year-old. For this reason the clinician might want to significantly truncate the number and variety of these questions when dealing with an older client. As in the other sections, this set of questions can be contracted or expanded according to the needs of the particular client and the goals of the examining clinician. Of particular interest are questions such as, "When did he (or you) begin to say his (or your) first words?" in relation to the question, "When did he (or you) first begin to have difficulties speaking?" Many times the parents, in particular, will report two or three years of remarkably fluent speech *prior* to the first observation of stuttering. This issue is explored further in later sections.

ACADEMIC INFORMATION

Obviously, parents of preschoolers are asked the most cursory question or two regarding schooling: "How does he seem to be doing in nursery school/the day-care center/prekindergarten program?" For the school-age child and teenagers in high school, questions in this area can be very informative. Many times the problems you observe in the diagnostic, for example, difficulties with oral reading tasks, receptive and expressive language, attention span, and so forth, are also apparent in school. Sometimes it becomes obvious that stuttering is the least of the child's concerns and that therapy for stuttering will have to be a lower priority to a number of other issues that must be worked out through the school system; for example, hyperactivity in the classroom, chronically wandering attention, acting out against other children, social immaturity, autism, and difficulties with reading and language to the point where the child is required to repeat the grade. The experienced clinician always wants to know something about the child's school experiences as well as the older stutterer's feelings and experiences with school since these feelings/experiences may continue into the present and influence social, employment, and communication experiences.

SOCIAL/BEHAVIORAL

Questions about the client's social life, maturity, and the like can provide the SLP with perspective. The SLP will hear such things as the following: "He frequently cries when he doesn't get his way," "is very much afraid of loud noise, fire and the dark," "has no friends his own age," "seems to be much less mature than other children his age," and "avoids conversations with people at all costs." While some of these observations can be attributed to a normal reaction to an abnormal situation, when a child *routinely* exhibits *strong* fears of the dark, loud noises, fire, or anything strange, the SLP may want to (1) monitor the evolution of these fears, and/or (2) make referral for psychosocial evaluation. A child who *routinely* exhibits *strong* fears of everyday events and objects may be a child whose sensitivities and emotional stability make it difficult for him or her to receive maximal benefit from speech therapy until such concerns are specifically addressed and mitigated.

The client or associate's response to the question, "Is there anything (other than speaking) that concerns you, in any way, about yourself or your child?" is particularly revealing. Sometimes the answer to this question suggests one of the main reasons the client is seeking services: "I can't hold or find a job" or "Billy has no friends," and so forth. Any consistent and/or strong concerns expressed by the client or associates in this area bear further exploration for they may be the "real" problem or at least significantly contribute to the person's inability to recover from stuttering.

HISTORY/DESCRIPTION OF PROBLEM (PAST AND PRESENT)

By this point in the interview the conversation between client and clinician should have put the client sufficiently at ease so the crux of the matter can be discussed: "Tell me about your speaking difficulties or problem." This question strikes at the core of the problem, and the clinician shouldn't be surprised that this core, like the center of the earth, is going to be fairly hot, particularly for older clients. These questions deal with the past as well as the present and are not always things the client and associates particularly relish discussing. A delicate, supportive approach on the part of the clinician will help ("I know some of these questions are going to be tough, but just do the best job you can").

There is a redundancy in the questioning here and it is for a purpose: to help the clinician get the clearest picture possible of the client's problem at present and from the beginning. Gathering this information is one of the

SLP's most important tasks because it will permit the SLP to decide if a problem exists and if so what course of action should be taken. Although previously discussed questions provide useful perspectives and supportive information, the SLP should try to keep in mind the purpose of the diagnostic and diagnostic interview: Does the person have a stuttering problem and if so what course of action should be taken?

SPEECH/LANGUAGE ABILITIES

Rationale for these questions would appear to be straightforward: Are there any other speech-hearing-language problems that contribute to or may need more immediate attention than stuttering? Although much is made of language development and difficulties with stutterers, it is our experience that articulation/phonological problems occur in approximately one-third of all children who stutter. Several studies (for example, Cantwell and Lewis, 1985; Riley and Riley, 1979; Thompson, 1983; Williams and Silverman, 1968; St. Louis et al., 1988; Louko, Edwards and Conture, 1988), based on actual or direct examination of young stutterers' speech behavior, report that between 24 percent and 45 percent of young stutterers exhibit articulation/phonology problems; this is much higher than the approximately 2 percent of the school-age population that has "extreme deviation" in articulation and others having "residual" articulation errors up through the third grade and beyond (Hull, Mielke, Timmons and Willeford, 1971).

At this point, the connection between speech articulation and speech fluency difficulties is unknown, but clinicians would be well advised to consider the implications of this connection on their diagnostic assessment and therapy plans when stuttering and articulation disorders are observed in the same child.

HISTORY/DESCRIPTION OF PROBLEM (ASSOCIATED BEHAVIOR)

If a problem with fluency is apparent, this section of the evaluation permits the clinician to assess the degree to which the client is presenting overt reactions to the problem and, with children, the degree to which this is bothersome to the parent. Often with children, it is their behavior, for example, head turning, blinking (both eyelids), facial grimaces, *associated* with their stutterings, rather than their stutterings per se, that convince the parents that the child needs help. As we have discussed elsewhere (Schwartz and Conture, 1988), while adults who stutter probably produce a larger number and greater variety of these associated behaviors than do children, young stutterers definitively exhibit a number and variety of these associated behaviors and it would seem that these differences are suggestive of different strategies for coping with stuttering.

ANXIETY/SITUATIONAL HIERARCHY

Brutten and Shoemaker (1967) were among the first to introduce the use of anxiety/situational hierarchies to stuttering theory and therapy. Erickson (1969) subsequently reported a scale for measuring the communication attitudes that distinguish stutterers from nonstutterers, and Andrews and Cutler (1974) revised this scale to measure change in these attitudes during the course of therapy. While the relation of stutterers' attitudes to changes in their speech as a result of therapy remains unclear (Ingham, 1984), Erickson's, Andrews', and Cutler's efforts in this area provide a solid beginning for the eventual development of an instrument for assessing stutterers' attitudes.

More recently, Hanson, Gronhond and Rice (1981) measured the speech-related attitudes of adult stutterers with a different but related form of speech situation checklist. However, for children who stutter, only Guitar's and Peters's (1980) experimental version of the Erickson Scale and Brutten's (1982) still-in-development Speech Situation Checklist for Children have been reportedly used to assess self-reports of school-age stutterers' speech-related attitudes. It is still unknown whether such a self-report questionnaire procedure could be readily and reliably administered to preschool/early elementary school-age children (between two and seven), the age period when most children actually begin to stutter.

Although my purpose for obtaining a "situational hierachy" differs from those of individuals eventually interested in systematically desensitizing the client to various environmental stimuli, the procedure is roughly the same. At present, however, it is most feasible to do this with adults. When done with adults an interesting observation may be made: Those adults who stutter who give the most detailed situational hierarchy—precise descriptions and a rank order, in degree of strength of perceived emotionality, of stimuli associated with stuttering—will often recover quicker and more permanently from stuttering than those who provide a less detailed hierarchy.

For most younger clients, some direct but simple questions such as, "When does he appear to stutter the most?" will elicit such parental responses as "When he is tired, excited, or in a hurry and asking questions." Sometimes no such connection between the environment and child behavior and stuttering will be reported. This observation is instructive, particularly if the clinician notices differences in the child's stuttering during different activities or when the child is feeling or behaving in certain ways.

This is also the area where questions regarding avoidance of persons, places, or things can be asked. Once again, avoidance is generally more pronounced or apparent in older stutterers, but it is wise to get some idea if avoidance, in any form, is beginning to be part of the problem, even in children.

HISTORY/DESCRIPTION OF PROBLEM
(WHAT PEOPLE HAVE BEEN DOING TO "HELP")

There is a line in a Marlo Thomas's et al. (1972) song ("Free to Be You and Me") that goes: "There is some kinda help which is the kinda help we can all do without." This is particularly true with stutterers and we, as clinicians, want to know as much about the past and present of these helping efforts as we can. In the main, suggestions to "Slow down and take a deep breath," or "Speed it up, I don't have all day," or "Relax and think about what you are going to say," reflect expressions of sincere concern as well as frustration on the part of the listener.

Whatever the case, it helps to know what kind of reactions, suggestions, assistance, and so forth the stutterer is routinely as well as occasionally exposed to. Having this sort of information is crucial in your attempts to help the client's associates adopt more facilatory reactions and minimize their apparently inhibitory reactions. It also gives you clues regarding what the client's associates as well as the client think have caused and perpetuated the problem. This too should be useful to you as you try to gather more objective, factual information about stuttering and what influences it.

FAMILY INTERACTION

While questions about family life are generally directed at the child or teenager living at home, they may also be useful for the older client still living at home or one who is married. With the child, we want to know all we can about the role speech and language has in the home, that is, its relative importance and value as well as the amount and kind routinely produced. It is not uncommon to find oral expression and speech highly prized in the home of stutterers and the child may be encouraged to recite orally for family, friends, and neighbors such things as nursery rhymes, speeches, memorized stories, or putting on little plays or singing songs. We call this "performance" (as in "command performance") speech. This is not unlike singing for one's supper or grandmother, as the case may be.

Routine "drill" with flash or cue cards where the child has to recite memorized numbers, objects, colors, or letters is also sometimes observed. Answers to your questions may also indicate that family dinners are spent with the television, radio, or stereo in the background in addition to mother, father, brother, sister, and the young stutterer talking all at once! Once again, the client is a person, a person living in some environment, and it behooves the clinician to find out as much as possible about that environment in order to understand more clearly the person's stuttering and what may be done about it.

SOCIAL/BEHAVIORAL

While tests like the Vineland Test of Social Maturity will help the clinician understand the child's social maturity, we also want to learn the client's ability to interact appropriately with individuals in and outside the home. Actually, this is related to questions regarding family interaction and academic experiences. Of particular note is the question: "What does he/she do that particularly annoys you or anyone else?" With an adult you might ask, "Do you know of anything that you do that might annoy your friends, relatives, or fellow workers?" Usually, both parents and adults will respond, "You mean besides speech?" and we say, "Yes, besides speech." Often, particularly with parents, the thing or things that annoy them about the child beside the child's speech are as much a reason to seek your advice as the speech itself. With children, we are especially interested in knowing about the number and ages of friends they have in the neighborhood and in school if they attend.

It is not unusual for parents of stutterers to say, "We don't want him associating with this or that child," or "We don't want him to get hurt, dirty, or in trouble playing outside," or similar words that indicate they are having trouble letting the child have the normal amount of independence all children need in order to develop. Many of these parents will be particularly concerned about sending the child to nursery school, prekindergarten, a baby-sitter, day care, or even kindergarten or first grade ("People will pick on him . . . he is not ready . . . some of those children play real rough and Todd is so gentle").

One response I make to these parents (when it is apparent that junior has what it takes to absorb the slings and arrows of outrageous fortune at the hands of his peers) is something like, "You want to know if it's all right if you keep him out of kindergarten and have him stay at home with you? Sure, as long as you plan on enrolling yourself in his school and sit next to him in kindergarten, first grade and beyond." This usually gets the point across. Yes, I know its hard to let go, but let go you must, at least a little bit now, unless you plan on having your child lean on you for life. More on this in the next chapter.

WRAP UP

As anyone knows who has attended a reception, leaving can almost be as awkward as arriving. The same is true of an interview. We have found that questions about things the client or client associates think need to be or can be changed is a good way to end. Talking about past or present services for stuttering gets people thinking about the role the present clinical services, if they are recommended, will play in their lives. Our last question is particularly instructive: "If you could wish for three things for yourself or your child—the sky is the limit—what would you wish for?" It is *not* unusual for speech language or any other aspect of communication to be excluded from this list. Such exclusion should tell the clinician something about priorities in the person's life. Although wishes do not necessarily reflect reality, wishes do tell us about a person's aspirations and desires. Knowing something about these things is not to be considered lightly.

ASSESSING COMMUNICATIVE AND RELATED BEHAVIORS

With the intake form and the results of the interview in hand, the speech-language pathologist may then turn to the third component of the evaluation: the actual assessment of communicative and related behavior. If the interview places a premium on appropriate questions and adequate follow up, the actual assessment of communicative and related behavior places a premium on rapid but careful observations and clear, precise note taking.

Of particular importance is the notion that behavior can be within normal limits but different from the mean. Again and again, the SLP will observe behavior that is different from the expected *average* or *mean*. The question, however, is whether this difference is appreciably or significantly different from the mean to warrant concern. Once again, I will point out that many readers of this book have an IQ that is different from 100, but is this cause for concern on their part? I think not. Most behavior seems to have a central tendency (mean, median, or mode) but "surrounding" that central tendency is a dispersion or spreading of values or scores (range, variance, standard deviation, and so forth) and trying to understand, recognize, and deal with the "normal" spread of human behavior is a task to which most clinicians devote a good deal of their time.

Table 2–1 shows a summary sheet that we routinely fill out during this portion of the diagnostic. Obviously, not every portion of this form will be filled out for every client, but we have found that assembling test results on one piece of paper makes the job of summarizing results much easier, quicker, and effective. Besides, when all information is in place, it significantly reduces the risk of losing information and the clinician is better able to relate findings in one area to those in another. Once again, such a form

TABLE 2–1. Syracuse University Fluency Diagnostic Summary Sheet. This form is provided as an example or a model for clinicians interested in developing their own diagnostic summary sheet. DOE = Date of Examination, DOB = Date of Birth, Re-eval = A re-evaluation assessment or diagnostic, Judges = Clinicians who are observing or assessing behavior, SSI = Stuttering Severity Instrument, SPI = Stuttering Prediction Instrument, CAI = Communication Attitude Inventory (after Andrews and Cutler, 1974), MLU = Mean Length of Utterance, TOLD = Test of Language Development, PPVT = Peabody Picture Vocabulary Test, S/Z ratio = length of sustained /s/ divided by length of sustained z (after Eckel and Boone, 1981), DDK = diadochokinetic or alternating motion rate assessment, and QNST = Quick Neurological Screening Test (after Mutti et al., 1978)

SYRACUSE UNIVERSITY FLUENCY DIAGNOSTIC SUMMARY SHEET   as of 6/1/89

NAME:_____

AGE:_____ DOE: _/_/_ DOB: _/_/_

OVERALL IMPRESSION:

Therapy____ Yes___ No___ When _/_/_ Other_____
Re-eval____ Yes___ No___ When _/_/_ Other_____

STUTTERING

FREQUENCY OF STUTTERING
	1	2	3	4	5	6	x
	(←---(Judges)----→)						
Mean (x)							
Range							

DURATION OF STUTTERING
	1	2	3	4	5	6	x
	(←---(Judges)----→)						
Mean (x)							
Range							

RANK ORDER OF DISFLUENCY TYPES
% of Total	1	2	3	4	5	6	Mean
	(←------------(Judges)-------→)						
SSR							
WWR							
SP							
PHR							
REV							
INT							
OTHER							

CHILD'S RATE OF SPEECH
	1	2	3	4	5	6	x
	(←--------(Judges)-----→)						
Mean (x)							
Range							

PARENT'S RATE OF SPEECH
	Mother	Father
Mean		
Range		

STOCKER PROBE
	1	2	3	4	5
TOTAL					
BREAKDOWN-					
RECOVERY-					

SSI
TOTAL
Freq-
Dur -
Physical

SPI
TOTAL
Hist -
Reac -
Rep -
Prol -
Freq -

CONSISTENCY
Inconst. -
Quest. -
Consist. -

CAI

OTHER

LANGUAGE/ARTICULATION/READING/RECEP. VOCAB.

M.L.U.
Mean
Range

GRAMMATICAL MORPHEMES

ARTICULATION ERRORS/
PHONOLOGICAL PROCESSES

WOODCOCK
READING TEST

TOLD

AMMONS and AMMONS

PPVT

OTHER

VOICE/ORAL MECHANISM/NEUROMOTOR

VOICE
Pitch
Intensity
Quality

S/Z RATIO

x = 0.99
SD = 0.36

ORAL PERIPHERAL
EXAMINATION

DDK

QNST

should in no way restrict or preclude the clinician from developing her own form; our form is presented as a guide rather than a prescription.

Fluency

Assessing the fluency of speech requires that the clinician consider some or all of the following:

1. Mean and range of frequency or number of *each* type of speech disfluency (for example, part-word repetition versus revisions) per 100 words or syllables spoken.
2. Mean and range of frequency of *total* speech disfluencies per 100 words or syllables spoken plus percentage of this total contributed by each disfluency type. For example, a client produces, on the average, a total of 10 disfluencies per 100 words and of these 10, 6, on the average, are sound prolongations suggesting that 60 percent of all disfluencies are sound prolongations.
3. Mean and range of *duration* of approximately 10 within-word speech disfluencies (a digital stopwatch is most useful for recording this temporal measure). Another related measure of duration is the average number or units of repetition per whole-words or sound/syllable repetition..
4. *Consistency* of instances of stuttering. For example, on reading one the client stutters ten times and on reading two, six times; how many stutterings on reading two were previously stuttered on reading one?
5. Average number and variety of nonspeech behaviors (for example, head turning, eyeball turning, eyelid opening and closing, facial grimaces, and so forth) associated with each stuttering.
6. Results of such tests as the Stocker Probe Technique, Stuttering Severity Instrument, and Stuttering Prediction Instrument as well as such severity rating procedures as The Iowa Test for Stuttering Severity.

Other behaviors such as stutterers' attitudes, rates of utterance, turn-taking ("turn-switching") skills, conversational overlaps between stutterer and listener, and so forth (cf. Conture and Caruso, 1987) are also important—and will subsequently be discussed.

Frequency of stuttering   While it is difficult to make hard and fast rules because we still lack adequate norms for speech fluency, our experience suggests that individuals who exhibit 3 or more *within-word* disfluencies per 100 words spoken (average across various types and complexities of speaking situations) have some degree of fluency concern (cf. Table 1-1). However, this frequency of within-word disfluencies in and of itself does not mean that the person is a stutterer. The younger the client, of course, the less reliable any such absolute percentages become because the young child's communicative skills are still developing.

Readers should be aware that other clinical guidelines exist with regard to frequency of stuttering. Although these guidelines suggest 10 disfluencies (of *all* types) per 100 words (Adams, 1980), we are advocating the use of 3 *within-word disfluencies* per 100 words. These apparent differences are, we believe, fairly easily reconciled since individuals who produces 10 disfluencies, of all types, per 100 words of speech are more than likely producing 3 or more *within-word* disfluencies as part of those 10. We have chosen to consider only *within-word* disfluencies since a great deal of research indicates that these are the type of speech disfluencies that listeners are most apt to consider as stuttered and are the type of disfluencies that stutterers appear to produce much more often than normally fluent speakers (for example, Zebrowski and Conture, 1989). A "count" rating sheet like the one shown in Table 2-2 is of value during on-line (while the client is speaking or reading) tabulation of number, type, and total of speech disfluency.

Sample size   The first issue concerning stuttering frequency is the sample size (that is, number of spoken or read words). In general, the sample size should be sufficient to permit averaging across several 100-word samples. We have found that a 300-word sample is sufficient for this purpose, but some might feel more comfortable obtaining 500 words. Obviously, with a very severe stutterer, the length of time he or she would take to produce 300 words is counterproductive to achieving the end goals of the diagnostic and a sample of 50 to 100 words might suffice (being supplemented, as soon as possible after the beginning of therapy, with a sample based on a larger corpus of words). Once again, stuttering is a behavior that varies, and the nature and extent of such variation can only be understood by the clinician if he or she collects a large enough sample to adequately assess variation.

Frequency not the only measure   The good news about stuttering frequency is that with a modicum of training, a clinician can learn to count reliably the number of times per conversation or reading passage a person stutters. (It is, however, another matter whether two different listeners can as readily agree on where in a conversation stutterings occur—the exact sounds, syllables, or words that were stuttered—as they can on the frequency or number of stutterings that occur during the conversation [cf. Young, 1984 for review of this topic].) The bad news is that stuttering frequency, while certainly one of several factors used in judging stuttering severity, is less than perfectly correlated with other measures of speech fluency, for example, duration. Thus, to "capture" the totality of the stutterer's speech disfluency problem several measures must and should be simultaneously considered.

Stuttered words versus syllables   Another issue pertaining to the measurement of stuttering frequency is whether it should be computed in terms of percentage of stuttered *words* or *syllables*. At present, as far as we know, there is no conclusive evidence published in refereed journals that indicates that one procedure—words or syllables—surpasses the other in terms of accuracy or precision in estimating stuttering frequency. We discussed else-

TABLE 2–2. Syracuse University Disfluency Frequency Count Sheet. This form is provided as an example or a model for clinicians interested in developing their own diagnostic disfluency frequency count sheet. SSR = sound/syllable repetition, WWR = whole-word repetition, PR = phrase repetition, A. PROL = audible prolongation, I.A. PROL = inaudible prolongation, INTERJ = interjection, and REV. = revision.

SYRACUSE UNIVERSITY
DISFLUENCY COUNT SHEET

as of 6/1/89

DURATION OF STUTTERING (Based on _____ stutterings)

MEAN _____
RANGE _____

OVERALL STUTTERING

SAMPLE #	1	_____	per 100 words
	2	_____	per 100 words
	3	_____	per 100 words
MEAN		_____	per 100 words
RANGE		_____	per 100 words

SAMPLE #1 (100 words)

SAMPLE #1

% OF TOTAL DISFLUENCIES (% T D)

Disfluency Type	Freq.	% T D
SSR		
WWR		
PR		
A. PROL		
I.A. PROL		
INTERJ		
REV.		

SAMPLE #2 (100 words)

SAMPLE #2

% OF TOTAL DISFLUENCIES (% T D)

Disfluency Type	Freq.	% T D
SSR		
WWR		
PR		
A. PROL		
I.A. PROL		
INTERJ		
REV		

SAMPLE #3 (100 words)

SAMPLE #3

% OF TOTAL DISFLUENCIES (% T D)

Disfluency Type	Freq.	% T D
SSR		
WWR		
PR		
A. PROL		
I.A. PROL		
INTERJ		
REV		

RATE OF SPEECH	CHILD'S	MOTHER'S	FATHER'S
MEAN			
RANGE			

Disf. Type	SAMPLE # 1	2	3	Mean	Range	MOST TO LEAST FREQ. OCCURRING DISFLUENCY TYPES
SSR						
WWR						
PR						
A. PROL						
I.A. PROL						
REV						
INTERJ						
OTHER						

where (Conture and Caruso, 1987) whether one would obtain *significant* differences in percentages of stuttering, across most stutterers, using one method versus another. As Andrews and Ingham (1971) have shown, one can convert percent stuttered words to percent stuttered syllables by multiplying the former by 1.5. While such conversion would, of course, only provide a rough approximation of stuttered syllables, it is probably sufficient for most clinical diagnostic assessment purposes. Ham (1986) provides an excellent discussion of this issue.

Disfluency types Once the clinician knows something about the client's stuttering frequency, he or she should attempt to compute the relative proportion of total disfluencies contributed by each disfluency type. This, in our opinion, is a most important measure. For example, we have shown elsewhere that the percentage of sound prolongations in a sample of stutterings is one important feature in distinguishing among youngsters who stutter (Schwartz and Conture, 1988). It will also be noted that the Stuttering Prediction Instrument for Young Children (Riley, 1981) measures the presence of "blocks" (which are essentially audible or inaudible sound prolongations produced by stationary or fixed articulatory postures) to predict chronicity.

It is our belief that some within-word disfluencies, to paraphrase George Orwell, are more equal than others in terms of implications for severity and chronicity of stuttering. As more and more empirical investigations of the association between other behaviors and stutterers' type of disfluency are undertaken, we expect to see *type* rather than *frequency* of disfluency become a more meaningful measure for both experimental and clinical purposes.

Typically, the client's speech disfluencies will consist of four to seven different types of disfluencies with one or two of them accounting for most observed disfluencies. Computing and reporting the rank order, from most to least frequently occurring, of each observed disfluency type as well as their proportion (0 percent to 100 percent) of the total disfluencies is, we have found, quite an important measure. With children, for example, the most frequently occurring type of speech disfluency is apt to be (a) sound/syllable repetition followed by (b) sound prolongation with (c) whole-word repetition coming in a close third. As mentioned in Chapter 1, we believe that these differences in the type of speech disfluency stutterers most likely produce have implications for etiology and at the least for stages in development of the problem and we would really like to see basic and applied research address such possibilities.

We will discuss in Chapter 3 how the most frequently occurring disfluency type is used as an index of where the child is in the development of the problem as well as what this means in terms of therapeutic approach. Typically, we consider a client who predominantly produces sound/syllable repetitions (that is, the beta phase of development) to exhibit a less developed, less established problem than a child who predominantly produces the cessation or fixed articulatory type of disfluency, for example, sound prolongations (that is, the gamma phase).

In recent years, however, we have become aware of yet another group of children who predominantly produce monosyllabic whole-word repetitions (we are uncertain, at this point, whether this finding can be extrapolated to teenagers and adults who stutter). How these children fit into the alpha-delta schema previously discussed is quite unclear, and empirical research is needed to determine whether these children have a problem whose origins and course of development are different from those children who predominantly produce either sound/syllable repetitions or sound prolongations. It is our guess, and it is only a guess based on clinical observations, that children whose first or second most frequent disfluency type is a monosyllabic whole-word repetition are more likely to have "pure" expressive language delays than phonological concerns. This hunch, however, needs empirical testing before we fully subscribe to its veracity.

Duration of disfluency The extent, duration, or length of stuttering is often measured and would appear to be one of several interrelated variables that contribute to perceived severity of stuttering. Typically, we measure the average (and range) of the child's stuttering duration across a randomly selected sample of ten stutterings. A related measure, the number of units of repetition per sound/syllable repetition (cf. Yairi, 1983; Yairi and Lewis, 1984), may also be used as or considered to be an index of duration. While it makes intuitive sense that the more units of repetition per sound/syllable repetition the longer the repetition, there are no published data, that we know of, that conclusively support this notion. That is, the *rate* of repetition could conceivably differ to the point where a three-unit repetition could take 1200 ms (400 ms per repetition) whereas another three-unit repetition could take only 600 ms (200 ms per repetition). The *rate* and *rhythmicity* (that is, temporal regularity) of the units of repetition would seem to be just as important as the number of units itself in determining the duration of the sound/syllable repetition as well as its contribution to judgments of the person's severity.

The best way, in our experience, to become sensitive to differences in durations of various disfluency types is to measure them. This is best done using a digital stopwatch; they are a bit quieter (particularly those without an audible beep when the start/stop button is depressed) and easier to read than the old-fashioned analog stopwatch with its audible clicking and sweep-second hand. If the clinician practices tabulating the duration of each client's stuttering (or at least a subsample of each) he or she will, after awhile, be able to approximate much better, *without* the use of a stopwatch, the difference between a 250 ms and 750 ms instance of stuttering. Understanding such differences not only makes the clinician a better diagnostician but helps him or her assess behavioral changes in therapy since the duration of stuttering is often one of the very first things to improve in therapy, even before frequency of stuttering and other such behaviors.

Becoming more sensitive to the temporal domain of each instance of stuttering also improves the clinician's ability to judge other aspects of timing relative to speech production, for example, number of words per minute and measures of alternating motion rate (diadochokinesis). Along these lines, Pindzola, Jenkins and Lokken (1989) have provided useful information pertaining to both speaking and articulatory rates of normally fluent children (ages 2 to 5 years) during conversation—such data should help clinicians compare young stutterers' rate of utterance to those of their normally fluent peers. As the clinician learns to appreciate the wide variety and number of fluent and disfluent events that occur under 1000 ms (1 second), he or she will be better able to identify quickly and precisely those behaviors that need change in therapy. Assessment of stuttering requires more than merely counting instances of its occurrence; it also requires some ability to judge its type and duration as well.

Consistency of disfluency   Consistency of disfluency—the tendency for the loci of stuttering to be constant from reading to reading of the same material—can be judged on an informal as well as a more formal basis (Johnson and associates, 1963, pp. 272–76, 292). Although we still don't know the exact clinical significance of consistency of disfluency, we use this information as one more piece of data indicative of the relative habituation and association of instances of stuttering with particular stimuli. Knowing something about the nature of the various types of stimuli (Bloodstein, 1987, pp. 250–61) allows the clinician to show the client that stuttering has some degree of lawfulness—that it is not a random event behaving helter-skelter like kernels of corn popping in a popcorn popper (cf. Tate and Cullinan, 1962; Cullinan, 1988, for an excellent presentation of issues relating to the measurement of consistency).

Once again, however, you must be cautious: Be prepared for individual differences. While this or that study may indicate that stutterers as a *group* are consistent in their stuttering, as we mentioned in Chapter 1, stutterers don't enter your clinical doors in a group; they walk in as individuals. Individual behavior varies around the group's central tendency (for example, mean), and it is not at all unlikely that one particular stutterer may show very little consistency (or minimal adaptation) but still be a stutterer and need your services.

Another thing to consider is how to measure consistency in a nonreader, for example a four year preschooler. Neelley and Timmons (1967) and Williams, Silverman and Kools (1969) utilized a procedure for collecting and measuring data on stuttering consistency in young children that we have used for years in our clinic. In essence, seven or so age-appropriate sentences (five years and under = three-to-five-word sentences; five years old and older = six-to-eight-word sentences) containing age-appropriate vocabulary, are read to the child one at a time, and the child is instructed to repeat the sentence back to the examining SLP immediately. Most children can and will tolerate three readings/repetitions of these seven sentences but, once again, individual differences in attention span, fatigability, memory for words, and the like may inhibit a child's ability to perform this task. Whatever the case, this procedure is easy to implement and takes very little time to complete and may, for some younger clients, be the only time you get a reasonably adequate index of their fluency.

Number and variety of associated behaviors   Sometimes that which is the most apparent is that which we know the least about. Although there is hardly a textbook on stuttering that doesn't mention *secondary* or *associated* or *concomitant* behaviors, there is actually very little objective information regarding the number and nature of these behaviors. While one can find no end to clinical observations and anecdotes regarding these behaviors, there are, to the best of our knowledge, only three published empirical studies of these behaviors, by Prins and Lohr (1972), Krause (1982), and Schwartz and Conture, 1988. We suspect that the paucity of objective information regarding behavior associated with stuttering relates to at least two factors: (1) Most such associated behavior is nonverbal and it is not clear how such behavior can be systematically and objectively analyzed, particularly by speech-language clinicians whose interests and training lie in the realm of oral communication (see Ekman, 1982, for discussion of such methodology), and (2) these associated behaviors are generally considered so idiosyncratic that little or no central tendency is assumed to exist. (However, preliminary findings by Conture and Kelly [1988] do suggest that certain nonverbal behaviors, for example, eyeblinking, are more apt to be exhibited by stutterers during stuttering than during comparable fluent utterances produced by their normally fluent peers.)

While such tests as the Stuttering Severity Instrument request, and rightfully so, the clinician to measure "physical concomitants" of each client's stuttering, it is not clear what numbers and varieties of these behaviors a clinician could expect to see across a number of people who stutter. It is entirely possible, as Schwartz and Conture's (1988) study of the associated behaviors of 43 young stutterers indicates, that there are commonalities in terms of the number and nature of these behaviors but only for "subtypes" or "subgroups" of stutterers. That is, some stutterers are very similar to one another but very different from all other stutterers in terms of their associated behaviors. It is entirely possible that these similarities within a group and differences between groups, in terms of associated behavior, have implications for (1) etiology of the problem and (2) remediation of the problem. It is also entirely possible that it is the number rather than nature of stutterers' associated behaviors that represents the main difference between them and the nonverbal behavior produced by their normally fluent peers during comparable fluent utterances. For example, a stutterer may produce three nonverbal behaviors during a stuttering—a head turn, an eye blink, and a raising of the upper lip—whereas a normally fluent speaker may produce only a head turn and an eye blink (see Stern, Walrath and Goldstein, 1984, for excellent review of measure and meaning of human eyeblinking). Thus, much of what clinicians call "secondaries" may be nothing more than more frequent and longer duration behaviors rather than different nonverbal behaviors from those observed during normally fluent speakers' fluent productions.

What makes these associated behaviors all the more difficult to assess objectively is their interdependence with speech or verbal behavior (Beattie, 1983). While we might like to separate, say, a speaker breaking eye contact with his or her listener from the speaker's words produced slightly before and during the break in eye contact, in reality these two events—verbal and nonverbal—are connected. Even if we greatly simplify the situation and assume that verbal behavior conveys mainly content while nonverbal behavior conveys mainly a social/emotional message, we realize that the two messages—content and emotion—are inextricably related during most of our communications. For example, a father, with a steady gaze and lowered eyebrows, states: "Johnny, come in here. I want to talk to you about this stain on the coffee table." While the verbal message is relatively neutral, the speaker's associated nonverbal behavior gives Johnny more than an adequate idea of how the father feels and what he might say.

We have only the most rudimentary understanding of the number and nature of nonverbal behaviors associated with stuttering. The reasons for these behaviors, their significance for etiology and treatment, and their relation to behaviors produced during normally fluent speech are far from clear. Furthermore, we have a very limited understanding of the role of listeners' nonverbal behavior during stuttering, particularly those of parents during the stutterings of their children; whether such behavior differs from that observed when listeners listen to fluent utterances; and whether such behavior has potential for exacerbating or worsening the stutterer's stuttering. As noted at the beginning of this section, sometimes that which is the most apparent is that which is easiest to overlook.

One of the more interesting phenomena with stuttering in our experience are parental reactions to their child's nonverbal behavior associated with stuttering. It is not unusual for parents to have their child evaluated only *after* the child begins to produce nonverbal behavior that the parent notices during instances of stuttering. The child may have been "stuttering" for 3 to 12 months *before* the parent started to notice these associated behaviors. It is our experience that parents react to these nonverbal behaviors for one or both of the following reasons: (1) The number and nature of the associated nonverbal behaviors appear, to the parent, to be different from those seen during fluency and are thus "abnormal," unusual, and undesirable, something to be stopped, minimized, or eradicated, and (2) these associated nonverbal behaviors suggest to the parent that the child is "aware" or "concerned" or "bothered" or "frightened" by his problem and such a reaction on the part of the child concerns the parent.

In the next chapter we discuss how to deal (or how not to deal) with associated nonverbal behaviors, but suffice it to say that they are a part of stuttering that gives us a number of clues as to the severity, chronicity, and possible etiology of the problem.

(In)formal tests of stuttering   We have discussed elsewhere (Conture and Caruso, 1987) our diagnostic use of such tests as the Iowa Scale for Rating the Severity of Stuttering (Johnson et al., 1963), the Stuttering Severity Instrument (Riley, 1980), the Stuttering Prediction Instrument (Riley, 1981) and the Stocker Probe Technique (Stocker, 1976). We typically use each of these instruments in our assessment of fluency but for very different purposes. For example, we (Conture and Caruso, 1987, p. 98 and fig. 1) use the Iowa Scale to provide loosely objective support for our "Tentative Diagnosis"; in this case an individual described as a "moderate stutterer" would have an asterisk (*) after the word "stutterer" and at the bottom of the first page of the diagnostic report a footnote would say, "*Rating = 4 on the 0 (no stuttering) to 7 (very severe stuttering) Iowa Scale for Rating the Severity of Stuttering (Johnson et al., 1963).

In our opinion, the jury is still out on whether the three above mentioned tests of stuttering severity are any more accurate than a quantitative as well as qualitative assessment of the client's frequency, duration, and type of disfluency. It is important to note, however, that the aforementioned tests are relatively easy and quick to use, help the clinician organize the salient measures, and provide some sort of "norms" or values to which the clinician can compare the client under evaluation.

The other test—the Stuttering Prediction Instrument (SPI)—is, in theory, an even more important test since it tries to predict the chronicity of the child's problem. That is, while a test of severity may tell us *today* about the severity of the client's stuttering problem, it really tells us very little with regard to whether the client will continue to stutter tomorrow. At this point, no one, to our knowledge, has independently validated the extent to which the SPI does what it purports to do: predict which children will become chronic stutterers.

For the present, however, the SPI and the other tests of stuttering severity provide us with the beginnings of an objective means for assessing the severity and chronicity of stuttering. All clinicians who manage stutterers of any age should be familiar with the rationale, administration, scoring, and interpretation of these tests. They are important adjuncts to the evaluation of stuttering in children, teenagers, and adults.

Articulation

Although we don't have the objective data to support such a claim, it is our belief, based on our clinical experience, that stutterers exhibit more concerns with articulation than they do with expressive/receptive language (certainly, Cantwell and Lewis's [1985] descriptive analysis of stutterers' speech would support our belief). While one may decide, for a variety of reasons, to approach a particular stuttering problem from a "language stimulation" or "language enrichment" point of view, the expediencies of a particular therapy approach or management decision should not blur the clinician's view of the realities of the stutterer's actual problem. As Bloodstein (1987) states, "There is hardly a finding more thoroughly confirmed in the whole range of comparative studies of stutterers and nonstutterers than the tendency of stutterers to have functional difficulties of articulation, 'immature' speech and the like" (pp. 219–20).

While distinctions between *articulation disordered* and *phonologically disordered* are still not clear, findings of several studies (Daly, 1981; Cantwell and Lewis, 1985; Darley, 1955; Johnson and associates, 1959; Morley, 1957; Schindler, 1955; Williams and Silverman, 1983; Thompson, 1983; St. Louis and Hinzman, 1988; Louko, Edwards and Conture, 1988) indicate that between 24 percent to 45 percent of stutterers also exhibit articulation difficulties. This suggests that approximately one-third of all stutterers have some sort of difficulty with speech articulation. McMillan and Pindzola (1986) also provide some intriguing findings, based on acoustic measurement of stuttering and articulation-defective youngsters' "accurate" speech, which suggests that both groups are similar to one another but different from controls in terms of initiation of articulatory movements for speech.

While some stutterers with articulation concerns certainly also exhibit difficulties with expressive/receptive language, we are unaware of any empirical findings that would suggest 24 percent to 45 percent of stutterers also exhibit language problems. Obviously, the nature and severity of these articulation concerns undoubtedly vary among stutterers, just as they do in the normally fluent population. However, if we make the reasonable assumption that between 2 percent to 6.4 percent of the school-age population has some degree of a problem with speech articulation (Hull, Mielke, Timmons and Willeford, 1971; Beitchman, Nair, Clegg and Patel, 1986), finding that approximately 33% of stutterers exhibit articulation problems is several times higher than would be expected. (There are, of course, as Beitchman et al. [1986] report, another 3 to 7 percent of children who exhibit both speech *and* language problems; however, it is very unclear how many of these children with both problems also stutter.)

We would suggest to the clinician, particularly in the diagnosis of the school-age child suspected or known to be a stutterer, to informally (or better yet formally) assess the child's speech sound productions. Typically, we use the "Sounds in Words" subtest of the Goldman-Fristoe Test of Articulation (Goldman and Fristoe, 1969) for any and all sounds we suspect are problematic. Besides noting the number and type of sounds in error, the clinician should also note the presence of any "unusual" phonological process, for example, a glottal replacement, such as, /be?/ for 'bed.' Edwards and Shriberg (1983) have extensively discussed these and other phonological processes and the clinician unfamiliar with phonological process analysis is well advised to read their discussion. In our experience, most (two out of three) school-age stutterers will exhibit speech sound articulation and phonological processes well within normal limits but the remaining one child out of three will exhibit delays and/or deviancies in speech sound productions that warrant further testing and documentations of the child's possible articulation or phonological difficulties.

As we mention below with regard to expressive/receptive language concerns, it is not at all unusual to observe that as a young stutterer becomes more fluent, the child exhibits concerns with articulation and vice versa. It is as if the child's previous stuttering problem obscured or made relatively unimportant his articulation concerns or vice versa. In some cases, however, we are not convinced that the therapy for correction or modification of the child's speech sound difficulties did not, in some as yet unknown way, contribute to the child's emerging speech disfluency problem. Given the possibility that some children seem to begin stuttering *after* therapeutic attention to their speech sound difficulties, we urge clinicians to use relatively low-key approaches to changing articulation; we urge these clinicians to *avoid* therapies that use a physically tense, posturally correct, and relatively rapid production of sounds in error.

Indeed, at this point we are just beginning to understand the complex relation between speech sound articulation and speech fluency and the clinician is best advised to proceed carefully, to use a supportive, gentle, and unhurried manner when correcting a child's speech sound problem, particularly when there are co-occurring speech disfluencies or the likelihood for such co-occurrences.

Expressive/Receptive Language

Language difficulties can also accompany stuttering; however, as mentioned above, the frequency and nature of such language concerns with stutterers are still unclear. We have observed that an occasional client, particularly a child, exhibits a length and complexity of language structures that are less than appropriate for their age. Still other children seem less than adequate for their age in sequentially relating a story or event to a listener.

Other children seem to persist in continuing to monologue ("to hog the floor") to the extreme frustration and boredom of their listeners. Some of these children also exhibit reductions in their receptive vocabulary which, of course, places added strain on their ability to verbally communicate their thoughts quickly and efficiently.

We typically assess our younger clients' mean length of utterance (MLU) in morphemes and document the presence/absence of any and all grammatical morphemes. If these relatively informal procedures suggest a problem, then we may also use formalized tests like the Preschool Language Scale (Zimmerman et al., 1979) or the Test of Early Language Development (Hresko et al., 1982). As we have mentioned elsewhere (Conture and Caruso, 1987), clinicians should try to distinguish between the receptive/expressive "language problems" that are (1) relatively separate from, although possibly contributing to, fluency concerns; for example, a client with a reduced MLU and a number of missing grammatical morphemes, and (2) those problems that are the result of or secondary to a fluency problem; for example, a client who habitually uses subtly and some not so subtly incorrect vocabulary in attempts to avoid production of certain sounds, syllables, or words.

With regard to vocabulary, there are two tests of receptive vocabulary we routinely use that provide norm-referenced measures: the Peabody Picture Vocabulary Test (PPVT) (Dunn and Dunn, 1981), and the Quick Test (QT) (Ammons and Ammons, 1962). The PPVT is more appropriately used with preschool and elementary-school children while the QT is better used for older children, teenagers, and adults. We have previously mentioned (Conture and Caruso, 1987) our use of the QT as a rough index of the older child's general intelligence. While we fully realize that informal/formal testing of intelligence is the province of the clinical psychologist, we need to know at the time of assessment whether the client's IQ is roughly within normal limits and hence our use of the QT in this regard. We base our use of QT in this way on the fact that the QT as well as WISC vocabulary subtest are both highly correlated with the full-scale WISC IQ.

As we mentioned above with articulation, sometimes as a client who stutters becomes more fluent, a language concern appears (cf. Merits-Patterson and Reed, 1981). As with an "emerging" articulation problem, it would seem that the previously severe stuttering hid or drew attention away from an already apparent language difficulty. Therapeutically, this may mean a switch in emphasis from stuttering to language; however, a somewhat better approach might be a blending of attention to fluency *and* attention to language issues right from the beginning of therapy.

With regard to receptive vocabulary, most clients who stutter will be within normal limits, but clinicians will want to note those clients who score six months or below age norms and possibly address this—in a physically and mentally relaxed, unhurried, and gentle fashion—through the use of activities geared to enrich and stimulate vocabulary development.

Voice

In the past 10 to 20 years, perhaps no area in the field of stuttering has received as much attention and stirred up as much controversy as speculation regarding how stutterers use their larynx for speech production (for example, Conture, McCall and Brewer, 1977; Conture, Schwartz and Brewer, 1985; Adams, Freeman and Conture, 1984; Starkweather, 1982; Conture, Rothenberg and Molitor, 1986; Borden et al., 1985). However, it must be noted that during speech stutterers and normally fluent speakers can use their larynx as either (1) an articulator (for example, to adduct or abduct the vocal folds to or away from midline for the purposes of beginning or terminating voicing, respectively), or (2) a phonatory vibrator (for example, vibrating the approximated vocal folds for the purposes of voicing). While the articulatory and vibratory aspects of the larynx are interdependent, it is the larynx as a vibrator that we are primarily concerned with when we discuss "voice" or "voice quality" and the larynx as articulator that we are mainly talking about when we mean "beginning with a hard attack" or "getting stuck on that sound."

First, with regard to voice quality, there is no published empirical research* of which we are aware that proves that the perceptually fluent speech of stutterers, young or old, is more apt to be associated with a different sounding voice or voice quality than normally fluent speakers or that stutterers are more apt to have voice problems than normally fluent speakers, for example, hoarseness, harshness, and breathiness.

One exception to this is Healey's (1982) empirical observation that stutterers' fundamental frequency is less variable than that of their normally fluent peers and this observation is consistent with our clinical experience that some stutterers, young as well as older ones, seem to exhibit a rather monotonous, inappropriately low-pitched voice. However, this low-pitched Johnny-one-note problem is not unique to stutterers; many normally fluent speakers—salespersons, teachers, business people—also exhibit such voice use. At this point, it is unclear if the low-pitched monotone voice of some stutterers results from a stuttering problem or if it is a separate issue altogether.

Another exception is the stutterer, typically a younger one, who presents a hoarse and/or breathy vocal quality seemingly in relation to hyperfunctional voice usage. These are the clients who frequently "sing" with loud music or noise in the background, frequently imitate or use "mon-

*St. Louis et al. (1988) report such differences; however, it is unclear from their published report whether the judgment of stutterers' voice quality was based on samples containing instances of stuttering. The act of stuttering itself involves disruption in laryngeal behavior that can in turn change perceived vocal quality. These changes during and surrounding stuttering, however, should not be viewed like those of a voice problem that would be pervasive throughout the entirety of the stutterers' speech, the fluent as well as the stuttered aspects.

ster" or animal, car, truck, machinery, etc. noises when playing, frequently yell inside and outside, frequently engage in loud talking, and so forth. When such problems as inappropriately low-pitched, hoarse, or breathy voice do occur in a person who stutters, it usually justifies a referral to an ear, nose, and throat specialist (ENT), particularly if the client or associates report that such voice quality is persistent.

One caution, however: Disruptions in voice quality *during* or *surrounding* an actual instance of stuttering should not be confused with disruptions in voice quality throughout the stutterer's entire speech, the fluent parts as well as the disfluent. Often, the very act of stuttering involves laryngeal disturbances that result in changes in voice quality during the stuttering, but these changes are not the same as an ongoing problem of hoarseness, breathiness, diplophonia, inappropriate low-pitch, and the like, that would be observed throughout the *entirety* of the client's utterances, the fluent and stuttered parts (cf. Conture, McCall and Brewer, 1977; Conture, Schwartz and Brewer, 1985).

Typically, we assess a stutterer's voice through informal testing of the ability to change pitch from low to high (and vice versa) in both discrete and continuous steps. This may have to be modeled or demonstrated several times since many naive speakers confuse changes in vocal level (loudness or volume) with changes in vocal fundamental frequency (pitch). These clients will attempt to "go up and down the scale" by merely increasing or decreasing their vocal level (getting louder or softer). In our experience, the client's "flexibility" or variability of pitch is far more important than his or her modal or average pitch in terms of predicting whether the client will be able to, if required to do so, quickly and efficiently modify inappropriate aspects of laryngeal behavior.

With younger clients, for whom low and high as well as pitch and loudness mean very little, we have found that using nonhuman or animal models (that they must imitate) works much better: "Make a sound like a baby kitty (or) Meow just like a baby kitty. . .now meow just like the daddy kitty." "Make a sound like a wolf howl. . .Like a siren." Having the young client imitate these models permits the clinician to assess the client's ability to quickly, efficiently, and smoothly change from low to high pitch and back again, a crude but reasonable index of the ability to do this in running speech.

Another procedure we employ that we previously discussed (Conture and Caruso, 1987) is the s/z ratio (Eckel and Boone, 1981). Our experience indicates that youngsters below seven to eight years of age have difficulty understanding and/or cooperating with the task; they don't seem able to prolong the /s/ and /z/ for sufficient durations. However, even if these preschoolers shorten the duration of these fricatives to three to seven seconds in length, the clinician should be able to calculate the degree to which the client's s/z ratio approximates the norm: 1.00 (with approximately $\pm 1\ SD =$ 0.37). The s/z ratio is computed by timing the duration (in seconds or milliseconds) that the client can sustain the /s/ on one exhalation and then dividing this duration by the duration /z/ was sustained on one exhalation. The client is given several chances to sustain the /s/ and the /z/, with the longest duration of each used to figure the duration, and the resulting s/z ratio representing a "rough" means of determining the client's efficiency of vocal fold approximation or functioning during phonation.

A point or two about technological approaches should be made. With the advent of the desktop computer and hardware/software specifically designed to analyze speech, the use of such devices as the electroglottograph or EGG for both diagnostic and therapeutic purposes is going to increase (cf. Childers et al., 1983, Colton and Conture, in press, on practical/theoretical aspects of EGG usage and interpretation). For example, Conture, Rothenberg and Molitor (1986) reported that young stutterers are more apt than their normally fluent peers to use atypical vocal fold adjustments during consonant to vowel and vowel to consonant transitions. (It is unclear whether these atypicalities are perceptible to listeners but many, we suspect, aren't.) At present we interpret this to mean that young stutterers are using one of several different available means—albeit less efficient and perhaps more susceptible to disruption under stress—to make vocal fold adjustments for speech production.

The use of the EGG and other such devices (for example, the Visi-Pitch) for the assessment and remediation of laryngeal behavior in stuttering and other disordered populations is almost certain to increase in the years to come, particularly as researchers develop a means to reliably digitize the EGG signal, thus making EGG information analyzable through convenient and reasonably priced desktop computers. We urge speech-language pathologists to consider these devices as adjuncts or supplements to, rather than replacements for, their trained perceptual judgments and to try to keep abreast of these kinds of technological developments since they will have important implications for the types of diagnostic assessments and therapy programs they will be performing in the not-too-distant future.

Hearing

While there is a great deal of speculation and empirical investigation about the role audition plays in stuttering (for example, Conture, 1974; Neilson, 1980; Blood and Blood, 1984; Neilson and Neilson, 1987), most clinicians do not seem to place a great deal of emphasis on the assessment of audition with the stuttering population. This is unfortunate because stutterers have just as much right as nonstutterers to have hearing difficulties. Ideally, a full-scale diagnostic for stuttering should include pure tone screening (air and bone) as well as speech discrimination testing or access to the client's most recent test records.

For children in particular, middle ear status should be, if at all possible, assessed by means of tympanometry, for example, static acoustic impedance measures (single peak tympanograms) reported in acoustic ohms. Of course, for some clients, it may not be possible to obtain "normal" tympanograms if the client appears to exhibit a cold or an allergy or if the client lacks sufficient cooperation to permit completion of testing. However, assuming that retesting at a later date is not possible, the speech-language pathologist should at least try to record the presence or the history of any such middle ear concerns as frequent earaches, ear-drum rupture, persistent fluid in the ear, surgically inserted pressure-equalizing tubes, frequency and kinds of medications used to treat these concerns.

The SLP should be aware of these concerns because they may mean that a client who stutters, who also has chronic middle ear problems, is not always going to have the best auditory sensitivity-discrimination. It may also mean that a child may be more tired and/or more prone to rapid fatigue as a result of frequent middle ear infections (and associated upper respiratory infections), the various medications used to remediate such infections, or the excessive postnasal secretion brought about by a client's allergy. Since certain phonological concerns have been shown to be associated with middle ear difficulties (for example, Paden, Novak and Beiter 1987) in children whose phonological concerns appear intertwined with stuttering, the presence of hearing/middle ear problems may delay recovery and/or actually contribute to difficulties the client is having with speech sound articulation and speech fluency.

Reading

It is interesting to note that while reading material is frequently used in the management of stuttering, clinicians often have little objective information about the stutterer's reading abilities. It seems obvious, however, that if a person who stutters has oral reading difficulties, these difficulties may contribute to the person's stuttering during reading. Although we and others using standardized tests of reading abilities reported no significant difference between the reading abilities of stutterers and nonstutterers (for example, Conture and van Naerssen, 1977; Janssen, Kraaimaat and van der Meulen, 1983), others studying eyeball movement associated with silent reading reported that stutterers produced more eyeball "regressions" (eyeball moving back over previously read material) than normal speakers (for example, Brutten, Bakker, Janssen and van der Meulen, 1984).

Where do these apparent differences in empirical findings leave us clinically? Uncertain. It is entirely possible, although probably not the rule, that any one particular stutterer being evaluated may also demonstrate reading concerns that warrant attention from a reading specialist before or at least during the time speech therapy is undertaken. The SLP needs to coordinate speech-language services with the reading specialist so that the two services—reading and speech/language—complement rather than compete with one another. For example, any reading program that places emphasis on *quick, precise,* and *physically tense* speech sound articulation of reading material is not going to be in the best interests of a child who stutters. At the least, the SLP should understand that a child who stutters who also has a reading problem might find speech therapy difficult if reading material is used as a means of remediating speech behavior.

Academic Abilities and Status

Related to reading concerns are the school-age client's academic development and achievement. Academic concerns can be a problem in speech therapy with a child who stutters if the child is having so much trouble with school subjects that he or she feels discouraged or lacks confidence and regards any new seemingly "academic-like" situation like speech therapy sessions as a threat. Furthermore, a child struggling with school work, particularly if that child is doing poorly, is a child who may be tired at the end of the school day. Such fatigue needs to be taken into consideration by the SLP planning therapy for that child. If at all possible, the SLP should try to obtain general as well as specific knowledge of academic performance to date through records and discussions with the client's teachers. Particularly with a school-age child, administering speech therapy without knowledge of the child's academic abilities, progress, and performance is like traveling through a strange land without a map.

Attention Deficit Disorders (ADD)

An important interaction with academic performance as well as speech therapy performance is attention deficit disorder (ADD) (cf. Riley and Riley, 1988, for discussion of its possible relation to recovery from stuttering). Although there are still unclarity and lack of agreement regarding the etiology, symptomatology, and management of ADD (see Krupski, 1986; Shaywitz and Shaywitz, 1985, for excellent reviews of clinical and research findings relating to ADD), the experienced SLP will recognize some of its more common symptoms: (1) failure to finish tasks once started, (2) inattention, easily distracted, (3) restless, overactive, and unpredictable behavior, and (4) disturbance of other children.

Shaywitz and Shaywitz (1985, p. 6) suggest the presence of ADD if three or more of the following interrelated symptoms occur for more than six months' duration and have begun before the child is 7 years of age: *inattention* (for example, does not finish what he starts), *impulsivity* (for example, is extremely excitable), and *hyperactivity* (for example, always on the go; would run rather than walk).

According to Shaywitz and Shaywitz, there are three to four criteria for diagnosing each of these symptoms (inattention, impulsitivity, and hyperactivity). For example, impulsivity is diagnosed when at least three of the following are observed: (1) child calls out in class; makes noises in class; (2) is extremely excitable; (3) has trouble waiting his turn; (4) talks excessively; and (5) disrupts other children.

In my clinical experience, it isn't that a child exhibiting ADD doesn't observe what is going on around him or her as much as the fact that he or she is observing everything going on around them and all at once. These children seem to lack the ability to selectively attend for a sufficient period of time to the task at hand before they are off onto a new and different task—but for only a while before they switch to yet another task. Obviously, if this sort of behavior persists in school and in therapy, the child is going to have trouble being successful.

Wherever possible, referral to a clinical psychologist, child psychiatrist, or pediatrician *familiar* with this problem (and its behavioral, educational, and pharmaceutical management) is clearly in order if the SLP suspects ADD. However, and this is very important, the SLP should realize that *all* children sometimes fidget, get distracted, become restless, disturb other children, and so forth.

Thus, it is not the mere presence of such ADD-like behaviors that warrant referral but their chronicity and predictability, that is, their frequent and consistent occurrence across a wide variety of situations. Furthermore, the SLP should realize that there is no published, empirical evidence to suggest that children or adults who stutter are more apt to exhibit ADD than their normally fluent peers; however, there is also no evidence to suggest that stutterers never exhibit ADD. It seems reasonable to suggest that a young stutterer who also chronically exhibits disruptions in attention regulation and activity modulation may, at the least, take a protracted period of time to recover from stuttering and, at the worst, unless ADD is ameliorated, exhibit little or no improvement in stuttering. Certainly, most children who stutter do not seem to exhibit ADD, but the SLP should try to recognize those who do and plan management strategies accordingly.

Neuromotor Speech and Nonspeech Behavior

Many normally fluent children occasionally exhibit what some would call neuromaturational signs or "soft signs" of minimal brain dysfunction (MBD), for example, slow and/or asynchonous difficulties with some or many fine and gross motor tasks. All too often, in our experience, professionals, when observing these so-called "soft signs," are quick to apply the label of MBD that implies structural central nervous system abnormality. And yet, even with a problem like ADD, which would clearly seem to be related to MBD or structural CNS abnormality, computed tomography (CT scanning) studies of ADD youngsters' cortical anatomy has proven normal (Shaywitz, Shaywitz and Byrne, 1983). In other words, let us continue to assess the neuromotor abilities of people who stutter, but at the same time be cautious when we interpret what "causes" the problems we observe in this area.

It is not uncommon for a child, teenager, or adult who stutters to demonstrate marginal skills in certain fine and/or gross motor tasks, particularly tasks that require rapid, sequential and coordinated touching, such as tip of thumb to each finger tip. Some clients who stutter will exhibit difficulty touching their tongue tip to either the middle of their upper lip or the middle of their chin, just below their lower lip. Some stutterers may show slow and/or awkward movements when trying to move their tongue rapidly from side to side. They also may demonstrate "overflow" in that their mandible moves with their tongue instead of remaining fixed or stationary. That is, they cannot maintain the necessary stabilizing "background" behavior, in this case a stationary mandible, to allow for the fastest and most precise "foreground" behavior, in this case, rapid side-to-side tongue movements. However, none of these skills, even for the normally fluent population, have been shown to relate to speech difficulties (see Hardy 1970, 1978). We are not denying the existence of neuromotor difficulties in people who stutter, but we are urging caution in terms of how we interpret their etiology and relation to stuttering.

Practically, rates of alternating oral motor movements (diadochokinesis) can be assessed for uni-, bi- and tri-syllabic productions and then compared to published norms (Fletcher, 1972). Riley and Riley (1986) have recently introduced the Oral Motor Assessment Scale (OMAS) that provides some norms against which to compare the client as well as a means to assess various aspects of oral motor coordination, that is, "accuracy" (precise production of target speech sounds), "smooth flow" (evenly spaced, correctly sequenced, coarticulated flow of syllable production) and "rate." At this point, is is still uncertain which of the three aspects—accuracy, smooth flow, or rate—of the OMAS are the most central to the diagnosis and management of youngsters' oral motor problems, but this test is a clear step in the direction of more quantitative, comprehensive testing of youngsters' speech motor abilities and development (cf. Peters et al., 1975, for examples of such clinical tests of youngsters' neuromotor development).

Another, more general test of neurological functioning is the Quick Neurological Screening Test (QNST; Mutti, Sterling and Spaulding, 1978). The QNST assesses gross and fine motor movement, balance, coordination, and related abilities. QNST scores individuals as "normal" (0–24), "suspicious" (26–35), and "impaired" (35 and above); however, the QNST can be difficult to administer in whole or in part because the tasks it requires the client to perform require a good deal of cooperation, attention, and energy— variables that are often in short supply in children under seven years of age, particularly at the end of a diagnostic. Like the OMAS, the QNST should be viewed by the clinician as a supplement to rather than replacement for the clinician's ability to judge oral motor proficiency. It should also be noted that the QNST's assessment of oral and/or speech motor movements is limited although it provides a fairly extensive assessment of basic hand coordination and movement and the client's ability to "translate" auditory and visual information/instructions into hand movement.

With regard to rates of alternating oral motor movements (diadochokinesis), clinicians will observe that some stutterers, particularly those who seem to have a more habituated, severe problem, will also stutter on the first mono-, bi- or tri-syllable produced in either an alternate or sequential diadochokinetic task. This stuttering usually takes the form of an audible or silent prolongation of the syllable-initial sound of the first syllable in the string, after which the client generally produces the remaining syllables in a fluent manner. If the clinician excludes the time taken up by this initial stuttered syllable, and computes the diadochokinetic rates based on the remaining fluent syllables, the SLP will typically find that fluent syllables are produced at a rate roughly within normal limits. It is our opinion that stuttering during the initial sound/syllable of these various diadochokinetic tasks suggests a very habituated problem and many times less than a positive prognosis. Such stuttering may also occur on the Word Attack as well as other subtests of the Woodstock reading test and can be similarly interpreted.

Word Finding

We have discussed elsewhere (Conture and Caruso, 1987) the difficulties of separating, in clients who stutter, those "latencies" of responding that are due to "word-finding" difficulties and those that are related to the act of stuttering itself. The general relation of word finding to language abilities has been adequately explored elsewhere (Kail and Leonard, 1986) and we will not repeat this coverage here. Suffice it to say, that German (1986) recently introduced the Test of Word Finding that is an objective means of assessing word finding and related abilities. To date, this test appears to be the best way of assessing word-finding abilities in children that we have used. However, we are still not sure that it can readily and reliably distinguish stutterers' response latencies due to difficulties with word finding from those due to stutterers' hesitating or pausing because of reluctance to say a particular sound, syllable, or word. Clearly, more empirical research is needed in this area to determine the nature of the situation.

Psychosocial Adjustment

The overwhelming evidence suggests that stutterers' psychosocial adjustment is within normal limits (Sheehan, 1970a); however, this does not mean that any one individual who stutters might not have psychological concerns. In our experience, psychological factors to be considered during the evaluation typically involve one or more of the following: (1) motivation for seeking services (a difficult but important variable to assess); (2) psychological aspects that may hinder or facilitate therapeutic progress; and (3) psychological considerations that warrant referral to other professionals, such as a clinical psychologist or a psychiatrist.

It is not particularly easy to assess a client's motivation for seeking services. One essential aspect of motivation is whether the client is seeking help him- or herself (internal prodding) or because others have told the client to get help (external prodding). External prodding, as from a parent or spouse, may get a person in the therapy door, but it will not provide the effort level, initiative, and insight necessary to successfully complete therapy.

Internal-prodding motivation may result from a variety of factors, for example, lack of satisfaction with employment ("If I could only speak more fluently then I could get a better job") or dissatisfaction with the social status quo ("If I could speak more fluently I could meet more people, have more friends, do more things"). Occasionally, external prodding comes from an employer; for example, "Bill, if you want to become sales rep for the district, you've got to stop stuttering. We'll help you pay for the services, but you are not going to go any further in this company until you speak better."

External-prodding motivation from parents comes from their sincere concern for the child's future in school ("We want to get this cleared up before he begins school and it becomes a problem and gets in the way of his schoolwork") and/or employability ("No one is going to hire him if he talks that way . . . he'll have real trouble finding a job"). Parents are also motivated, as mentioned previously, to seek help for their child when the child's problem continues longer than they think it should, when the child starts to exhibit nonspeech behavior in association with the stuttering, and when they believe the child is starting to become "aware" of his speaking difficulties. In truth, the SLP can only guess at these various forms of motivation; however, the guess can be quite educated and should help in the planning of therapy and information sharing that must take place during the diagnostic and during therapy itself.

Psychological concerns can hinder therapeutic progress when the client is: too subjective about the problem (or unable to be relatively objective about the problem even with the SLP's help), too nonassertive, passive, and/or consumer-oriented ("looking for the cure"), too intellectual in his dealings about the problem ("deny emotions and explanations for behavior"), prone to project his feelings onto others ("Every time I open my mouth you think I'm stupid"), and so forth. We become particularly concerned during the diagnostic, if during some preliminary exploring with the client or his/her parents, we broach a seemingly reasonable explanation of a behavior or aspect of behavior that needs changing and the client or parent does one or both of the following: (1) categorically or flatly denies that the reason or explanation has any validity or relation to their problem, or (2) provides a myriad of excuses for why the behavior occurred or is necessary or important. Our experience suggests that the denial and/or excuse means of coping with a problem is a very counterproductive mechanism and is, in our opinion, an indicator of less than positive prognosis.

Recently, Healey, Grossman and Ellis (1988) had a psychologist observe the psychological characteristics and associated behaviors of 15 adult stutterers who exhibited minimal improvement in speech fluency through a variety of therapies. Some of the common traits observed among these stutterers were (1) self-critical behavior; (2) perfectionistic attitudes toward performance; (3) extreme resistance to change; (4) low self-esteem and self-confidence; and (5) denial of increased fluency. While these observations are of interest, we still do not know whether these traits would also be exhibited in adult stutterers who *did* increase their speech fluency as a result of therapy.

Andrews and Craig (Andrews and Craig, 1988; Craig and Andrews, 1985; Craig, Franklin and Andrews, 1984) have tried to do just that: study differences in psychological and related characteristics between those adult stutterers who do and do not relapse after therapy. Among other variables, they assessed locus of control, that is, the extent to which a person perceives events as being a consequence of his or her own behavior (internal control) and therefore potentially under personal control versus the extent to which a person perceives events as resulting from luck or environmental influences outside his or her control (external control). Andrews's and Craig's (1988) measures of locus of control, taken together with indexes of stuttering frequency and attitudes toward communication (Andrews and Cutler, 1974) indicate that 97 percent of those adult stutterers who did not relapse (relapse = stuttering greater than 2 percent stuttered syllables at ten months post-treatment) exhibited internal locus of control, "normal" communication attitudes, and no hint of stuttering on a telephone task at the end of therapy. Conversely, there were no adult stutterers who were fluent ten months post-treatment who obtained none of these goals—internal locus of control, "normal" communication attitudes, and no stuttering on telephone task—at the end of therapy.

Hence, we have some evidence that certain psychological constructs, in this case locus of control, when taken together with other more typical measures of fluency and related attitudes, might help us predict long-term recovery from stuttering, an observation that bears continued investigation with stutterers of other ages and in different therapy settings.

As Vaillant (1977) shows, *all* people have problems. What differs among people is the means—the psychological coping mechanisms—they use to deal with these problems and these differences in coping mechanism make all the difference in the world in terms of people's satisfaction and success in dealing with personal as well as work-related issues. In later chapters we discuss the relevance of these coping mechanisms to stuttering therapy, but for now suffice it to say that during the evaluation it is as important to understand the nature and number of psychological coping strategies as it is to understand the nature and number of problems the stutterer and associates are coping with.

Some stutterers (5 percent to 15 percent of all stutterers?) exhibit psychological concerns of a kind and severity that warrant professional evaluation and counseling by trained psychiatrists or psychologists. Some of these clients, as Van Riper (1973) so aptly put it, seem to stutter "with a gleam in their eye," with our only problem, as clinicians, being able to recognize that gleam. For these clients, who seem to represent only a very small percentage of all stutterers, the stuttering problem and all its manifold aspects seem to fulfill unmet needs, and this group of clients would appear to need referral to a professional counselor.

With children, who cannot as easily articulate their psychosocial concerns, one may have to look for behavioral indexes. The following is a partial listing of behavior to look for.

1. A child that other children routinely shun or avoid
2. A child that other adults report that they can't manage or won't allow in their home
3. A child who refuses to speak to the SLP, no matter what the topic or approach, after 30 to 90 minutes of trying, but who readily talks to mother/father once the SLP leaves the room
4. A child who routinely acts out against other children
5. A child whose strong fear of fire, loud noises, the dark, and anything strange is so routine and long-term as to disrupt home life
6. Any combination of (1) through (5)

Once again, it is the frequency and predictability of these behaviors not their mere presence once in a while that is of concern.

It should also be recognized that it is not uncommon for a stutterer, who is already receiving psychological counseling for other concerns like depression or compulsive-obsessive behavior, to also seek out the services of an SLP; however, it is important to understand the reasons such a client might want the services of an SLP and to make sure that the two forms of therapy complement rather than contradict each other.

While there is little objective evidence to suggest that psychosocial concerns *cause* stuttering, it is quite possible that stuttering itself might lead to psychosocial adjustment problems and that psychosocial difficulties may exacerbate an already existing stuttering problem and/or make recovery from stuttering more difficult. As previously discussed, we feel it is unwise to view stuttering from either a nature *or* nurture perspective; we prefer to view it as resulting from nature *interacting* with nurture. (At this point, the reader, particularly the beginning SLP or student clinician, might want to read Appendix E, which contains a sample of an entire diagnostic report.)

WHO IS AND WHO IS NOT REFERRED FOR THERAPY

After collecting some or all of the above information, we come to the moment of truth: Does the client have a problem and if so, is therapy warranted and what should be its form? Figure 2–1 shows the three possible decisions and their resulting consequences: (1) Yes, the client has a problem; (2) we are uncertain if the client has a problem; and (3) no, the client does not have a problem. Note that with categories (1) and (2) we are suggesting, for many of these cases, a follow-up evaluation (we typically request such reevaluations about three to six months after the initial assessment).

Some clients, particularly children, even those with obvious speech fluency concerns, may improve significantly enough in three to six months simply as a result of information sharing and counseling at the time of initial diagnostic to preclude actual therapy. Of course if the client still has a concern at the second diagnostic, then therapy is clearly recommended. Sometimes fools rush in where angels fear to tread; the mere presence of stuttering, particularly in younger clients, is not, in and of itself, sufficient to warrant the

DIAGNOSTIC DECISIONS

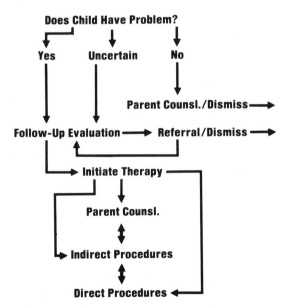

FIGURE 2–1. Diagnostic decision flowchart. A flowchart depicting the threefold diagnostic decisions—yes, no, or uncertain (an individual stutters—and the possible relation these have to management strategies. Note that therapy does not always follow a "yes" decision; a follow-up evaluation may occur first. There is nothing fixed about the number of these decisions—they could be expanded into five: yes, probably yes, uncertain, probably no, and no; or even seven: yes, probably yes, maybe yes, uncertain, maybe no, probably no, and no. Parents Counsl = Counseling of parents about their child's problem and/or what they can do to help.

time, energy, and expense of speech therapy until the clinician knows more about the entirety of the client's abilities and environmental interactions and is able to observe these over a modest length of time (say three to six months).

While we clearly do not want to deny services to anyone who needs them, we certainly don't want to make rushes to judgment and administer therapy to everybody who asks for or whom others say needs help. We have an obligation to our clients to be as discriminating as possible in delivering our services because if anyone can get them then no one really needs them.

Children

With children, as with adults, there is no *one* behavior or test result that we use to decide on therapy or no therapy. Typically, we recommend therapy if we note two or more of the following: (1) sound prolongations (audible and/or inaudible) that constitute more than 25 percent of the total disfluencies produced by the child; (2) avoidance of or averting eye contact with listeners more than 50 percent of time during conversations; (3) frequent and/or unusual phonological processes; (4) instances of sound/syllable repetitions or sound prolongations (silent or audible) on the first mono-, bi- or tri-syllabic production of diadochokinesis tasks; (5) OMAS scores and/or QNST scores indicating delays in speech and nonspeech neuromotor development; (5) Stuttering Prediction Instrument (SPI) score of 18 or above.

We become increasingly concerned if the parents of such a child talk too fast (190 to 200 words per minute or faster), frequently use complex vocabulary/linguistic structures that are too sophisticated for the child's level of development, and frequently exhibit brief (0.5 s or 500 ms) "turn-switching" or turn-taking pauses (Jaffe and Feldstein, 1970). Such parental behavior does (and did) not "cause" the child's stuttering, but it is quite likely that such parental communication may exacerbate, aggravate, perpetuate, or worsen the child's speech disfluencies and/or make it difficult for the child to maintain and/or become more fluent.

Parents and Relatives of Children

Whether we recommend immediate therapy, reevaluation, or no therapy, we counsel the parents. At the end of the diagnostic, we spend some time talking with the parents, even the parents of children who are doing nothing more than is typical for their chronological and developmental level. We have found that time spent with parents at the time of the diagnostic in counseling and information sharing regarding normal childhood development and behavior is well spent. With some of the parents, particularly where no apparent stuttering problem exists, other concerns are the real concern; for example, inability to tell time and be punctual; inability to keep a tidy room; inability to read, write, and count; inability to be as athletic as dad or an older brother or sister; and the you-can't-sit-down syndrome that may or may not indicate ADD.

Some of these parental concerns, we have observed, indicate that the parents are trying to speed up the pace of their child's developmental clock, as if they could bring about maturity and adult-like behavior in a five-year old. This parental concern is not helped as they continue to "look laterally" at their relative's or neighbor's child who is always going to do this or that earlier or better than their child. Sometimes, stuttering may be the name of what the parents say their concern is, but the real game is that they are worried that their child is "less than perfect." LeShan (1963), in a marvelous book discussing such typical parental concerns, says much that is of assistance to clinician and parent alike in understanding and dealing with these matters. It's not easy being a parent. There are the most minimal entrance requirements and it is little wonder that parents become concerned. If we want the parents of the young stutterer to become part of the solution rather than problem, we are going to have to spend time information sharing and counseling parents on what stuttering is and is not as well as on those things that will facilitate change in their child's speech and related behavior.

Older Clients

With older clients (say 16 years and older), the decision trilogy mentioned above—yes, uncertain, and no—becomes confounded with the notion of "benefit." Even with the older client who definitely appears to stutter, the SLP must consider whether the client can actually "benefit" from speech therapy. And if he or she can benefit, will that benefit last for more than a few weeks or months after the termination of therapy? While some might say it doesn't matter because therapy can't hurt, we would like to see more SLPs ask the question: Can therapy, of any form, actually help? There are no straightforward, simple answers to this question. It is a challenge to decide who might benefit from our services.

As in all matters, honesty is truly the best policy, but particularly with the older client, who may have experienced several other forms of therapy before coming to you, it is important to lay all your cards out on the table: "Yes, you have a problem. And yes, you are going to need help to change that problem. There are many things that can be done to help you become as fluent as it is possible for you to become. But let's be clear. You have been doing this for many years now, and some of these behaviors and attitudes are well learned, ingrained, and established. Changing these behaviors and attitudes will neither be easy nor quick. We are happy to be your guide as you make these changes, but you will be the one who has to do the changing. It can be done and we'll help and support you as much as we can but you're the one who'll have to do the work. . ." And so forth.

With the uncertain category of older clients, those whose problem and need for therapy are uncertain, you will note the fluent or relatively fluent stutterer whose presence is an everyday reality in a college or hospital clinic. Although some of these clients appear essentially fluent, they are very concerned about their speech and their ability to interact with others, particularly through verbal communication. These individuals will frequently complain that speech is not automatic for them (as it is for other people), that they have to think about speaking all the time, and that this lack of automaticity is one of the main reasons they want therapy. Sometimes with careful, detailed visual and auditory observations of these people while they are talking, you can spot or hear the brief, subtle things they seem to do to avoid, change, or stop saying particular sounds, syllables or words, for example, use subtly inappropriate vocabulary. Some of these individuals have no apparent speech-language problem, but because they adamantly believe they have a problem, they have one.

I have found that adult group therapy is beneficial for this type of client. It provides a forum to compare and contrast other problems as well as learn more about speaking and gain more reasonable standards for fluent verbal communication. Some of these clients also benefit from groups like Toastmaster's International. Like many adult stutterers, they find the contact and collegiality of self-help groups to be of benefit (more about self-help groups in the chapter on adults).

A third category of older clients (and this also applies to younger clients) may have a problem but their problem is not stuttering. Their problem may be speech apraxia, dialectical speech and language usage, psychoneurotic concerns, employment concerns, and so forth. We should not dismiss these other concerns out of hand, but instead make the proper referrals to agencies and professionals more equipped and trained to deal with them. Obviously, building up a pool of agencies and professionals to whom you can make such referrals takes time, effort, and experimentation, but there is no way we can overstate the importance of making appropriate referrals to agencies that can help your client with problems that are outside your professional purview and expertise.

SOME PARTING THOUGHTS

Thus, we can see that for both the child and the adult who stutters, deciding who is a stutterer, whether the person, once labeled a stutterer, needs therapy, and what form the therapy should take is not a black and white decision. There appear to be three points on the diagnostic continuum for dealing with this challenge:

1. Few clients receive therapy: Therapy is recommended for very few clients. Instead the SLP concentrates on thorough information sharing at the time of

evaluation when the client and associates are essentially told not to be concerned, that many "normally fluent" people do the same thing, and so forth

2. Some clients receive therapy: Therapy is recommended on the basis of a differential diagnosis whereby a certain percent receive therapy immediately, another percent are reevaluated until it becomes clear whether therapy is appropriate, and another percent receive no therapy

3. All clients receive therapy: Therapy is recommended on the basis that it is good, can do little harm, and acts as a preventative for some clients.

We advocate the middle position—some clients receive therapy—since it is our experience that frequently there is the marginal situation where therapy may or may not be of assistance. Furthermore, we believe that if everyone can receive our services then no one actually needs them, a situation that is clearly not the case.

We would like to see, particularly for the marginal client, more recommendations for "trial therapy" of three to six weeks in duration to see if remediation has a chance of being beneficial. Particularly with children, who are constantly changing along so many different dimensions, therapy immediately after the diagnostic may have little chance of being successful; perhaps in three to six months it might be more effective. However, to make these sorts of decisions the SLP must have conducted a thorough evaluation. Indeed, remediation presupposes a thorough evaluation, and only by so doing can the SLP understand and weigh all factors in coming to an informed decision for or against therapy.

In this chapter we have explored some of these factors, their relative importance to the evaluation of stuttering, and how they may influence our decision about whether therapy is needed and, if so, what kind. In subsequent chapters we discuss the remediation of stuttering and we hope that the reader will come to better appreciate how our regimens for remediation flow or follow from our approaches to evaluation. We take the first step down the road to remediating stuttering when at the beginning of the diagnostic we ask the client or his or her associates, "What can we do to help you?"

We should not view evaluation as a messy detail that must be gotten through prior to the "good stuff" called therapy. Rather, the diagnostic is part of therapy, the investigatory part, but a part nonetheless. To begin therapy with little or no attempt to evaluate is like setting out to sea without knowing a great deal about the waters upon which you are going to be sailing, sort of like the captain of the *Titanic*. It is better, as the Boy Scouts would say, to "Be Prepared."

SUMMARY

Assessment and evaluation of stuttering involves two general procedures: (1) interview of client and associates regarding attitudes, feelings, beliefs, and history concerning the problem and related matters, and (2) objective and subjective assessment of speech fluency and related behavior, for example, speech sound articulation, speaking rate, expressive and receptive language usage, voice quality, word finding skills, audiometric findings, and so forth. Additional aspects such as reading, academic standings and progress, social maturity, gross/fine motor skills for speech and nonspeech behavior, cognitive abilities, attentional deficit disorders, psychosocial adjustment, and so forth should be evaluated according to the dictates of each individual case. The fact that an individual is or is *suspected* of being a stutterer should not distract the clinician from considering other speech and nonspeech behaviors and their possible contributing role to stuttering. Assessment and evaluation is a very important aspect of the remediation of stuttering since the nature of the client's problem will often times dictate procedures used to remediate it; even though trite, it is nevertheless true that evaluation is the first stage of remediation and should neither be casually nor quickly undertaken.

Stuttering primarily involves a disruption in the temporal aspects of speech production. Typically this is manifest by a reiteration or cessation of forward-moving speech production or a disruption in the relatively rapid, smooth, and coordinated speech production movements. These reiterations and cessations typically occur at either the initiation of speech or during movements from one speaking posture to the next. Indeed, recognizing typical and atypical temporal aspects of speech production is essential when assessing and evaluating stuttering. Stuttering is typically not a problem in speech intelligibility, voice quality, or correct semantic or grammatical usage; it is primarily a disturbance in the temporal domain of speech production.

Thus, any and all factors, whether external or internal to the client, that contribute to the client's temporal disruptions in forward moving speech production are something the clinician must assess and then evaluate regarding their potential contribution to the client's stuttering. The clinician will want to become aware of and be able to assess such temporal components of speech as: duration of each instance of stuttering, number of words or syllables spoken per minute by client and/or parents, length of time from the end of the client's statement to the beginning of parent's reply ("turn taking" or "turn-switching" pause), the frequency of simul-talking or the extent to which the client and associates talk while the other is talking, and so forth. The clinician will also want to develop skills at differentiating *between-word* (for example, phrase repetitions) from *within-word* (for example, sound repetitions) disfluencies and be able to determine how many of both occur per 10 or 100 words or syllables spoken. Furthermore, the clinician must be able to assess and evaluate other problems—for example, delayed phonological development—that may co-occur with stuttering and require significant adjustments to therapy. Indeed, successful assessment and evaluation of stuttering requires the clinician to simultaneously take several different perspectives on the problem to ensure the most complete understanding and hence the most appropriate therapy.

THREE
Remediation:
Children Who Stutter

STUTTERING IS A DISORDER OF CHILDHOOD

It has been said that stuttering is a disorder of childhood (Bloodstein, 1987). This notion seems to be related to the fact that stuttering not only begins, for most individuals, during the early years of childhood but that the number of individuals who continue to stutter into their teen-age years and beyond drops off by 50 percent or more (Ingham, 1985; Sheehan and Martyn, 1970). These facts, as well as common sense, would seem to suggest that much of our research and remediational efforts with stuttering should be directed toward children who stutter; however, common sense is not all that common among both clients and clinicians.

CLINICIAN/CLIENT RELUCTANCE TO DEAL WITH CHILDHOOD STUTTERING

First, speech-language pathologists, until recent years, have directed much of their research attention to adults (cf. Conture, 1987, for further discussion of this topic). While there are numerous reasons for this, one major reason is that adults who stutter are simply more cooperative and can participate in more complicated studies than young children. A second reason is that one can be fairly certain that a 20-year-old with a history of 10 to 15 years of stuttering *is* a stutterer while it is far less clear that a 4-year-old with a six-month history is or will remain a stutterer. And finally, the caution that parents shouldn't openly discuss or call undue attention to the child's disfluent speech left many SLPs very hesitant to rush in where angels apparently were afraid to tread.

Second, the clients themselves. We daresay that when the reader was three, four, or five years old, the last place on earth she or he wanted to spend a sunny afternoon was in a clinician's office. Playing was next to godliness for all of us as children and "working on our speech" was not particularly high on our priority list. Furthermore, while adults who stutter generally seek out our services on their own, children are typically brought by their parents. Indeed, the problem is generally a problem for the parents long before it is a concern for the child. So, it is not surprising that some young children who stutter are eager and ready for speech therapy while others hang back and appear to resist the SLP's every effort. Some of these youngsters appear receptive to our therapeutic efforts and readily make and implement necessary change while others appear uncertain and confused about almost everything that goes on in therapy. Likewise, some children who stutter easily leave mom and dad and proceed into the therapy room while others kick and scream as if being led to the gallows.

It is small wonder, therefore, that beginning clinicians encountering such experiences with children who stutter are less than eager to repeat the experience and may be more comfortable with the relative cooperation of older clients who at least seem more motivated than the average four-year-old to sit down and work. However, children who stutter and their families can and should be helped, even though understanding the dynamics by which young stutterers can be helped, motivated, and made to benefit from speech and language remediation is as complicated as it is with older stutterers.

KNOWING LITERATURE PERTINENT TO CHILDREN WHO STUTTER

SLPs who manage young children should be aware of literature specifically addressed to remediation of young children who stutter (Ainsworth and Fraser, 1988; Conture and Caruso, 1987; Cooper 1978, 1979; Luper and Mulder, 1964; Luper, 1982; Conture, 1982; Rustin, 1987; Wall and Myers, 1984; Williams, 1971; Van Riper, 1973; Zwitman, 1978).

Likewise, the SLP should be aware of and be prepared to share with parents publications that are specifically addressed to parents of stutterers (Johnson, 1946; Cooper, 1979; Ainsworth and Fraser, 1988; Guitar and Conture, 1988). These publications can be given to parents to elaborate upon, reinforce, and clarify points made by the speech-language pathologist in counseling sessions. Of course, such publications are not always completely read or understood by the parents, but with the SLP's encouragement and guidance, as well as further or repeated explanation and answering of questions, parents can be helped to gain valuable insights from reading this material. We have found that the SLP should be thoroughly familiar with the contents of these self-help publications—these publications should never be handed out until read by the SLP—and the SLP should be ready and willing to help parents grasp, critique, and implement their contents. Similarly, since many children who stutter will be initially assessed and/or referred by the family doctor or pediatrician, the SLP should be aware of articles on stuttering published in medical journals (Cooper, 1980; Conture, 1982; Guitar. 1988). The SLP can cite these medical journals when interacting with pediatricians or family practitioners and the contents of these publications can provide a basis for informed discussion between the SLP and the physician.

Remediating Children May Mean Involvement with Their Parents

While perhaps obvious, another reason that remediating stuttering in children differs from remediating stuttering in adults is that the SLP will many times have to deal with the child's parents. And parents, like their children, come in a variety of sizes and shapes, and their personal idiosyncrasies will influence therapeutic success. To make the situation even more challenging, parents are often unclear regarding their role in remediating young stutterers. Some parents see little if any purpose being served by their involvement (for example, a mother might say, "Bobby is the one with the problem not me").

Parents themselves, of course, are not the only problem; sometimes the SLP is responsible for unduly engendering guilt, concern, or confusion in parents regarding their contributions to their child's speech and language problems. Parents of young stutterers need support, encouragement, and advice on ways to explore and make changes that will facilitate their child's speech fluency. What they don't need are additional lectures, sermons, reprimands, and chastisements for past and present, real and imagined transgressions against their children. Many of them already feel bad enough; they don't need our help to feel any worse.

LeShan (1963) discusses the role of parental guilt in the upbringing of children, and LeShan's thoughts are well worth reading by SLPs who may need to consider parental guilt and what should and should not be done about it. While the SLP will strive to do nothing to increase and everything to decrease parental guilt regarding their child's stuttering, the SLP must recognize that in many cases all the good that is done in therapy can be offset, in a relatively short time, by parents who cannot or will not understand their role in their child's speech and language development. This does not imply that the child's parents *cause* stuttering, but that some of the things they do may be *maintaining, perpetuating, aggravating,* or *exacerbating* the child's problem.

Talking to Parents about the Cause of Stuttering: Their Own Behavior as *Causal* versus *Maintaining* Agent

The SLP wants the parent as an ally not foe in the war on the child's stuttering. One of the easiest ways to make an enemy out of the parent is to explicitly or implicitly indicate that the parents *cause* their child's stuttering. Once this is done, the war is generally lost before the first battle has even begun.

Far better, the SLP should help the parents understand the difference between agents (behaviors, factors, or variables) that may (1) *cause* versus (2) *maintain* stuttering. This is no intellectual shell game; there is a difference. To begin, we tell the parents, no one knows what *causes* stuttering. We may discuss some of the possible causes, but repeatedly explain that no one can be sure which one, if any, of these possibilities applies to their child. However, we go on to explain that there appear to be a variety of things that parents do that may contribute to a child's speaking difficulties once they begin and that these *maintaining* (or aggravating, contributing, or perpetuating) factors may need to be explored and possibly changed.

One analogy we use is a knife (Figure 3–1). The knife blade causes the wound while the salt rubbed in the wound a*ggravates* or *contributes* to the discomfort. The salt may hurt but it didn't cause the wound. The knife is the reason for the wound and, as we say to parents, we are not sure what knife caused their child to stutter, but we do have some information about the types of salt that may be perpetuating the problem.

Talking to Parents about the Cause of Stuttering: Nature versus Nurture

Closely related to parents' concern that they, by something they did, "caused" their child to stutter is the issue of inheritance. It has become increasingly clear that genetics play some sort of as yet imprecisely defined role in stuttering (for example, Kidd, 1983; Cox, 1988). However, if for some stutterers stuttering is "inherited," it does not happen in a straightforward Mendelian genetic way like eye or hair color or height. Furthermore, if 50 percent of the relatives of stutterers also stutter, this means that 50 percent of the relatives don't. Clearly, environmental or nongenetic factors must play a role (Cox, 1988), if only a partial one, and it will be some time before we know the relative contributions nature and nurture make to the onset, development, and perpetuation of stuttering for stutterers as a group or for any one individual person who stutters.

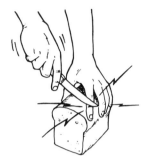
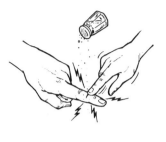

Knife CAUSES cut and pain

Salt rubbed into cut
MAINTAINS the pain

FIGURE 3–1. Knife and salt analogy. Here the knife originally *caused* the cut and pain while salt rubbed into the cut *maintains* the pain. Just as the child's abilities may originally cause too frequent production of within-word disfluencies, environmental issues (for example, parents who expect and demand quick, precise and mature speech from a 4-year-old) may *maintain* or *aggravate* the child's speech disfluencies.

Indeed, knowing that their child may be predisposed to react to psychosocial or communicative stress by ceasing or reiterating speech sound production (that is, stuttering) should make the parents work all the harder to minimize those elements in their interactions with the child that may be contributing to their child's tendency to stutter. The possibility that a child is predisposed to stutter should not mean that the parents and SLP must throw up their hands, give up, and "let nature take its course." Perhaps, what is inherited is a generally slow-to-develop system for fluent speech production and knowing this, the parents can be more supportive of and tolerant for the longer-than-normal time it will take their child to reach fully mature speech production.

Whatever the case, the SLP should be prepared to discuss with the parents the possibility that genetics plays a role in stuttering (and at this point in our knowledge this is a strong possibility, not an absolute certainty) and, present evidence that would support and refute such a possibility. The outcome of such a discussion should neither panic the parents into having tubal ligations or vasectomies nor should it absolve them from their responsibilities to change behaviors of their own that may be exacerbating their child's problem.

While lay people may believe that stuttering has either a nature *or* nurture cause, the SLP should realize that the probability is much greater that nature *interacts* with nurture to cause and perpetuate the problem. The SLP should also realize that predispositions to behave in a certain way do not mean that such behavior cannot be mitigated or modified or that the child is preordained to behave that way for life. Indeed, parents should be helped to understand that things that are inherited, for example, intelligence and physical size and abilities, are not immutable; environmental factors can and do influence many things that are inherited and this is also probably true with inherited predispositions for disfluent speech. Furthermore, many times, by the time the SLP meets the child who stutters, the causal agents have long since disappeared with a host of perpetuating events now much more salient to the child's remediation. It is the SLP's job to help the parents focus on the present and future while understanding, but not dwelling, on the past.

Parents Generally Want to Do the Right Thing

Shortly, we are going to discuss our approach to remediating stuttering in young children. Part of this approach involves talking and working with parents and, because of this, some preliminary words are in order. Previously, we have discussed the issue of parental attitudes and behavior as *causal* versus *exacerbating* factors and we won't reiterate that discussion. However, we do want to stress that it is our experience, despite the impression one gets from reading the daily newspaper, that the vast majority of parents love their children. Most parents want to do the right thing by their child, but sometimes they just don't know how to go about doing it. For the most part, parents' intentions are excellent; it's just their methods that need modification.

Since parents, like all of us, want to do the right thing, with our expressed respect, support, and a little guidance they can be helped to do more and more of the the right things for their child and themselves. Parents need respect and support for their attempts to understand and deal with their children, not reprimands, lectures, and threats. Perhaps some will take longer than others to see the error of their ways but few will even look if they feel they aren't being treated with respect or are being told that their intentions are all wrong. Just like their children, parents respond best when it is their behavior rather than themselves that is being critiqued.

THERAPY: WHEN TO START, HOW LONG, AND HOW OFTEN

Once the clinician decides that the child has a stuttering problem or a high probability for developing one *and* that the child needs therapy, he or she must decide about the nature of the therapeutic intervention. Bound up in this latter decision are three nitty-gritty questions: (1) When should therapy start? (2) How long will it take? and (3) How often per week? Unfortunately, there are, at least to my knowledge, no fixed guidelines to help the clinician decide.

Starting therapy generally involves some compromise between the parents' urgency to begin therapy yesterday and the clinician's ability and/or willingness to begin immediately. It must be remembered that many times the parents have, for one reason or another, waited 6, 12, 24 months or (many times) even longer to bring the child in for services and in many of these cases an additional wait of 1 to 6 months is probably going to be of little consequence. As shown in Figure 2–1, reevaluation *prior* to the start of therapy is many times a viable alternative, but this doesn't preclude the clinician from talking with the parents in some detail, about the child's problem, things they can do at home to help, things they might change that would help their child, providing appropriate literature, and so forth.

As mentioned in Chapter 2, our clinical experience indicates that therapy should start as soon as possible if (1) the child is producing two or more sound prolongations per every ten instances of stuttering, (2) the child breaks eye contact with his or her listeners more than 50 percent of the time during conversation, and/or (3) the child exhibits concomitant speech sound articulation problems (particularly if exhibited phonological processes are indicative of delays or deviations in phonological development). Children who stutter, but who exhibit none or only one of the above, can probably be more appropriately put on a waiting list and/or reevaluated, but this period of time should probably not exceed six months.

The length of time therapy takes depends as much on the child and his/her parents as it does on the therapy they receive. Our experience indicates that most children take approximately 20 weeks of once-a-week therapy before they are ready to be dismissed. Some children are quite successful after only 10 weeks, but some still require therapy after 30 or more weeks of therapy. It has been our experience that parents need to be told of the average length of time therapy may take as well as the low-end (for example, 10 weeks) and high-end (for example, 30 or more weeks) possibilities. While some youngsters who stutter will improve simply with parental counseling (either in person or over the phone), many will require visits to an SLP for some period of time. The length of therapy will also be influenced by the inclusion of maintenance or follow-up sessions and, once again, the parents should be informed, right from the beginning, of the approximate number and nature of these maintenance or transfer sessions.

How often therapy occurs (on a weekly basis) is a question open to debate. There are pros and cons, in our opinion, to both intensive (for example, everyday, all day for three weeks) and extensive (for example, once a week for a six month period) approaches to therapy. There can be little doubt that intensive therapy brings about relatively quick behavioral change, but we question whether there is enough time to make the types of attitude, feeling, and life-style changes that are sometimes necessary to support long-term behavioral change. Conversely, extensive therapy provides the time necessary to make needed attitudinal, feeling, and life-style changes, but behavioral change is relatively slow, occurring over a matter of weeks and months rather than days.

At present, we have little empirical data that would allow us to answer the most important question regarding this topic: Are there significant differences between intensive and extensive therapy with regard to *long-term* improvement or transfer? Until we know that children who stutter are more likely to *remain* fluent not just *become* fluent as a result of intensive versus extensive therapy, clinicians will select one or the other approach based on their experience, philosophy, and clinical schedules.

THERAPY: THREE ISSUES ALL CLINICIANS ENCOUNTER

No matter which approach is used, the SLP who services youngsters who stutter will, sooner or later, have to deal with three issues in the earlier stages of therapeutic intervention: (1) mentioning the label *stuttering* in the presence of the child and/or the parents of the child; (2) talking to the young child, in clear, nonpejorative, but nevertheless direct terms, about talking in general and his/her talking in specific (for example, Williams 1971); and (3) the age of the child. The first two issues, we are cautioned by some, are better not broached since they are counterproductive to successful remediation. Conversely, some appear to feel that little or no harm will be done by calling the child a stutterer and directly talking and dealing with the child about talking. Once again, there is little empirical evidence to support either approach and the clinician must sort out for her- or himself which of the two dueling theories makes most sense.

Saying the "S" Word

Our experience suggests that when trying to *describe* the child's speech, we want to do just that. The only effective means to describe something is to use the most descriptive terms you know that you think the client and associates will understand and relate to, for example, descriptive terms like "hard" or "easy" or "smooth" or "gentle" or "repeating" or "stopping." A term like stuttering, for all its common use by the lay public, is simply not as descriptive, tells neither the child nor parents precisely what the child is *doing* and thus doesn't tell them what must be *done* to change. However, putting a bell and cowl on the word "stuttering" and treating it like a leperous entity is patently silly. It makes little sense to go out of your way not to say the "s" words if the parents and/or child have already been using "stuttering" or "stutterer" to talk about the child or his speech. Instead, be realistic and try to help the parents understand the difference between descriptive and nondescriptive terms and how their usage can help or hinder therapeutic progress. When the nondescriptive "s" words come up, deal with them as matter-of-factly as possible, but resume usage of their descriptive counterparts as soon as you can.

Talking to the Child about Talking in General and the Child's Talking in Specific

This issue is a variation on the concerns about saying the "s" words. However, we are concerned not only about making the child's problem worse, but also whether the young child can understand what we are saying. At the least, we would hope that our words are (1) as descriptive as possible and (2) at a level of abstraction (Johnson, 1946) that the child can understand and relate to. While it may be most parsimonious and correct to describe the things the child does as "cessation" and "reiteration" of speech production, it is probably better to use terms like "stuck" and "bouncing." We'll come back to this issue later when we discuss the specifics of indirect and direct therapy.

The Child's Age in Relation to the Type of Therapy Prescribed

It is our experience that the child's age is an important consideration when planning the length and type of therapy but that age has little relation to the nature of the child's stuttering problem. That is, a four-year-old has just as much right as a six-year-old to be a severe stutterer. Although the developmental sequence of stuttering is not yet clearly understood, we know the *rate* and *nature* of this development vary widely from one young stutterer to another. Furthermore, the time of onset, for example, an onset at four years versus six years of age, interacts in a complex way with the speed and type of development of stuttering. Some children rapidly move from producing mainly sound/syllable repetitions to sound prolongations while others take several months if not years to do the same thing. Some children steadily increase the frequency and duration of their instances of stuttering while others exhibit a herky-jerky progression, now more and longer stutterings, now fewer and shorter stutterings. Age, therefore, is a variable in planning therapy. For example, with very few exceptions, we have found it unwise to group seven-year-olds with four-year-olds; however, age per se has a far less than perfect relation to the quantity and quality of the child's stuttering problem.

THERAPY: DIRECT VERSUS INDIRECT APPROACHES

One general consideration is whether speech therapy with the child who stutters should be direct or indirect. Van Riper (1973) and others have already covered this topic, but it is a topic that continually seems to plague SLPs who manage the young stutterer. By *indirect* we mean any approach that does not explicitly, overtly, or directly try to modify or change the child's speech fluency in specific, and oral communication skills in general. With an indirect type of therapy, the focus is on the child and the child's environment, particularly parents. Thus, indirect therapy many times also involves information sharing and/or counseling of the parents in addition to remediating the child through a variety of relatively low-key, play-oriented activities where speech and speech-related activities are not the obvious focus. With an indirect approach, explicitly talking about the child's actual talking behavior is kept to a minimum and the focus is more on relatively relaxed, enjoyable communication between clinician and client.

Conversely, a *direct* approach involves explicit, overt, and direct attempts to modify the child's speech and related behavior. Parents may still be involved but not to the same degree as with the indirect approach. Directly talking to the child about his or her talking, the "bad" as well as "good" parts, is often part of a direct approach.

Now that we have distinguished between direct and indirect therapy approaches to childhood stuttering, which approach do we take? Once again, we find there is no easy or simple answer to what seems to be a rather straightforward question. While the indirect approach may be quite feasible for some, the direct procedure makes more sense for others. It is not too hard to decide about children at the extremes: indirect approaches for a child who is just beginning to stutter versus a more direct approach for a child who has been stuttering for three or four years. But how to decide about the many children in between these two extremes? Clearly, an indirect approach will have minimal impact on a four-year-old's stuttering if that child is producing 30 percent disfluent speech with 90 percent or more of those disfluencies being sound prolongations.

The child's chronological age is not as significant a factor in making this decision as the nature of the child's problem and both his and his environment's awareness of /reaction to it. This does not mean age is of no consequence in the planning of therapy. Indeed, we would not want to use the exact direct procedures for a four-year-old that we would employ with an eighteen-year-old; we would want to temper, modify, or drastically change certain of these procedures to make them more suitable for the younger client.

After years of evaluating young stutterers or suspected young stutterers, we have come to the conclusion that the nature of therapy, that is, indirect versus direct, is more related to the nature of the child's problem than to the child's chronological age. For example, we have just evaluated a 5.5-year-old girl whose problem is easily as severe as that of the typical 10-year-old. Certainly, experience has shown us that we don't want to group 7-year-olds in with 4-year-olds, but we also don't want to assume that the 4-year-old's problem is less than that of the 7-year-old's. There is a fine balancing act the clinician must perform here: gearing the approach so that the child isn't underwhelmed or put off by the seemingly "juvenile" nature of the therapy versus overwhelming the child with tasks that he perceives to be or actually are beyond his or her level of development.

FOUR CATEGORIES OF CHILDREN
WHO RECEIVE OUR SERVICES

In the first edition of this book (Conture, 1982, pp. 42–44) we discussed three groupings of children whom we typically remediate. We have expanded this trilogy somewhat to include the following four groupings: (1) children with no objective-subjective-communication whose parents are reasonably to quite concerned; (2) children who exhibit stuttering but whose parents are minimally or completely unconcerned; (3) children with some stuttering whose parents are also concerned; and (4) children with some to a great objective-subjective-communication problem whose parents are reasonably to quite concerned.

Young Children with No Communication Problems
Whose Parents Are Reasonably to Quite Concerned

When a child is essentially fluent, that is, when the child's type and frequency of speech disfluency are within normal limits for the child's chronological and developmental age level, remediation of the child's speech fluency is contraindicated. While this may seem like a reasonable decision based on the facts of the matter, sometimes the child's parents see things otherwise. That is, the child's parents or other important adult listeners explicitly, insistently, and/or strongly state their belief that the child has a stuttering problem and that the child is a stutterer. In many of these cases, the parents are raising their first child, and they are generally, but not exclusively, younger parents (30 years old and younger). Parents who deny the "normalcy" of their child's fluency are the exact opposite of a different group of parents (whom we discuss later in this chapter) who deny the "abnormalcy" of their child's fluency. Both parent groups provide the clinician with a challenge.

One caution is in order: It is possible that the parents are seeing and hearing aspects of the child's behavior that the SLP has missed during the diagnostic. This possibility points out two important things: (1) the SLP's need to conduct her own, independent assessment of the child and not merely take the parents' or other lay person's diagnosis, and (2) the SLP's need to sample the child's fluency in as many situations as possible.

It is important for the SLP to realize that she doesn't have to observe the child at his or her worst (and the parents need to be told this); she only has to observe the child speaking in enough different situations during the diagnostic to answer the question: Would the observed speech disfluencies increase in frequency and duration (and perhaps change in type) given more environmental stressors? If the answer is yes, then the child needs some form of intervention; however, if the answer is no, then intervention may not be required. Before disregarding a parent's claim that their child stutters, the SLP should be as sure as she can be that her sampling procedure was as varied and thorough as possible. If there are doubts, it is very reasonable to reevaluate the child in three to six months and see if the child's behavior has changed and/or whether the parents are still concerned (cf. Figure 2–1).

Parents who seemingly insist, despite evidence to the contrary, that their child stutters generally appear to want the best for their child. They also seem to expect, in a number of areas, that the child will achieve high levels of performance, regardless of the child's ability. We believe that the intentions and motivations of many of these parents are fine; it is just their methods of interacting or dealing with their child that may need some modification. Such parents seem to fall into three different, but not necessarily mutually exclusive, camps:

1. Why can't Johnny be perfect (as I was)?
2. My husband (wife) is wrong and he (she) thinks I'm wrong about how we raise our child.
3. These problems run in the family.

Parents' Concern: Why can't Johnny be perfect (as I was)?   The first camp—why can't Johnny be perfect?—comprises parents who seem to want their child to be perfect and are frustrated because the child, like most humans, cannot achieve such perfection (many of them are perfectionists concerning their own behavior). These parents may tell you that they want their five-year-old son to be a doctor, a rocket scientist, or some other professional. These parents often see the world in black and white terms: either all good or all bad. And because of this, they may consider their child as either all right or all wrong. That is, they appear to believe that either their child's behavior is all right or their child's development is all wrong. These parents seem to have trouble believing that their standards for their child may need modification; rather, they tend to see the problem as being produced or caused by the child.

Many times these children are heavily monitored in their communication, social, and academic development, and the parents may be less than flexible in their standards for child behavior. These parents need assistance to assess objectively their standards for child development and performance in light of what is typical for children of the same chronological and developmental age. Such parents must be patiently, but firmly, instructed to evaluate and adjust their expectations for their child's behavior in general and speech and language development in specific. Many of these parents are also apt to do a lot of telling rather than showing the child what they want. Or, as Bettelheim (1985) states, many parents are "ready to teach their child (but). . .are less ready to accept the idea that they can teach only by example," and that children "are influenced less by what (parents) tell them than they are by what (parents) do" (p. 57).

These parents, like many others, can be helped by discussing with them booklets like those developed by Cooper (1979) and Ainsworth and Fraser (1988) so that they will have a better understanding of typical speech and language development as well as stuttering. We have found that these parents can be helped if they will listen to reason: If they will entertain the notion that their standards for their child are less (or more) than desirable and that these standards need reevaluation and change. Sometimes, referrals to psychologists and psychiatrists who specialize in child-family counseling may be the only way such change can be made. We have often observed that the child's "problem" is generally resolved when the parents' concerns and standards for the child's behavior are modified and brought into line with what is considered reasonable for their child's chronological and developmental age.

Parents' Concern: My husband (wife) is wrong and he (she) thinks I'm wrong Related to the why-can't-Johnny-be-perfect situation, is the situation where the parents think the other is wrong. This is most commonly manifested by the mother's *frequently* and *consistently* stating that the father is "too strict" with the child and/or the father's stating just as *frequently* and *consistently* that the mother is "too lenient" with the child or "lets the kid get away with murder." Neither parent seems to agree with the other on the way in which the child should be raised (such disagreements are generally noticed when discipline is an issue) or how a child their son's or daughter's age should speak, think, read, write, behave, play, and so forth.

These parents not only disagree in private, but also openly and frequently disagree about the raising of the child in front of the child. This particular parental situation, like most other parental concerns, is only a *dilemma* if it occurs frequently and consistently. That is, if arguments between parents are the rule, rather than the exception, then the parents may need more than simple information sharing and informal counseling by the SLP. Perhaps the child is the focal point for difficulties the mother and father have between themselves. They may be taking out their frustrations and anger with each other on the child. In some of these cases referral to appropriate psychological services may be appropriate. (Interestingly, we think, that mothers seem to be somewhat more receptive to such referrals than fathers.)

We have found, however, that most parents will listen to reason and seriously try to minimize their differences when they are helped to realize that their difficulties may be adversely influencing the child. As we have said before, the vast majority of parents love their children and have excellent intentions, but just need to reconsider and modify their actual approaches to the raising of their children.

In such cases, where one of the parents is quite convinced that the child has a communication problem, whereas the other is just as firmly convinced that no problem exists, the clinician should avoid giving the appearance of choosing sides. Persistence on the part of the clinician in helping the parents to see their child as he or she really is, not as they idealize him or her, is important. Continued reiteration of basic child development information is important: just becoming a parent does not mean that someone is automatically bestowed with rich insights as well as a full understanding of the complexities and long-term process of child behavior and development. The SLP must persevere in these matters if he or she expects to move these parents in the right direction.

The plain truth of the matter, as we discuss throughout this and subsequent chapters on remediation, is that *real* changes in such parental attitudes and behavior may take more time than any of us would like. The clinician should try to (1) be as persistent as possible without being obnoxiously repetitious; (2) convey respect for and listen to the opinions and ideas of parents (they have perspectives that any clinician, no matter how wise or experienced, can learn a great deal from); and (3) explicitly express to the parents the fact that the clinician knows that the parents love their child, and have the best intentions for the raising of their child. If the SLP can do all three of these things, at least some of the time, it is amazing the change parents can and do make and the degree to which the parents can come to see the realities of their child's behavior.

Parents' Concern: Stuttering runs in the family   Once you've experienced a car accident you realize they can happen even to you. You become a bit more cautious, a bit more wary. The old saying of once bitten, twice shy applies here. Likewise, in a family where Uncle Fred stutters or even mother or father, it is not hard to see why parents would be on the lookout for their offspring to begin doing the same thing. The SLP must walk a thin line with these cases and their families. While the SLP doesn't want to deny the real possibility that stuttering tends to "run in families"—for example, at least 50 percent of the relatives of stutterers also stutter (Johnson et al., 1959)—the SLP must realize that this tendency doesn't absolutely dictate the fact that the child will also stutter. Yes, there is an increased probability that the child may be a stutterer and will continue to stutter, but this is not an absolute certainty. The sun's coming up tomorrow is a certainty; picking the winner of the Kentucky Derby based on bloodlines, trial runs, and the like involves probability.

Related Parental Concern: Looking for and thus finding stuttering   Many times these parents give the appearance of waiting for the other shoe to drop; they sometimes seem to have been looking for signs of stuttering since the child began to speak, and, to paraphrase an old saying, "look and they shall find." Many times one or both parents will mention the horrible stuttering problem of an Uncle Ralph or sister Kate and how they hope that their Johnny will not end up the same way their poor relative did. Some of these parents also seem to have high, relatively unreasonable expectations for their child's speech, language, fluency, and behavioral development even when confronted with the fact that their child is developing at his or her own normal, albeit slow, pace.

Like many other parents, these parents will have numerous old wives' tales about what causes stuttering and/or what makes it better or worse. They are likely to bring up the issue and want to know your opinion of whether stuttering results from: (1) a physical flaw *or* (2) a psychological problem ("Is this something he was born with or did we cause the problem?"). Some of these parents may begin to shop around from one SLP to another until they find one who will agree that their child has a stuttering problem.

It is important, particularly with this type of parent, to quickly establish your credibility and concern for their child while at the same time conveying your respect for and willingness to listen to their opinions. You may find your patience being tested since you will have to continually reiterate what you believe the facts of the matter are and what you think the parents need to consider to make appropriate change.

Counseling the parents and keeping in touch   When all is said and done, counseling parents about their child's apparently nonexistent stuttering problem is both remediative as well as preventive. You try, through information sharing, discussion, and counseling, to help the parents provide for their child a home environment conducive to optimal development of speech fluency and related behavior. For example, you help them make changes in their own speech behaviors, communicative interactional styles, emotions, feelings, attitudes, and so forth. During this time, the parents may want you to "therapize" the child and the degree to which they insist on this therapy may be an indirect measure of the degree to which they are abdicating their responsibilities for helping their child. Perhaps, if you bring the child in for informal play therapy or for general speech and language "enrichment" or "stimulation," you may assuage the parents while you continue to discuss with them what they may do to change their interactions with and expectations of their child (for example, Axline, 1947; Murphy and FitzSimmons, 1960; Van Riper, 1973).

Many times, immediately after the initial evaluation, when the parents have just been interviewed and the problem is fresh in their minds, is a good time for a 30 to 60 minute information sharing session. Sometimes, as we and others have found, this initial post-evaluation findings and recommendations session is all some parents need to significantly diminish their concerns (for example, Johnson and others, 1959). It helps to make sure, before these parents leave the first time, that they have written down somewhere your office phone number and address and that they truly feel that that they can call you (we specifically tell them, "Feel free to write or call me") if they have further questions or concerns. It is very important to give these parents the impression that the door to your clinic, office, or school is always open to them. Try not to let the parents feel they are "locked" out from further contact. Instead, let them know that you want to and expect to maintain contact with them and will welcome their calls. (Since some parents are not aware of how busy the average SLP's schedule can be, I tell them that sometimes they won't be able to get me immediately but that I'll get back in touch with them if they leave their name, number, and a time when it is best for me to call them.) We try to provide these parents with a sense that someone is available to help and that the parents themselves have the ability to change the situation.

When counseling parents, one point that most professionals seem to agree on is the need *not* to make parents feel guilty (or at least any more guilty than they already feel) about their child's behavior. LeShan (1963) writes about this point at length, and we believe it is important to remember and consider in parental counseling. Instead of engendering feelings of parental guilt, we, as SLPs, should try to provide parents with objective information about speech and language behavior in general and stuttering in specific and listen and thoughtfully respond to their questions. We should try to support parents in their attempts to understand and explore their feelings, concerns, and thinking about their child, and their role in their child's general and communicative development. Such exploration may take many meetings with you, depending on the nature and type of parental feelings and concerns.

Although much is written about the individual nature of the child, we often forget that parents are also individuals. Too often, because of the quick pace and relative brevity of the clinical day and our many clients, we tend to deal with all parents in fairly similar ways. That is, we tend to gloss over individual differences and try to talk to and handle each parent as though the parent is the "typical" parent of a "typical" child who stutters. This is not an inherently evil practice; indeed, some degree of commonality must exist among these parents for us to develop an effective remediation regimen. However, when we routinely and consistently counsel each and every parent in the same manner, we run the risk of overlooking some individual parental differences that may make a significant difference in terms of the particular child's progress. For example, we may become concerned if the parent routinely uses the "s" word when talking to his or her child, but become more relaxed when another parent talks about talking to the child using such terms as "hard" and "easy" speech.

And yet, the specific words used may not be as important as the manner in which the parent uses them. As Neill (1960) suggests, "it doesn't matter what a parent says to a child as long as the parents' feelings towards the child are correct," and, we might add, the child recognizes the appropriateness of such feelings. The point here is that we sometimes give patented or standard responses and recommendations to parents without carefully considering the individual nature, needs, and concerns of parents and their child. It is the wise clinician who can detect and differentially respond to those aspects of the parents of young stutterers that are typical as well as those that are unique.

Recognizing the individuality of each parent and attempting to avoid increasing parental guilt must be done within the broader construct that these parents are raising children in a highly technical, competitive society. Too often, clinicians, particularly clinicians without sufficient experience interacting with a variety of parents, misinterpret a parent's remarks that "Johnny can do better in school" or "Sally isn't very careful in her work" as meaning the parent is too demanding, perfectionistic, rigid, insensitive, or sets too high standards. While recognizing that some parents of stutterers do seem, as Neill (1960) puts it, to "want to speed up the pace,"* this does not mean that *all* such parents are too demanding or time urgent or that even those parents who are somewhat demanding are necessarily demanding about every aspect of their child's behavior every hour of the day. Clinicians should work to understand the difference between normal parental concern and those concerns that frequently and consistently occur and that seem to be less than desirable in terms of fostering the type of environment where a child's speech fluency can positively develop.

Finally, and at the risk of stating the obvious, parents are people and as the song goes, "people with children" (Thomas and others, 1972). Many of us will eventually become or already are parents, and we should recognize that parents encounter many of the same problems that SLPs, as people, encounter in daily living. When we clinically interact with the parents of stutterers we try to do so within the perspective that we are dealing with people who happen to be parents. We try not to be too willing to cast the first stone at parents who, after all, are people like the rest of us, with all our human foibles and fortes.

Reevaluation of the child and keeping in touch with the parents   With the child with no apparent problem but whose parents are quite concerned, we generally set up, at the end of the initial evaluation, a reevaluation. Such reevaluations permit us to maintain contact with the parent, monitor the parents' actual ability to positively change, and to assess changes in the child's speech and related behaviors over time. Maintain the contact with

---

*A. Neill, *Summerhill: A Radical Approach to Child Rearing* (New York: Hart Associates, 1960), p. 253. Reprinted by permission.

these parents, not as a means of extending your professional preciousness, but as a way for these parents to contact you at times when they are concerned (and having a scheduled reevaluation, which they are told they can cancel any time, gives them the security that something is being done while at the same time seeming to make it easier for them to call in with "interim" reports).

Keeping in touch with these parents reduces their feeling of helplessness, frustration, and "being alone in the boat"; your suggestions and insights may well be the only voice of reason the parents hear, and, as I can attest, these parents need that. Besides, the parents know, at some level, that you are not emotionally involved with their child and that you can be as objective as possible in your suggestions.

When helping these parents, we also feel it important for the SLP to know what parenting books the parents have and/or are reading. The young parent raising a first child usually reads such books as those by Spock and Rothenberg (1985), Brazelton (1974, 1983), those published by Gesell and associates (for example, Ilg and Ames, 1960), or one of the many "how to" parenting books like Dodson's (1970). The SLP should read and be familiar with these books and develop an understanding of the types of written inputs many parents routinely turn to when they have questions and concerns about the general well-being of their child.

Children with Some Stuttering and Whose Parents Are Unconcerned

If you establish that the child is producing a frequency, duration, and type of speech disfluency that puts him at risk for becoming a stutterer, then you have to tell this to his parents, guardians, or adult associates. However, no matter how patiently, clearly, and sensitively you express your belief, some parents are simply not going to accept your findings. While some of these parents may appear as if they don't respect your opinion, clinical acumen, and experience, most of them are actually hoping against hope that the child's problem will go away with time and/or denying the reality of the situation.

Some of these parents will shop around until they find some professional who agrees with their feeling that the problem will resolve with time and/or that there is no problem. Others will simply wait several years and eventually come back to you with the simple statement, "I guess he didn't outgrow it."

The most difficult of this lot are the parents who intellectually know that there is a problem but emotionally seem to deny its existence. These parents find a variety of reasons why they can't meet scheduled appointments, why scheduled appointments conflict with the all-important tuba lessons, and why therapy, although necessary, may actually be "harming" the child. Such parents need time to think the situation through and most of them, with sufficient support and the right kind of gentle but firm advice that the child's problem is not getting any better, can come to see the reality of the situation. Remember, most parents want to do the right thing; it is generally only their approach or methods that need change.

Who knows who will become fluent and who will stay a stutterer?   To make this situation even more of a challenge, the child's actual speech behavior appears, to the parents, to support their belief that the child will get better by himself or that there is no problem. It is not hard to see why parents think this way when we consider the following types of behaviors exhibited by many of these youngsters. First, these children generally, but not always, exhibit no apparent awareness of a speech disfluency problem. Second, the child's speech disfluencies are marked by unpredictable cyclical changes of indeterminant length; one day (or week or month) the child is "good" (that is, the child does not stutter) and the next, "bad" (that is, the child stutters quite frequently). Third, most of these youngsters' speech disfluencies are "easy" in that they are associated with little sign of physical tension and are generally only 250 to 1000 milliseconds in duration. Fourth, the child is still relatively willing to talk in a variety of situations about a variety of topics. In essence, the child is often just as fluent as disfluent, seems to have little awareness of a problem or concern about talking, and exhibits disfluencies that are generally short in duration and appear associated with minimal physical tension. Given this sort of picture, it is small wonder that some parents believe that there is no problem and/or that the problem will resolve by itself. And, of course, a percentage of these children do become better with time, with or without therapy.

The only problem with all this is that no one, to my knowledge, can accurately and reliably determine which of these children will and will not resolve with time. The two extreme ways of dealing with this uncertainty are (1) telling all such parents that their child will "outgrow" the problem and (2) telling all such parents that their child has a problem and needs remediation as soon as possible. Both approaches would appear to be playing the odds: The "he'll outgrow it" approach will certainly work for a percentage of the children, but for another percentage therapy will eventually be necessary. The "everybody-gets-therapy" approach will provide therapy to those who need it, but probably needlessly remediate a percentage who don't. What is needed, in my opinion, are more clinical investigations that try to uncover reliable indicators, no matter how subtle, that a child (1) has a stuttering problem and (2) that the problem will probably not resolve with time. At present, no such indicators exist; however, many researchers are working in this direction and someday this area will be far clearer than it is at present.

Our own rule of thumb is that a child has potential for becoming a stutterer if he or she exhibits (1) 3 or more *within-word* disfluencies per 100 words of conversational speech, (2) 2 to 3 sound prolongations per 10 instances of stuttering, and (3) delay in and/or unusual types of phonological processes. We explain these findings to the parents as clearly as we can—pictures or tables like Table 1–1 (page 11) help in this regard—but still some of these parents disregard these observations.

Sad to say, but you are going to lose a percentage of these "discussions" with parents. That is, some of these parents will keep their child out of therapy until such a time that the child's stuttering has become so obvious and pervasive as to make its remediation very problematic. Likewise, some of these parents, for a variety of reasons, will not follow up on your suggestion that the child needs help from other professionals, such as a psychologist, and wait until related problems become far more pronounced or pervasive or other agencies, like the school system, literally force them to take action. Fortunately, in our experience, the percentage of parents who continually deny or disregard our assessment or referral is relatively small, while most of the rest of these parents, after some degree of discussion with us, begin to see that their child indeed needs some form of professional intervention.

Concomitant speech and/or language problems exhibited by children who stutter somewhat   It is not uncommon that a child with an incipient stuttering problem, whose parents believe has "no problem," also exhibits other concerns, such as language delays and phonological difficulties. Such co-occurrence obviously confounds the situation but, with some patience and thought on the part of the SLP, can be dealt with quite constructively. Patience, however, is the watchword here and it is particularly unwise to rush in and remediate one part without considering its influence on the whole of the child's speech abilities and language development.

It must be emphasized that development of speech fluency is not an isolated phenomenon; it is connected in intimate, if poorly understood, ways to the child's overall development of language and phonology as well as related processes. If, for example, one were to remediate a young stutterer's phonological difficulties by employing repetitive drill that emphasizes overly precise, rapid, and physically tense articulatory postures and gestures, the child's speech "sounds" might indeed improve, but it would have a less than desirable long-term influence on the child's fluency problem. But we get ahead of ourselves.

USING A CONCOMITANT PROBLEM TO GET THERAPY GOING

Sometimes a young incipient stutterer's concomitant problem can be used to advantage, particularly if the parent believes there is no concern. It is not uncommon for these parents to be more receptive to therapy focused on language or articulation concerns. We would still tell the parents that the child is or has potential for becoming a stutterer, but that other problems co-occur and probably need more attention at this point. If the parents agree to such a strategy, then we proceed to "work" on the child's language and/or articulation problem but at the same time discuss with the parents their child's behaviors (and changes) just as we would if the child were being remediated for stuttering. If asked by the parents why they have to, for example, slow down their rate when talking to or in the presence of the child, we explain that this sort of change makes it easier for the child to verbally interact with the parent and puts less time pressure on the child to communicate—changes that should help every aspect of verbal communication, not just fluency.

DEALING WITH DELAYS IN LANGUAGE IN A CHILD WHO STUTTERS

Delays in language development (for example, Johnston and Schery, 1976) do occur with some children who stutter—whether or not their parents think they stutter—and as such, these problems need to be assessed and possibly remediated. Sometimes a child's speech disfluency problem seems secondary to delays and deviance in language development and when this is the case the child's language skills need attention prior to remediation of fluency. This is particularly true when the speech disfluencies are of the easy (that is, physically non-tense), relatively brief duration part- and whole-word repetition variety.

However, we have noticed that some children whose language seems delayed and/or deviant in development may actually become *more* disfluent when their language actually improves and this observation is supported by an empirical study of the impact of language therapy on a child's speech disfluencies (Merits-Patterson and Reed, 1981). We have noticed this association between positive change in language and increases in speech disfluency to be particularly apparent in children around five to six years of age. We are not sure what this means or its long-term implications for recovery from disfluency. We are inclined to speculate that increases in the length and complexity of verbally expressed languages increase the opportunities for instances of disfluency to emerge and is probably a natural byproduct of improved but still unstable expressive language skills.

Some children who stutter may have a mean length of utterance (MLU) (Brown, 1973) roughly appropriate for his or her chronological age, but whose mastery of particular grammatical morphemes (that is, morphemes whose main purpose is to modify meaning of content words or to more specifically indicate relation of content words) is less than appropriate for this stage of language development. For example, the use of "be" as a copula verb (the "is" of "She is tired" and the "are" of "You are captain") may be omitted by some children who stutter who are at Brown's stage IV of language development.

It should be clear, however, that we are not saying that all of these children who stutter have language problems, or that they all exhibit the same type and severity of language difficulties, or that language problems cause stuttering. It is a challenge to decide which problem—a language delay or stuttering—needs more immediate attention; however, therapy oriented to modification of language seems most appropriate if the child's speech disfluencies are of a physically easy, relatively short duration and consist mainly of part- and whole-word repetitions.

Conversely, therapy should probably be more oriented to modification of stuttering if the speech disfluencies are associated with visible and audible signs of physical and psychological tension, and are relatively longer in duration and of a sound prolongation (audible and inaudible) type. Of course, both problems—language difficulties and stuttering—can not be simultaneously dealt with in the same session; the clinician will probably focus at least 60 percent of his or her attention on one problem and 40 percent on the other and change these proportions as the child improves in this area or the problem changes.

DEALING WITH ARTICULATION CONCERNS IN A CHILD WHO STUTTERS SOMEWHAT

We know now that difficulties in speech sound development frequently occur in children who stutter. Williams and Silverman (1968) reported that 24 percent of 115 elementary school-aged stutterers had associated articulation defects compared to 9 percent of their normally fluent peers. Riley and Riley (1979) reported that 33 percent of 100 young stutterers also exhibited articulation difficulties. Daly (1981) reported that 58 percent of a subgroup (n = 25) of young stutterers—taken from a larger sample (N = 138)—evidenced articulation disorders. Thompson (1983) observed a 35 percent to 45 percent incidence of "suspected (articulation) deficits" in two samples (n = 31 and n = 17) of young stutterers. Cantwell and Lewis (1985), in a large clinical investigation of the psychiatric and learning disabilities in 600 children with speech and/or language disorders, reported that 30 percent of the 40 stutterers in their sample also exhibited an articulation disorder. Thus, from a low of 24 percent to a high of 45 percent, several studies, of relatively large sample sizes, indicate that stuttering and "articulation" difficulties co-occur for a sizable proportion of children who stutter.

Obviously, 24 percent to 45 percent is far greater than the approximately 2 percent of the school-age population who have articulation concerns, as reported by Hull, Mielke, Timmons and Willeford (1971). These findings do not mean that one problem causes the other but that the two problems frequently—we estimate about 33 percent of all young stutterers exhibit some form of articulation concern—co-occur and that the SLP should be prepared to handle such co-occurrence (cf. Feinstein 1970 for an overview of general topic of co-occurring disorders).

Of course, there are articulatory problems, and then there are articulatory problems. A slight distortion of an /s/, or perhaps an /l/, is probably no real problem and can generally be ignored as the SLP proceeds to help the child modify his or her disfluencies. However, multiple articulation errors with omissions and substitutions, as well as distortions, are problematic, particularly if the child also exhibits any "unusual" phonological processes, for example, glottal replacement: /be?/ for "bed" (Louko, Edwards and Conture, 1988). Evidence of these frequent, multiple articulation errors, with or without unusual phonological processes, in a child who is also stuttering is not cause to panic, but it is cause for caution and adjustment of therapy to the particular child's needs and abilities.

The child who begins to stutter AFTER therapy for articulation problems. SLPs who work with children have, sooner or later, heard about or actually observed a child who began to stutter *after* therapy for remediation of a speech misarticulation problem. While no one, at this point, knows what the precise relation between articulation and stuttering is and whether therapy for one helps or hinders the other, it is apparent that some, albeit unclear, relation exists between speech fluency and speech sound production. In my opinion, what seems to happen with these children is that they begin therapy too early for their "articulation problem" with the result that even though their articulation improves, they learn their problem sounds and realize that they have to "work" or be careful to produce these sounds correctly, precisely, and quickly. This sort of approach is, in our opinion, counterproductive to facilitating children's speech fluency and, in some cases, may actually exacerbate their stuttering problems.

As an apparent antidote, these children need experience with speaking in a physically relaxed, relatively slow-paced atmosphere where communication is made an enjoyable, interesting, and shared activity. Phonetic placement drills or direct remediation of these youngsters' speech fluency and articulation are secondary; the SLP must first help the child come to realize that speech isn't such a chore—that it can be fun and done in a relatively physically easy, unhurried manner.

The young stutterer who stutters and exhibits speech sound problems. A child who hasn't had any form of therapy who exhibits both stuttering and articulation concerns presents a slightly different problem. First, carefully think through the *relative* importance of modifying the child's articulation problem versus his stuttering problem. While the child may indeed be misarticulating some sounds, is it not possible that, although delayed, these problems will gradually resolve by themselves? If this doesn't seem to be the case, then remediation of these sounds-in-error may be necessary. Second, realize that these children do not need further instruction in which sounds are problems or difficult for them to produce. That is, no matter what the approach to their articulation concerns, these children do not need further instruction in how to work at, force out, or be careful or cautious in the production of their "problem" sounds. They do not need to learn concern, fear, fright, avoidance, and struggle when confronted with the production of certain sounds. Indeed, some of these children already seem to have these ideas or are at least on the road to developing such notions.

Third, it is better that these children receive no speech therapy rather than one that exaggerates, emphasizes, or stresses "overarticulation" of speech sounds and/or physically tense speech articulatory musculature and posturing. Too many of these children, without our help, are unfortunately developing a strategy toward speech production that we interpret as "speech is hard, speech takes work, and thus I'll use force (or avoid) to speak" (Bloodstein, 1975). It seems that sometimes our good intentions to assist some of these children with their articulation difficulties backfire on us when the youngsters just learn more sounds to fear and more and better ways to physically tense up and push out speech segments (cf. Dell, 1980, for further discussion of ways to deal with these issues with the school-age stutterer).

In essence what appears to be needed for these children is assistance in helping them develop a physically easier, less hurried or rushed means of initiating and maintaining speech rather than very careful, cautious, physically precise, and overarticulated productions of sounds.

The young stutterer who is almost or completely unintelligible.   Assuming that about three young stutterers out of ten have some articulation concerns, we speculate, based on our clinical experience, that about one of these three children will be nearly, if not completely, unintelligible. "Working on articulation" is not a question; something needs to be done to help these youngsters become better understood by their listeners. However, all the cautions raised above—when remediating the articulation concerns of children who stutter—still need to be considered. These children also need experience with physically easy, unhurried, and enjoyable forms of communication. Of course, it is difficult for these children to experience "enjoyable" communication when their listener is continually asking them to "Say that again" or "What did you say?" or "Huh?" (The situation becomes even more problematic if the listener has unreasonably high standards for the child's speech or is so perfectionistic that any and all of the child's speech errors are corrected or criticized.) We have also found that some of these children may begin to stutter for awhile as their articulation improves. We are not sure why but suspect with these cases that the entirety of their speech sound production development is delayed and that the "normal" period of disfluency is also delayed in onset. Thus the period of disfluency typically observed around three or four years of age, is now being produced by these children, when they are about five or six. Much more needs to be explored in this area but for the present, the SLP should approach these children somewhat differently than the typical child who stutters.

DEALING WITH VOICE PROBLEMS IN CHILDREN WHO STUTTER

As mentioned in the previous chapter, as a rule, children who stutter exhibit voice usage roughly or grossly within normal limits. When concerns with voice usage are present, however, the two most common, based on our experience, are: (1) inappropriate low-pitched, monotonous or restricted pitch range and/or (2) hoarseness related to hyperfunctional voice use. The low-pitched, Johnny-one-note problem seems to be far more common than hoarseness.

While this is an area in need of a great deal of empirical study, we can share some of our clinical observations regarding how to best handle these problems. As mentioned in Chapter 2, it should be noted that the very act of stuttering, for example, tensely posturing the vocal folds in an adducted position, influences the vocal quality associated with the instance of stuttering. We are not discussing changes in vocal quality associated with the actual instance of stuttering; rather we are discussing differences or changes in vocal quality throughout the entirety of the child's speech, the fluent as well as disfluent aspects.

We have no empirical evidence to support us, but we speculate that the low-pitch, monotonous voice of some children (and teenagers and adults as well) is somehow related to the child's stuttering problem. That is, the child may be lowering his or her pitch and restricting pitch variations in an attempt, albeit seemingly maladaptive, to avoid or minimize stuttering. This would suggest that the stuttering precedes the low-pitch, monotone; however, as we said, we have no evidence that this is the case, but we think it is highly likely. It is also possible that the low-pitch monotone reflects overall delays and/or difficulties the child is having with speech motor control and is also reflected in the child's stuttering.

Whatever the cause, we have found that the stutterings of a child who also exhibits a low-pitched, monotonous voice can be readily remediated—providing there are no other concerns—with the "voice problem" being essentially ignored. We don't know what influence increased fluency would have on the child's voice usage, but we have observed children begin to use a wider range of pitch as they become more fluent. Once again, however, this is an empirical issue in need of investigation.

The other kind of voice problem—hoarseness—presents us with a slightly different challenge. Frequently, upon questioning, the parents will tell you that the child who is hoarse does one or more of the following: (1) yells excessively inside and outside of the home, (2) habitually talks loudly inside and outside the home, (3) frequently imitates animals, machines (for example, trucks, cars, planes) or makes "monster" noises, (4) sings frequently in accompaniment to loud background music or noise, and so forth. Of course, one might naturally expect and not be concerned if one noticed some hoarseness or change in vocal quality associated with a child's cold, laryngitis, flu, or other upper respiratory infection; such changes are usually temporary and resolve with the illness.

However, in the absence of such an illness and/or where the hoarseness becomes or seems to be more persistent and chronic in nature, a referral to an ear, nose, and throat specialist would appear justified. Asking the parents to have the ENT send you a copy of his or her findings and recommendations would be very helpful to the SLP in planning therapy. Sometimes these children will be asked to (1) minimize the kinds of vocal abuse mentioned above and/or (2) to give their voice some degree of vocal rest. However, it is our experience that both the parents and child will need more than a one-time lecture in this regard and will need the help and support of the SLP in making such changes.

Therapy for stuttering can be conducted concomitantly with therapy for voice problems as long as the cautions described above (for example, emphasizing physically relaxed, relatively unhurried, and enjoyable forms of verbal communication) are heeded.

DEALING WITH OTHER PROBLEMS IN CHILDREN WHO STUTTER

While an occasional child with cerebral palsy or cleft palate will also stutter, we have not had enough repeated experience with these types of children to warrant any meaningful generalizations. What appears to be the case is that each of these children presents a relatively unique situation that must be dealt with individually. Furthermore, the relation between the other problem and stuttering is not particularly clear; what is needed, it seems, are published reports of detailed case studies of these children to increase our understanding of the nature and means of remediating the special problems and needs these youngsters appear to have.

A seemingly more common "other" problem is psychosocial adjustment. However, in our experience, there are very few children who stutter who also exhibit clinically significant apparent psychosocial adjustment concerns. This does not mean that youngsters who stutter and their families don't have psychosocial concerns, but the *origin* or *cause* of such concerns for different stutterers may be quite different. Clinicians must try to distinguish between young stutterers whose emotional concerns are seemingly normal reactions to abnormal situations (that is, being unable to produce speech fluently) from young stutterers whose stuttering appears related to a more basic psychosocial adjustment problem.

We believe that it is a sign of psychological intactness for a child to become concerned about and hesitant to do that which he or she cannot do very well. Of course, such concerns, on the part of the child, increase the complexity of the child's stuttering problem, but these concerns relate directly to the child's speaking difficulties and are not caused by other, more deep-seated psychological issues. Generally, many of these concerns will disappear or at least significantly diminish as these children become more fluent. These children need support and understanding for their concerns, but basically they need assistance in becoming more fluent.

Another group of children, who we estimate number only 5 percent to 10 percent of the stuttering population, have a *real* psychosocial adjustment problem. Some of the behaviors we believe suggest at least a referral for a psychological evaluation are the following (it is possible that a child can exhibit one or more of these behaviors in a variety of permutations):

1. Children who routinely demonstrate strong and persistent fears of fires, loud noises, the dark, and anything strange. Many children do this on occasion or for brief periods of time during their development, but when the fears are chronic, strong, and predictable, when the child spends parts of every day or week openly discussing, worrying, and asking parental reassurance that, for example, his bedroom won't catch on fire, a psychological evaluation is not inappropriate; that is, when the child is obsessed with these concerns and compulsively repeats activities in relation to them, a referral for psychosocial evaluation would appear appropriate.

2. Children who are acting out physically against other children either at home, at play, or at school. Once again it is the frequency and persistence of these physical acts that are important. An occasional slap or punch is one thing; *daily* or *weekly* punching, kicking, pushing/pulling, slapping, or pinching other children, particularly for no apparent reason, is something that should not be overlooked. This problem is particularly noticeable in the child who is not getting any positive attention for school achievement, that is, he is failing or not mastering his school assignments. These children seem to opt for the idea that attention, of any type, is better than no attention at all.

3. Children whom other parents routinely refuse to let their children play with, or whom other adults or school personnel report they are having trouble controlling or dealing with. Some of these children are also acting out physically against other children.

4. Children who appear to have large amounts of anger and hostility stored within them which they cannot appropriately channel or express. These children may be quite tenacious in their refusal to discuss themselves or their feelings, even when such discussion would appear to be an appropriate part of therapy.

5. Children who refuse to talk to the examining clinician but readily talk to parents *once* the clinician is outside of the room. We are not talking about 5 to 15 minutes of reticence to communicate with the clinician because of shyness or the like. We are not talking about a child who stops talking because of momentary embarrassment or fatigue. Here we are referring to the child who will not talk to us

after 45 to 90 minutes of our trying, the child who seems to purposely refuse to talk to us, but will readily talk to mother and father when we are not in the room. While the examining psychologist may have better luck than we have in getting such a child to talk, it is our experience that the reasons these children refuse to talk is not solely related to stuttering and that family counseling may be a better place to begin than therapy for stuttering.

Many times, with a child who stutters and who exhibits real or apparent psychosocial adjustment problems, the question comes up: Which came first, the stuttering or the psychological problem? In reality this is often difficult to tell, but most of the time, even as the child becomes more psychologically intact, the child's stuttering remains. Both the parents and psychological therapist should be made aware of such a possibility at the beginning of psychotherapy, so that their efforts can be focused on helping the child to develop in a more appropriate fashion psychologically and not be too concerned that the child's fluency is not also improving.

Children Who Exhibit Some Stuttering but Whose Parents Are Minimally or Completely Unconcerned

When confronted with these children and their parents, we have found that we have three choices: (1) observe the child through periodic reevaluations until such time as the child has no problem and/or the parents change their minds; (2) bring the child in for individual speech therapy; or (3) bring the child in for parent/child fluency group. We have found neither options (1) or (2) are completely satisfactory, and at present we tend toward option (3), the parent/child fluency group, an option that has been detailed elsewhere (Conture and Kelly, 1988b) and that we will only briefly mention here.

With the first approach—periodic reevaluation—the SLP runs the risk of having the child's fluency problem and/or environment deteriorate; however, with the second approach—individual speech therapy—the SLP runs the risk of boring the child and the parents with therapy since improvement may not come fast enough or be of sufficient quality and quantity to maintain motivation and satisfaction with therapy. If a parent/child fluency group is not a realistic or desired approach, one compromise between options (1) and (2) is to bring the child and/or his or her parents in for a period of trial speech therapy of, say, three to six weeks.

It must be stressed, however, that *before* this trial period begins the parents should be clearly and explicitly told that this will be a trial and that it will last for only so many weeks. Thus, if the child and parents seem to benefit from this trial therapy, fine; it can be extended and/or modified as need be; if not, we cancel the trial therapy and put the client and family into a hold pattern during which time we observe through periodic reevaluations, phone calls to parents and school, or school and home visits (if possible).

Even when parents are relatively unconcerned about the child's problem, it is all too easy to make a rush to judgment and initiate therapy with the child. Before we begin therapy with any child (or teenager or adult, for that matter) we must try to make professional decisions whether the child is emotionally, socially, physically, communicatively, and otherwise ready for therapy. Therapy started before the client is ready to benefit from it is not only counterproductive in the short run but in the long run has the real potential for turning the client off from therapy at a point when he or she is ready to benefit ("I already had speech; it didn't help").

THE PARENT/CHILD FLUENCY GROUP

We and others believe that involving parents in the therapy process, although adding to the complexities of the process, also increases our effectiveness and the child's chances for long-term recovery (for example, Bailey and Bailey, 1982; Rustin, 1987). Of course, if the parents are unconcerned and/or resistant to therapy in any form, then they will not be involved with a parent/child (P/C) fluency group; however, some of these parents also will not allow their child to be involved with this or any other form of therapy. While we are presently talking about parents who are unconcerned, we have found that the P/C group is equally effective for children whose parents *do* express concerns about their child's speech and related issues (these children and their parents will be discussed in the next section).

The rationale, logistics, and difficulties of conducting such groups have been discussed elsewhere (Conture and Kelly, 1988b); however, we will cover the essential aspects of these groups. In our opinion, the logic behind these groups is relatively straightforward, but it can be modified, simplified, or made more complex as the need arises. Typically, the parent/child group meets once a week for approximately 45 to 60 minutes with the parents meeting in one room and the children in another. Groups generally meet in the late afternoon (3:00 P.M. to 5:00 P.M.) after school, and weekly sessions are arranged in 10 to 12 week blocks with about 3 "blocks" arranged per calendar year.

The typical child is involved with the P/C group for 2 10-to-12-week blocks with some children requiring only 1 block and some 4 or more blocks. We are beginning to find that 10-week blocks are better for the child and parent; 12 weeks seems to be 2 weeks too many and both parents and child seem to get stale and/or bored with the process.

While some might be concerned that there are approximately 4- to 8-week breaks between each 10-week block, we have found this to be an excellent "living laboratory" for assessing the child's ability to transfer change during a period of nontherapy. If a child cannot maintain his or her improved fluency during scheduled breaks from active therapy, we have found that there is little chance that the child will maintain improvement once therapy is discontinued.

Arranging groups by age   Before proceeding with details of the P/C group, the ages of the clients within each group should be discussed because it is quite crucial when bringing children together as a group. Children, if at all possible, should be grouped together with other children of a comparable age. In this way, the clinician maximizes the chances that the children will neither feel patronized nor overwhelmed by the level of activities. Once again, with children, the *form* of the activity is many times more important than its *content*. While the content, rationale, and purpose of activities may be the same for a group of 5-year-olds versus a group of 7-year-olds, the form should be adapted to the level of each group's development.

Logistics   A typical group session begins with the parents and children being separated into two rooms. Sometimes the parents and a clinician spend the entire session discussing parental questions and concerns and the parents minimally observe their children. Other times, the parents observe the entirety of their children's group, but only enter the children's group in the last ten minutes. As we have found it beneficial, we are trying to include the parents in each and every group during the last ten minutes, but sometimes it is difficult to get parents to terminate their own group discussions in time to participate in their child's group.

The child's group   After the children and parents have been separated, the children (two to six age-comparable youngsters) are paired with one or two clinicians. In our setting, one clinician acts as group facilitator while a second clinician assists with the demonstration of group activities and helps the facilitator with "crowd control." However, we believe that one *experienced* clinician should be able to run such a group just as effectively, although such groups should probably not exceed four or perhaps five children.

Each child has his or her own small rug (labeled with his or her name to avoid dickering over whose rug is whose and conserving precious therapy time) that they sit on; they are arranged in a circle on the floor. If chairs are used, each chair would likewise be labeled with each child's name. While we don't want the children to feel that they are in church neither do we want them to develop the relative laissez-faire attitude typically exhibited on the school playground. They are in the group to have a good time and to enjoy themselves, but they must be reasonably well behaved and attentive during the activities.

In essence, the child's group has two goals: (1) help the children change speech production behaviors that inhibit fluency and increase those behaviors that facilitate fluency and (2) help the children change those communicative interactive behaviors that inhibit fluency and increase those communicative interactive behaviors that facilitate fluency. Each group session, therefore, combines therapy approaches that try to help the child speak more fluently as well as to develop communicative interaction behaviors that will facilitate this fluency.

As mentioned in Chapter 1, we believe that stuttering relates to a complex interaction between the child's abilities and the child's environment and some of that environment is "created" by things the child does during speaking that are not directly related to speech production, for example, interrupting people when they talk.

Changing speech production behavior It must be remembered that on the whole the child's group approach to changing stuttering is indirect, that is, the clinician is not directly, by word or by deed, trying to modify the way the child talks. Instead, the clinician is trying, through play, game, and modeling, to get the child to speak with more appropriate levels of physical tension and at rates of production that are reasonable given the child's level of development. As shown in Figure 3–2, we do this by demonstrating, identifying, and trying to produce the temporal difference between "turtle" (slow) versus "rabbit" (fast) speech and the physical tension difference between "scarecrow" (relaxed) and "tinwoodsman" (tense) speech.

However, one caution: Some of these children, regardless of apparent intellectual and social readiness, may not understand the concept of "same" and "different." Thus, it is not a bad idea to include throughout the first two to five group sessions, examples of same/different (for example, pipe cleaners of various colors, textures, and lengths) so that children get a more concrete example of this concept.

Another caution: The clinician should be ready and willing to demonstrate and use rabbit, turtle, scarecrow (or Raggedy Ann) or tinwoodsman speech. The clinician should be adept at *showing* and should minimize *telling* the children what she wants them to do. This is also true with the parents.

Changing communicative interaction behaviors Although becoming more fluent is the ultimate goal of any therapy with stutterers, there are a number of related behaviors which, in our opinion, if left unchanged, have the real potential for making it difficult for the child to maintain his or her fluency. It is not at all unusual to observe children who stutter interrupt people while they are talking, exhibit difficulty waiting their turn to talk, and in general being less than attentive listeners. Accordingly, we use a number of play-

WHAT HAS TO BE CHANGED

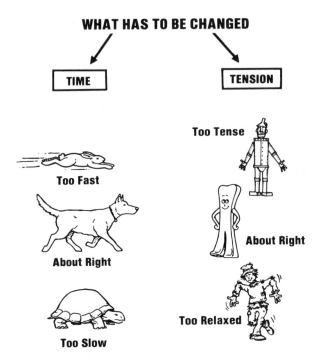

FIGURE 3–2.   Time and tension are the two elements of speech production that need to be changed to become more fluent. Children have little appreciation for the abstract, complex concepts of time and tension, and need to have these ideas made more concrete and tangible. With regard to *time*, overly rapid speech is represented by a rabbit, and a turtle obviously represents speech that is too slow. Regarding physical tension, a tinwoodsman is too tense while a scarecrow is too relaxed. The "happy medium" in terms of time is represented by a trotting dog, while "about right" tension is depicted by the bendable, rubber stick figure. Fluent speech, therefore, is not overly slow and flaccid but moves along at a reasonable pace with a degree of relaxed tension or tonus in speech and related musculature.

oriented activities, games, and models to show the children how to (1) *listen* (when someone else is talking), (2) *wait* (your turn), and (3) *don't talk* (when someone else is talking). Sometimes, getting children who stutter to obey or at least observe these rules more frequently is all that is necessary for them to become more fluent.

It would seem that it is difficult for anyone to speak with optimal amounts of fluency if they are always trying to "get a word in edgewise" and reluctant to wait to talk until it is their turn. Our clinical experience suggests to us that speaking rapidly, exhibiting minimal or very short turn-switching pauses, interrupting, and/or not listening to speakers when they talk are behaviors that *stress* young stutterers' abilities to achieve and/or maintain fluent speech.

The parents' group The parents of the children are seen separately but simultaneously with group therapy for their children. While the group has a variety of functions, each group is a mix of (1) discussing concerns general to all parents and their children and (2) discussing concerns specific to one or two parents and their children. As in all groups, some parents are better than others at understanding how general concerns relate to their own situation or how someone else's problem, seemingly different on the surface, may actually be similar to theirs. For the SLP, the hardest skill to learn is the ability to talk the fine line between closing one's mouth and listening versus opening one's mouth and conversing. Neither too much listening nor talking will be effective; there is a need for some mix of both.

Parents have a natural curiosity about the past and what may have caused their child to stutter and their role in it. As we have already discussed this issue, all we will now say is to answer their questions on this subject politely and respectfully, but steer them, as best you can, away from a relatively fruitless dwelling on the past and concentrate on how things can change in the present and future. While we can understand their curiosity and desire to make sense of the past, once it has been made clear to them that the past is over and done, that we have told them our best guess about what may have happened and that we can change only the present, it is time to move on. Unfortunately, some parents remain fixated on the past and their possible role in their child's stuttering and fail to come to grips with what they may be able to do to change the present. For these parents, group therapy, while not a waste, probably has minimal influence.

Parents learn many things in a group setting, and not just from the SLP. From the other parents they learn that they are "not alone in the boat," that other parents share some but not all of their same concerns, and that other parents can and do change and that such changes do help their children. The SLP provides the parents with objective information about children in general, stuttering in specific, up-to-date, and hopefully more accurate, perspectives with which to view themselves and their children, and the means by which they can change their own speech and related behaviors in order to facilitate their child's speech fluency.

Much of each parent group involves talking—either by the parents or SLP. While these discussions can and do also take the form of information sharing and counseling, they can also take the form of parental venting. That is, one or two parents will raise a concern or problem that is particularly vexing or frustrating to them and other parents will identify with the problem and add their own feelings. In these situations, it is best for the SLP to listen and try not to be too directive or defensive, particularly when parents are being critical over apparent slowness, lack of progress, or apparent slippages/regressions in their child's fluency.

Sometimes these parental venting sessions are based on misinformation on the parents' part about what should be taking place at a particular point in therapy. However, other times a parent's concerns are based on accurate perceptions that things are not going as well or as quickly as they should for their child. If the clinician believes that a particular parent is getting out of hand with his or her critique, that parent should be gently but firmly told so but, and this is extremely important, out of earshot of the other parents. One of our cardinal rules for conducting this or any group is: *Praise in public and criticize in private.* A group leader violates this rule at his or her own peril.

Maintenance therapy In past years, once a child had successfully maintained normal or near normal fluency for the last half (four to six weeks) of a block of the P/C group, we would dismiss the child and parents and have them return in about six months for a reevaluation. While a number of these children maintained or transferred their fluency, a disturbing number of them didn't.

Now, to alleviate that problem, once a child achieves normal or near normal fluency during the P/C group, we set-up a "maintenance program." While the specifics of this maintenance program vary somewhat from child to child, we typically continue to have the parent and child come to the P/C therapy group for approximately one more year—twice a month for the first 10-week block, once a month for the second 10-week block, and 2 or 3 times for the last block. In this way we can better monitor the child's ability to transfer and at the same time get the child, and particularly the parents, gradually used to doing things on their own. We have found this maintenance schedule to be a very important facet of our overall P/C group approach.

Children with Some Stuttering
Whose Parents Are Also Concerned

Children in this category can certainly be initially placed in the P/C group and, if they are not successful, after say two or three blocks, individual therapy can be started. Some other children, for scheduling or other reasons, may need to begin with individual therapy. Whatever the case, some involvement with the parents, particularly in the beginning to keep them informed as to the type and progress of the child's therapy, is strongly recommended.

Getting therapy started Much of the first individual session with a young child who stutters is spent getting to know the child, setting down rules of the road for the therapy sessions (and for the parents, if they are involved), and trying to develop some procedure for the first and subsequent therapy sessions whereby the SLP can assess whether the child's speech disfluencies warrant therapy. This last task—developing a strategy to assess progress or lack thereof—is often overlooked. All too frequently, SLPs will assume that the fluency achieved in the clinic is also manifest outside the clinic, without either asking the client or the client's parents or testing themselves. Many times it seems that therapy begins without much thought given to when the SLP will know that therapy should be terminated.

As with the P/C group, if at all possible, we like to have and think it instructive for parents to observe us playing and talking with their child. An ideal number of observations would be once every other session, but even once every ten sessions would be better than none. Although parents frequently say, "I simply don't have the time to spend playing with Bobby that you do," or "We don't have *all those nice toys at home*," or "I don't like to play with children," we try to emphasize to the parents the *quality*, rather than the *quantity*, of our play interactions with the child. Although the wise SLP would never say this directly to a parent who complains about not enough time, the issue is not really the *amount* of time, but the parents' willingness to *take* whatever time they can to interact with the child ("it's boring to play with him"). We are not talking about hours and hours here but 5 to 30 minutes a day. We can't state this strongly enough: It is not the amount of time but priorities for spending what time is available. While the parents clearly need time to relax and unwind themselves, they are, like it or not, parents also and must be helped to see, in firm but gentle ways, that some fairly brief but daily time spent interacting with their child should receive a reasonably high priority.

We also try to quickly point out that it is not the toys themselves that determine what their child gets out of playing with them as much as it is how the child and parent actually play with the toys. A cardboard box can, and very often is, a more attractive toy to a young child than the latest Death-Ray-Stun-for-Fun-Dream-Laser-Beam Gun. We try to point out to the parents such things as a clinician's unconditional, positive regard for the child, the clinician's attempts to listen to the content of the child's utterances, the clinician's clear but firm setting down of rules for communication as well as general behaving, and the clinician's showing as well as telling the child how to do a particular task. All too often, we find, parents will tell Johnny to do something like make his bed and think their mere telling him this is sufficient even though they have never really spent time instructing and showing Johnny how to actually go about making his bed (cf. Bettelheim, 1985).

Introducing concept of hard and easy speech   Although these children may be relatively inconsistent in the production of their stutterings, if the situation strongly suggests that there will be continued negative development (that is, greater numbers and varieties of stuttering), we become fairly direct in our approach. Elaborating upon Williams's (1971) concept of *hard* (that is, physically tense and relatively rapid) versus *easy* (that is, physically relaxed and relatively slow) speech, we start by having the child identify hard and easy speech in our speech. We then progress to having the child listen to the tape recordings of others, to listening to tape recordings of himself, and finally to the stutterings in his own speech *as* he or she is actually producing them. The terms *hard* and *easy* speech are nice, simple terms with minimal negative connotations associated with them (Williams, 1971). These terms may be used by the SLP to help children identify instances of hard and easy speech as well as describe speech targets that the child can aim toward. As the child demonstrates increased ability to quickly and accurately identify hard and easy speech, we then help the child learn strategies to facilitate (1) increased production of easy speech and (2) ability to change from hard to easy as needed. In essence, as will be seen, this sequence—identification preceding but being overlapped with modification—provides the foundation for all of our therapy procedures with children, teenagers, and adults.

Parents' role in hard/easy speech   One caution, however, is that some parents, once they hear and understand the terms *hard* and *easy* speech, rewrite or rephrase these terms into their own vocabulary and usage, employing these terms in statements like, "Stop that hard speech!" (We have a similar problem with some parents in the P/C group with the terms *rabbit* and *turtle* speech.) We never cease to be amazed at how some parents can continually and consistently selectively attend to only the negative aspects of their child's behavior. Ironically, these same parents will ask us whether they should or can say to their child in nice, positive tones, "That's it, that's good easy speech," while never once asking us whether they should say "Stop that hard speech this instant!"

While we certainly don't want to continually make a big deal out of the child's fluency and thus indirectly highlight the "terribleness" of the child's stuttering, we tell the parents that a little praise now and then, anything that builds their child's positive self-image, must be correct and should be good for them to do and for their child to hear.

As we've said before, parents want to do the right thing; it's just that their methods are not always the most appropriate. Likewise, parents are anxious to help their child, and typically view such help to be active, direct involvement with their child. They want to *do* something to help their child. Such parents find it difficult to accept the fact that sometimes the best thing they can *do* to help their child is *not to do* anything more than being a loving, attentive listener. Surely, they ask, there must be something I can *do* or say to help my child (there must be some *action* I can take)?

Unfortunately, no matter what we say, some parents can and do sometimes take things into their own hands. As mentioned above, these parents may simply substitute the word *hard* for the word *stuttering* and then proceed to reprimand, correct, nag, or badger the child regarding his continuing production of hard speech. As should be obvious, such usage by parents defeats the purpose of the term and its use with the child; this is a good example of the child's parents doing something they think will help their child but which is clearly not helping. That is, the parent's advice to the child becomes part of, rather than solution for, the problem. Parents must be assisted to understand that such active helping on their part may have to wait until both they and their child have progressed to a more advanced state of therapy.

Nature of communicative interaction between clinician and client   Van Riper (1973) and others have discussed the benefits of engaging the young stutterer in low-level types of verbal conversation. We are particularly receptive to Stocker's (1976) notion of level of demand in which she has developed five categories of questions that require different levels of linguistic and cognitive formulation (see Conture and Caruso, 1978, for review of this procedure). Surely, future work will refine these levels of demand and probably expand their number and quality; however, for the present, the idea of systematically controlling the child's utterance by the nature of the question one asks has intuitive appeal. This is very similar to the notion that stutterers' "demands" exceed their "capacities," an idea that appears to have received its first theoretical elaboration by Andrews and his colleagues (Andrews and Neilson, 1981; Andrews, Craig, Feyer, Hoddinott, Howie and Neilson, 1983; Neilson and Neilson, 1987) and more recently by Starkweather (1987), who has amplified and refined this concept and discussed its clinical application.

Of course, one would not want to restrict an entire therapy session to questions of only one type, for example, "Is the ball big or little? blue or red? hard or soft?" Instead, we would vary the nature of our questions and comments to the child so as to positively control, influence, and shape the child's fluency as well as reinstitute fluency after a period when the child has become disfluent and/or to elicit speech from the child once the child is talking. By experimenting with each individual child, the SLP may even be able to find types of questions that routinely elicit, for that child, fluency or disfluency and instruct parents in the use or avoidance of such questions, as the case may be.

The child's communicative interaction abilities   While we first and foremost want to modify the child's disfluency, positive changes in fluency are often impeded by difficulties children appear to have with verbal expression or communicative interaction abilities. *Verbal expression*, for lack of a better term, is used here to describe such things as the amount of time spent talking, the precise moment to begin talking, logically organizing thoughts into language, knowing when it is a good time to interrupt people who are talking, and knowing how to appropriately achieve listener attention. While some of these issues were previously discussed in our coverage of the P/C fluency group, these subtleties of verbal expression need to be discussed further since they are seemingly difficult for some young children who are beginning to stutter (see, for example, Bates, 1976, and Rees, 1980, for an overview of the pragmatic aspects of language).

Some of these children may:

1. monologue at the dinner table (to everybody's discomfort and utter boredom)
2. seem to "put the cart before the horse" in many of their verbal expressions
3. not wait their turn, but repeat sounds, syllables, words, and phrases in seeming attempts to gain listener attention, hold the floor during a conversation, or interrupt an already ongoing conversation (and yet seem to expect no one to interrupt them after they have begun to talk)
4. use long, relatively complex utterances in situations that really require shorter, less cognitively or linguistically involved replies

Now, before the reader begins to say, "Where are the data?" let me reiterate that I said *some* and not all children who stutter exhibit such verbal interactions; furthermore, these are clinical observations that require empirical, objective investigations in order to refine, refute, or support their veracity.

It should be pointed out that many other children who do not stutter also do these things, but, at this point, we are not sure what the frequency and consistency of these behaviors are in the nonstuttering population. Furthermore, in terms of parental reactions to their child's undesirable verbal expressions, we are certain that some parents have a shorter fuse than the average parent. Likewise, siblings who are also trying to gain the speaking floor and their parents' attention may not be too tolerant of a brother or sister who takes up more than his or her fair share of "talking time." These same brothers and sisters may not appreciate a sibling who takes what *they* think is too long a time to begin speaking or to get to the point of their speaking. (This can sometimes lead to criticism, mocking, or teasing by brothers and sisters, an issue that will be discussed in another section below.) Sometimes these siblings cause the young stutterer more problems because the siblings themselves use more than their fair share of talking time, take too long to get to their point, make inappropriate interruptions of the speaker who has the floor or speak for the young stutterer.

If at all possible, the SLP should try to address and change these verbal annoyances, at least those exhibited by the young stutterer. At the very least, the parent should see if these problems exist and if they do, how the various members of the family may be reacting. The problems some young stutterers have in this area leads, in my mind, to one of the many Catch-22s of stuttering. For example, the child who takes too long to get to the point of his or her topic or the child who tends to monologue, once he or she does get the speaking floor, becomes the child that other children, parents, and adults find less and less enjoyable to interact with verbally. However, if this child is continually told to be quiet or to "shut up," the child will get less and less opportunity to practice verbal expression, and his or her skills in this area have less chance for being exercised. The end result is that the child will remain even more undeveloped in these areas. All of this means that the child is still called on less frequently to speak.

Such vicious cycles, with which the problem of stuttering seemingly abounds, should be identified at an early age and mitigated, as much as possible, before they develop into consistent, undermining problems that contribute to the maintenance and perpetuation of stuttering.

Parents' reading to their children   In general, we believe that parents of young stutterers should be encouraged to talk and read more with their children. However, as Van Riper (1973) notes, there are some cautions, particularly with parents' reading to their child.

Let me first say that it is my experience that with patience, persistence, and support on the part of the SLP, that most parents can learn, and even come to enjoy, reading to their children. Reading to their child can become a family ritual or tradition that closes out the day in a relatively relaxed, mutually satisfying way. The parent has a chance to talk to the child, and the child has an opportunity to listen to and ask questions of the parent.

Problems in this area do exist, as Van Riper noted, and the SLP should be familiar with them if this sort of home suggestion is to have a positive or facilatory influence on the child and his fluency. First, too much of a good thing is bad. The child can be verbally interacted with to the point of fatigue, satiation, and unnecessary stimulation. The child, like all of us, needs quiet times, to think, day dream, or just plain rest. Likewise, reading to a child who is obviously more interested in playing with his toys or coloring in his coloring book is going to be a frustrating experience for everybody involved. Thus, not only the amount of time the child is read or talked to must be monitored, but the timing of when to talk and read to the child must be assessed. Some parents will need help with this assessment. Parents' reading and talking with their child should be an enjoyment rather than a regimen. The parents should be helped to select books and stories that the child can understand, relate to, and enjoy.

Reading for content versus reading for development of oral reading skills   It is also very important for parents to understand that besides companionship and parent-child sharing, reading has at least two other related but different functions: (1) It provides the child with cognitive, language, and vocabulary enrichment and stimulation, and (2) it provides the child with a model of speech production that she or he can use when starting to read aloud.

Many parents will opt for what I call fairy tales from the old country type of books. These are books that are long on intellectual content, moral messages, and imagination, but present a model of oral reading well beyond that which the typical child could be reasonably expected to follow. Instead, the parents should be encouraged to mix, blend, or interchange their reading material, sometimes reading for content, for example, the Babar the elephant series, and other times reading to provide for the child an obtainable oral reading model, for example, reading such books as *Go, Dog, Go* or *Left Foot, Right Foot.* Both types of books—those high on content and those providing an obtainable model of oral reading—have a place. Parents need to understand that one is not better than the other. Instead, the two sources of reading material just have different functions. Both functions, it should be pointed out to parents, are important in helping their child learn to love reading as well as love to learn how to read.

Third, it really does little good to read or talk if nobody is listening. One mother of a five-year-old stutterer we remediated could not understand why her son seemed bored with her reading a *National Geographic* article on the Apollo space mission. These parents need help in learning what kinds of stories, print, and pictures a child of their child's age might understand and enjoy. Dodson (1970) presents a comprehensive listing of books and stories appropriate for various ages of children. Fourth, as obvious as this may be, try not to give parents the impression that they must buy all these books themselves; encourage them to visit local libraries and to take their child with them. Be patient and supportive, and tell them that with time and experience their child will select books independently, but that in the beginning the parent will have to do much of the selecting.

Fifth, pick the parent, whether mother or father, that you think has the most patience for and interest in reading *aloud* to the child. The athletic, frenetic father or the extremely quiet mother who is impatient with mistakes may not be your best bet; try to figure out who would be the better (but not perfectionistic) out-loud reader and who would have the most patience and interest in reading aloud. Sixth, and this is quite important, help parents learn that when they read to their child that they should do so in as calm, physically relaxed, and unhurried a fashion as possible. Parents should be told to expect, and even encourage, the child to interrupt and ask questions or make comments. Indeed, if the parent simply cannot tolerate the child's interruptions for questions and comments about text and pictures, that parent is a poor risk for a reader and maybe other types of opportunities for parent-child verbal interactions should be sought. Most of the time, however, we have been able, by employing patience and persistence, to help parents like this learn to modify their behavior in this area so that they can become good, or at least, adequate oral readers. While we encourage parents to read to their children every day, we try to make it clear to them that it is certainly all right to skip a day or two when they or their child are just not in the mood.

We have found parental reading to their children to be an excellent vehicle for parent-child sharing, for providing the child with an obtainable adult model of physically relaxed, unhurried speech production, and for giving the child practice in listening to an adult speaking to him or her for a period of time (the very thing children experience in school classrooms every day). It is clear that such reading is also a stimulant for the child's vocabulary development, and that it also helps the child to learn that reading can be enjoyable and entertaining. If we can believe what we read about television's being a less than positive influence on our children (Winn, 1977), then the more reading we expose our children to and that they do themselves, the better.

Deciding when a more direct approach is warranted   The indirect approach is mostly suited for the child who is producing, albeit quite frequently, relatively physically relaxed ("easy") sound/syllable repetitions, appropriate eye contact with listeners, and appears essentially unaware of his or her speech problem. Of course there will be children who fall in the cracks, children for whom the above approach will not be specific or direct enough to achieve improvement in speech fluency, but for whom more direct approaches seem somewhat inappropriate. It is not always easy to identify these children prior to therapy and many times their needs only become apparent after 3 to 12 months of seemingly appropriate but relatively ineffective remediation.

We have developed through experience three relatively gross behavioral guidelines that we have found helpful in deciding whether a particular child needs a more direct approach: (1) The child makes sound prolongations that comprise 25 percent or more of all speech disfluencies; (2) the child makes eye contact with his or her listener less than 50 percent of the time; and (3) the child exhibits concomitant speech and language problems, for example, delayed and/or unusual phonological development.

However, children exhibiting this many sound prolongations with such reduced listener eye contact and concomitant communication difficulties will generally be "picked up" at the time of initial evaluation and more direct therapeutic regimens will be recommended. A far more challenging situation is the child who exhibits some sound prolongations, reduced but not seriously diminished eye contact, and some but not many signs of awareness of a problem. These latter children are in-between and it is difficult to be sure which way they are going to progress and whether indirect approaches are sufficient.

What is desperately needed are empirical investigations to assess which speech and related variables predict positive, negative, and minimal change in speech disfluencies. Why implement direct therapy regimens when with time and positive parental intervention some of the children initially evaluated, who are just beginning to stutter, will become more fluent? Conversely, why implement indirect therapy regimens and significantly involve parents when the child needs specific and direct modification of inappropriate speech and related behaviors? Unfortunately, at present, we are still missing the empirical evidence that would allow us to make such decisions based on a more solid foundation.

Children with Some to a Great Deal of Stuttering and Whose Parents Are Reasonably to Somewhat Concerned

These children are frequently and routinely producing within-word disfluencies (probably in excess of 6 within-word disfluencies per 100 words spoken), and adults (most likely, but not necessarily, the parents) explicitly notice and report these disruptions. Interestingly, parents appear most concerned about (1) the child's sound/syllable repetitions and (2) concomitant nonspeech behavior, particularly facial gestures. Facial grimaces and bodily movements many times seem to be the final straw that makes parents (and other professionals) call and set up an evaluation for their child. Furthermore, some parents seem to breathe a sigh of relief when their child begins to prolong more than repeat, particularly if the prolongations are silent and the child's mouth is closed or nearly so. Such parental acceptance is in opposition to our clinical intuition and experience that suggest that when a child begins to prolong more (that is, changes from reiterative or oscillatory speech gestures to more fixed or stabilized gestures) that the child's stuttering problem is worsening.

Of course, it is a waste of both the parents' and clinician's time to try to convince or persuade the parents to be less accepting of physically tense sound prolongations and more tolerant of physically easy sound/syllable repetitions; however, some of these parents may have to be told firmly but gently that as the child becomes more fluent he or she may resume repeating, at least for awhile, sounds and syllables, but that this is expected and not a cause of concern.

Unfortunately, some professionals, who do not have enough experience or interest in stuttering, will use up precious time in the early stages of the development of the child's stuttering problem and only refer to a more qualified professional when the child is showing signs of a worsening and, generally, more habituated speaking problem. Or, sometimes, when the child begins to frequently exhibit facial grimaces, some clinicians may stop trying to remediate the fundamental problem—the child's speech disfluencies—and instead focus on changing the child's facial grimaces and eye contact. This is most unfortunate since these problems will remain, albeit in different forms, until the child becomes more fluent. However, our observations of these sorts of problems are included to merely serve as a comment on their all too frequent occurrence and a hope for a better tomorrow for children who stutter and their families.

Try not to bug the children just as their parents do   A child who is frequently stuttering, to the point where direct, individualized therapeutic intervention is necessary, needs the most supportive and encouraging therapy environment as possible. We cannot emphasize this point enough. The SLP should not pester, cajole, nag, or otherwise harry the child in the same way as the parents and other individuals may be doing. All too often we tend to communicate with children who stutter in an "old wine in new bottles" vocabulary that does little more than change the name while the game remains the same: *Stop that stuttering!*

Many youngsters who stutter are not particularly eager to hear, see, or feel what they are doing when they stutter; some of them may be afraid to closely examine their stuttering or may be denying the fact that they speak differently from their friends. Whatever the case, however, many of them will appear to want to avoid all mention of and confrontation with it as if they are ostriches with their heads in the sand. These youngsters' reluctance to examine their stuttering on any level is, of course, a frustrating situation for both clinician and parent alike. Getting them to do these things will take patience, time, and encouragement.

These children, because they are human, would ideally like some procedure, technique, passive cure, or device that they could use, wear, or ingest that would take their stuttering away from them (or in the words of the old pharmaceutical advertisement, "Relief is just a swallow away"). In the beginning of therapy, the child and parents are particularly receptive to anything and everything that promises to lift the burden of stuttering off their backs. It is the role of the SLP to gently but firmly disabuse the parents and child alike of such get-fixed-quick notions.

Helping the child accept a more active role in the changing of his stuttering The SLP can help the child accept a more active or doing role in changing his stuttering by helping the child, right from the beginning of therapy, to understand that there are different ways we can begin and continue to speak and that there are ways to produce speech that make it sound and feel better than others. We like to use analogies with our clients—children, teenagers, and adults alike—by breaking the complex task of speaking down into terms and objects that make sense to them. We like to explain the child's problem on a level they can relate to so that they can begin to understand and *do* something about their own behavior. Not only do analogies help them understand their role in their problem, but it takes some of the fear and mystery out of the situation and treats their speech in a more matter-of-fact or objective manner.

Speech production is such a complex act, involving changes in muscular tensions and structural movements through time and space, that it takes years for even the speech scientist to gain some familiarity with its many activities and functions. Therefore, the SLP should not be surprised that the the lay client has difficult grasping what he or she is *doing* to interfere with normally fluent speech production.

Helping parents understand that many aspects of speech are out of sight and, therefore, out of mind The first analogy, which involves the activity of your heart, is really more for the benefit of the SLP and the parent. Its purpose is to make the SLP and parent understand that (1) most people take speech production for granted, (2) that the location of the speech musculature deep within the vocal tract obfuscates the nature of its structure and function and (3) speech production behavior is unknown because of (1) and (2).

This analogy (see Figure 3–3) is particularly useful in explaining to parents why their child seems unable to identify and/or modify clearly inappropriate behavior. It also helps, we believe, the SLP to better understand why the child is having such difficulty doing what clearly needs to be done. We start by asking ourselves or the parent: "What is your heart doing right now?" To which most people say, "I don't know." Hammering the point in a bit further we ask, "Where is your heart, exactly? What does it look like? Is it contracting or expanding right now?" and so forth and so on.

Most people have little or no clear idea regarding the color, shape, structure, or function of their hearts, nor should they. I mean, after all, why should they know about something that is always there when they need it? Why should they be concerned with something that takes care of itself? Why should they worry about fixing something that is not broken? Clearly, there is no need to know about the heart since it is taking care of itself just fine.

But what of their child's speech production system? It is not performing as it should, but everyone is treating it like the heart: out of sight and out of mind. The parent is helped to understand that some rudimentary understanding of speech production is necessary for the child to make a lasting

OUT OF SIGHT, OUT OF MIND

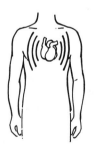
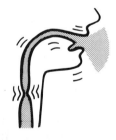

Heart beating/movements   **Speech structural movements**
deep within chest cavity   **deep within vocal tract**

Figure 3–3. Out of sight, out of mind analogy. The heart's shape, size, and function are "out of sight" and thus "out of mind" for most people. Likewise, the shape, size, and function of the person's vocal tract is out of sight, thus out of mind for most people. While most people need not concern themselves with cardiac structure and function, the stutterer with a problem that requires direct intervention must gain some rudimentary understanding of vocal tract structural movements in order to effectively change inappropriate to more appropriate speaking strategies.

change in his or her stuttering, but that since the child (and parent) have little understanding of the nature and function of the speech production mechanism that this understanding will not come easily. While speech behavior, just like cardiac function, may be taken for granted, that doesn't mean that children have to relinquish their ability to change their behavior. They may not be able to change the size or shape of their speech production mechanism, but they can influence its behavior even though they can see very little of its actual movement. This ability to change will not come overnight, but it will develop.

Helping parents understand what it feels like to stutter   To individuals who are normally fluent, the act of "being stuck," of being unable to move on to the next sound even though they know what they want to say, is relatively foreign. And probably there are no words or analogies that can adequately or completely describe the frustration, embarrassment, and fear associated with the act of stuttering. We believe, however, that some attempt must be made if the normally fluent parents of a young stutterer are to gain some degree of reasonable empathy for their child's problem.

The feelings of stuttering involve a number of levels of experience, and certainly when talking with parents it is not necessary to go into all these levels. Instead, we concentrate on the feelings of "unexpectedness," "suddenness," and "startle." The two analogies we use are (1) jumping into a swimming pool and (2) touching a hot burner. Both analogies, we think, help parents better appreciate what the act of stuttering sometimes feels like to their children.

JUMPING INTO A SWIMMING POOL

We tell the parents to imagine jumping feet first into a swimming pool that they thought was warm or at least room temperature (see Figure 3–4). As their stomach and chest hit the water, however, they discover that the water is like a liquid ice cube, that is, very cold. They are shocked at the unexpected cold water's temperature. The suddenness of the experience is even a bit scary especially as their head sinks below the water as their body descends into the water. The unexpected, startling nature of the experience may even "take their breath away" to which they may respond with a forced inspiration.

This unexpected, sudden, startling, and maybe even scary experience leads people to respond with a quick, forced inspiration and to try to make every effort to get out of the water. The unexpectedness, the startling quality of the experience, and the forced inspiration and attempts to "leave the scene of the crime" are somewhat akin to their child's feelings during the act of stuttering. The child's unexpected feelings, forced inspirations, and feelings

BODILY/PHYSICAL REACTION TO THE UNEXPECTED/UNPREDICTED
Example 1

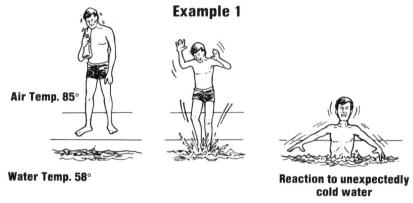

Air Temp. 85°

Water Temp. 58°

Reaction to unexpectedly
cold water

FIGURE 3–4. Bodily reaction to unexpected circumstances. Example 1: On a hot day in early summer a swimmer might forget that the water is still quite chilly and be surprised (if not shocked) when hitting the cold water. Sudden gasping, inhalations, and/or muscle tensing might all be exhibited by the surprised swimmer, much like the sudden gasping, inhalation, or muscle tensing exhibited by a stutterer when attempting to produce a sound, syllable, or word he suddenly and/or unexpectedly finds difficult to produce.

of wanting to escape when he or she can't move forward are no more "willful" than the parents' reaction to the ice cold pool water.

TOUCHING A HOT STOVE BURNER

We ask the parents to imagine a stove top with four electric burners (see Figure 3–5). We then ask the parents to imagine running their hand across the top of the stove looking for some utensil but all the while assuming that all burners are turned off. To their surprise and shock, one of the burners has been left on. Recoiling in fear of being burned, the parent may take a sudden, forced inspiration. Here, we explain to the parent, the recoil, the pulling back or backing away from something feared while taking a sudden, forced inspiration is similar to some of their child's instances of stuttering. While the intensity of the fear or depth of inspiration might not be as great or identical to that which their child experiences in each and every stuttering, there is some degree of similarity in the two situations.

We try, with these analogies, to help the parents understand the suddenness, the unexpectedness, the fear, and the out-of-control feelings of stuttering—the startle-like need to take a deep breath and/or escape the situation by whatever means necessary. In this way we try to help the parents better empathize with what their child may be experiencing and get them to realize that what may at times appear inappropriately purposeful on the child's part is often a normal reaction to an abnormal situation.

BODILY/PHYSICAL REACTION TO THE UNEXPECTED/UNPREDICTED

Example 2

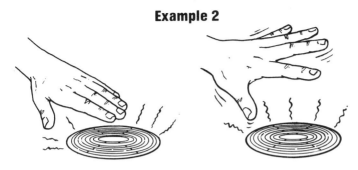

Hand exploring stovetop   Hand unexpectedly touching lit burner

FIGURE 3–5. Bodily/physical reaction to unexpected circumstances. Example 2: A person exploring a stovetop with his hand unexpectedly touches a lit burner. The person reacts by pulling the hand away and perhaps by gasping, sudden inhaling, and tensing muscles up in the hand, arm, and elsewhere in the body. Likewise, a person who stutters *may* react to the sudden, unexpected inability to say a sound, syllable, or word by physically pulling back the tongue, jaw, head, neck, or shoulders while simultaneously gasping or inhaling.

These analogies should never be used to scare or admonish parents for their apparent lack of understanding or concern, but as a way to increase their appreciation of the challenge their child faces and to provide a better basis for our communication with them.

THE GARDEN HOSE ANALOGY

One analogy we like to use with youngsters is what we call the garden hose analogy (see Figure 3–6). Most children have played with and used a garden hose with a nozzle at one end and a faucet at the other, and thus the analogy generally works. I explain the three parts of interest: the faucet on the side of the house, the flexible or bendable garden hose itself attached to the faucet, and the nozzle on the end of the hose. We begin by describing the garden hose and its parts and how the parts work separately as well as together as a unit to either (1) permit the water to flow out of the hose, (2) minimize the amount of water that flows, or (3) completely stop the water from flowing out of the hose.

As Figure 3-7 shows, we could turn the water off completely, or slow down its flow by turning the faucet at the house, or we could bend the hose, or we could turn or twist the nozzle. After the child seems to understand how a faucet, garden hose, and nozzle arrangement works (using a real nozzle attached to a short length of real, flexible hose makes this more alive, but

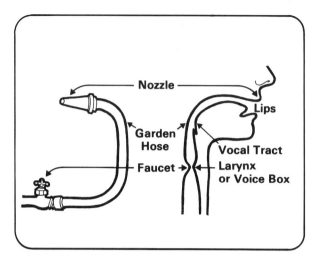

FIGURE 3–6. A lateral view of the supraglottal and glottal structures with their analogous parts of a garden hose-nozzle-faucet is presented. The lips are equated with the nozzle of the hose in that both can be constricted to stop or modify airflow (lips) or water stream (nozzle). The vocal tract is analogized with the flexible, bendable garden hose in that both can be manipulated in such a way (the garden hose can be kinked or bent, and the vocal tract can have the tongue partially or completely occlude airway) as to impede or modify the airflow or water stream. Finally, larynx or vocal folds (housed in voice box) are equated with the faucet in that both can be constricted or adjusted to stop or modify airflow or water stream. This analogy helps the young child identify the nature and function of each part of the vocal mechanism and the means by which his or her strategies to interfere with speech take place.

FIGURE 3–7. The four aspects of this figure (A, B, C, and D) depict the nature and function of the vocal tract during fluent and stuttered speech. The smooth, easy flow of air (A) for fluent speech strategies also shows how water flows through a garden hose in such a procedure. Naturally, during normal speech, the state of affairs depicted in A would be continually changing, but the idea of smooth, sequential movement from one speech posture to the next to produce a continuous flow of speech would still be apparent. In the first interfering situation (B), the client contacts long and with too much pressure on the lips and dams the airflow in much the same way as the nozzle on the hose when tightened would stop water flowing from the hose. In the next inappropriate strategy (C), the person is seen contacting the hard palate with too much tension for too long which dams airflow in an analogous way to a kink in a garden hose blocking water from flowing. Finally, the vocal folds can be constricted (D) in such a way to impede airflow, much like turning a faucet off will impede water from flowing from the vocal tract. What is not easy to analogize is the inappropriate laryngeal strategy of opening the vocal folds (see Conture, McCall, and Brewer, 1977; Conture, Schwartz, and Brewer, 1985). It is also possible for the three inappropriate strategies (B, C, D) to be combined in a variety of ways to interfere with speaking. In fact, such combinations of strategies are probably closer to the reality of the situation than the present examples, which were independently presented for the purposes of clear explication.

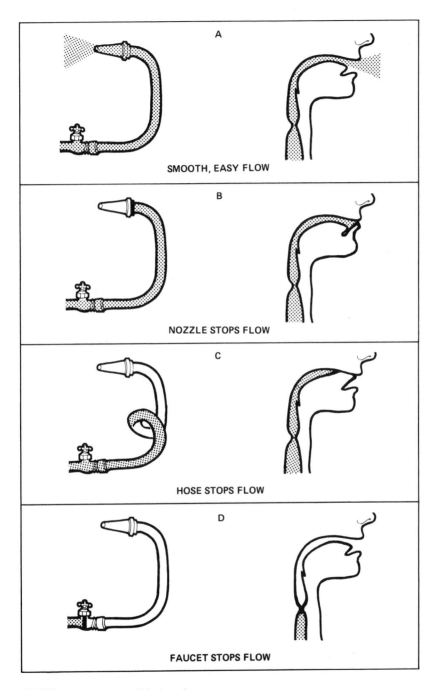

A

SMOOTH, EASY FLOW

B

NOZZLE STOPS FLOW

C

HOSE STOPS FLOW

D

FAUCET STOPS FLOW

FIGURE 3–7. (see page 132 for legend)

some youngsters may become overly attentive to the hose—this calls for clinical judgment), we begin to discuss the similarities between the garden hose and our speech production mechanism. Our larynx (voice box) becomes the faucet, our throat and tongue the garden hose, and our lips the nozzle. We then practice—first us and then the children—closing off the water (air) with our voice box (faucet), tongue (garden hose), or lips (nozzle).

As we mentioned above, for lay people, especially children, much of their speech production mechanism is out of sight and out of mind, particularly the voice box. Thus, it is hard for them to visualize, realize, or feel exactly what they are doing with the parts as well as whole of their vocal tract when they stutter. We have found, however, that children can come to some appreciation for the way they (mis)use their larynx by having them take a deep breath and then hold it with their mouths open. This gives them the idea of how they can use their "faucets" to stop air from flowing. Conversely, having them take a deep breath and then hold it with lips closed and cheeks puffed out gives them the idea of the way they can use their "nozzles" to stop air from flowing. Having them hold the /s/ and then gradually stop air flowing through the constriction by raising the tongue and finally totally occluding airflow by touching their hard palate gives them the idea of how the "hose" can slow down and then completely stop flow (they can, although it is harder for them at first, do the same thing with /z/ by gradually closing the vocal folds to minimize and then completely stop voicing/air flowing). We play with these hose parts until we think that the child has the idea or has had all the fun that he or she can stand.

AIR STOPPERS

We then introduce the idea of *air stoppers* in the children's actual speech by having them observe us slow, restrict, or stop the airflow through the vocal tract through the use of the nozzle, hose, or faucet (see Figure 3-7 on page 133). We encourage the children, at this point, to do the same as we are doing on selected words, sounds, or syllables. For example, the word-initial /b/ in the word *ball* could be used to demonstrate air stoppage at the level of the nozzle; the word-initial /k/ in the word *key*, for the level of the hose; and a word-initial vowel like /i/ in the word *eat*, or a sound like /h/ as in the word *hot*, for the level of the faucet.

As mentioned earlier, of the three levels—lips, mouth, or larynx—laryngeal constriction or its converse, abduction, is a most difficult concept to get across to children (or adults, for that matter). One way to reinforce or explain the idea of air stopping at the larynx is to have the children hold their breath, after taking a deep inhalation, with the mouth open. (Another way is with a blown up balloon, an analogy we detail below.) It must be emphasized that since the laryngeal area is not particularly rich in sensation, it is difficult to visualize its activity. Its activity is invisible to the naked eye, and children do not have a good picture or mental image of what the larynx looks or acts like. This vagueness makes this task all the more challenging.

Unfortunately, for some children whose stuttering is a real problem and concern, laryngeal involvement is a major aspect of the peripheral manifestations of their stuttering. Indeed, the careful observer will note that some of these children, in the interim between the listener's questions and the child's response, seem to take a quick, deep inhalation and hold it with the larynx (the mouth may or may not be open) as if to prepare themselves for the task of speaking. This seems to be a bit like when you take a deep breath and hold it in order to prepare yourself for the task of lifting or moving a heavy piece of furniture. To these children, the sensation in their throat will feel like being "stuck" and for many of these youngsters the resultant and/or associated oral and nonoral movements observed during the stuttering seem to be their attempts, albeit inappropriate, to "free" themselves or "release" or "work through" or "break through" the "block" they sense occurring in their throat. This initial response—to "break through the block"—must be mitigated if the child is to have a chance for significant improvement.

TIGHTNESS DUE TO AIR PRESSURE VERSUS MUSCLE TENSION

Laryngeal, vocal tract, or lip closure during speech probably leads to some degree of aerodynamic back pressure (Netsell, 1973) as well as normal feelings of muscle tension-tonus. Obviously, when these closures are held for too long or too tightly, associated aerodynamic back pressures and muscle tensions will be noticed and not felt to be appropriate. It is important for the SLP to be clear on the difference between aerodynamic back pressure and muscle tension since (1) most lay people who stutter confuse the two, and (2) changes in one—muscle tension and movement—many times must precede the other—aerodynamic back pressures—before positive changes in fluency are achieved.

We speculate that the "feelings of pressure or tension or tightness in the chest" that children and adults who stutter many times report result from these unusually high levels of air back pressures. Not only must these aerodynamic events be separated from muscle movements and tensions, but they must also be distinguished from those autonomic events associated with sympathetic nervous system discharge, for example, heart palpitation, feeling of lightness or heaviness in the stomach, flushed feelings, and sweating palms (see Guyton, 1971; Turner, 1969; Brutten and Shoemaker, 1967). The reason we try to help the child understand the nature of these feelings of pressure (besides helping to take away some of the mystery of the problem) is to enable the child to realize that these feelings result from something he or she is *doing*.

We revert back to the garden hose analogy and say that a quick closure of the nozzle makes the garden hose stiffen and even jump in our hands. The stiffening or movement result from water pressure or the fact that the water is suddenly dammed up and has nowhere to go so it pushes out the sides of the flexible garden hose. We explain to the child, if this seems appropriate, that the water in the hose behaves in much the same way as the air flowing up from the lungs that can suddenly be dammed up or closed by the child using the "faucet," "hose," or "nozzle." This "dammed" volume of air below the larynx, mouth, or lips exerts some degree of pressure within the respiratory and vocal tract and causes feelings of tightness or tension or constriction.

BLOWN-UP BALLOON ANALOGY: "IT'S STUCK DOWN HERE"

One excellent way to help the child understand tightness resulting from aerodynamic back pressure is by using a blown-up balloon with the thumb and index finger of one hand on the balloon's neck to stop the flow of air out of the balloon (Figure 3–8). Blow up the balloon and have the child feel the taut or tense sides of the balloon and explain this is a bit like the tension created by air pressure in the lungs and vocal tract. Have the child gently squeeze the side of the balloon and feel the changes in pressure on the sides of the balloon. Have the child him or herself hold the neck of the balloon and feel the pressure against the "laryngeal-fingers" as you squeeze the sides of the balloon. Have the child figure out the best way to let the pressure out of the balloon, for example, by (1) pushing hard on the sides of the balloon, (2) squeezing the thumb and index finger together, or (3) slowly releasing the air through slightly separated fingers and thumb. With some imagination, this analogy can help the child see the various reasons why he or she feels tight and constricted in various places in the vocal tract and how these feelings of physical tension can be changed by doing different things.

LILY PAD/BARREL BRIDGE ANALOGY: CHANGING AND MOVING FORWARD

If the child seems to get the general gist of what he or she does that interferes with speaking, seems to be able to describe and identify the interfering behavior, and appears willing to make at least some of the necessary changes, we move on to the next stage. Here too, we use analogies to help the child (and parents, if necessary) understand what the child must do to increase speech fluency. Two analogies we use at this point operate on the same theme: Speech involves a movement from one sound to the next.

The first analogy (Figure 3–9) involves pretending a frog or the child is jumping from one lily pad to the next to cross a stream. We pretend that each

"PERCEIVED INCREASE IN AIR PRESSURE"

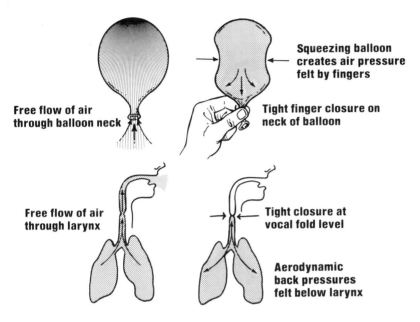

Squeezing balloon
creates air pressure
felt by fingers

Free flow of air
through balloon neck

Tight finger closure on
neck of balloon

Free flow of air
through larynx

Tight closure at
vocal fold level

Aerodynamic
back pressures
felt below larynx

FIGURE 3–8. Balloon analogy to the tight closure at laryngeal or vocal fold level. Since it is difficult for most clients to visualize and understand vocal fold structure and function, some "real-world" analogies are needed. Here a blown-up balloon is squeezed and the aerodynamic "back pressures" are felt by the fingers holding the balloon neck. Likewise tight vocal fold closure can create aerodynamic back pressure felt at and below the larynx, trachea, and chest. Some of the "tension" that stutterers frequently mention in their neck and chest is undoubtedly due to these aerodynamic back pressures resulting from laryngeal and, at times, supraglottal constriction.

pad is a letter of a short word like baby and that we must hop from the bank to the first pad, then to the next pad, and so on until we reach the other bank. We explain that we will get wet, go the bottom of the creek, and have to climb out and start all over again if we stand too long on any particular lily pad or if we jump on one of the lily pads real hard with both feet (that is, if we prolong the sound). Just as the frog would have trouble smoothly and easily getting across the stream, the child might have trouble easily saying the word. Likewise, if we hop up and down on the pad (that is, repeat the sound) rather than moving on to the next pad, we will also get wet, possibly go to the bottom of the creek, and have to climb out and start over again. In other words, we'll have trouble getting across the stream smoothly and easily, or saying the word. In either case, we explain to the child, we won't be able to

FORWARD VS. DISRUPTED SEQUENCING OF MOVEMENT: Example 1

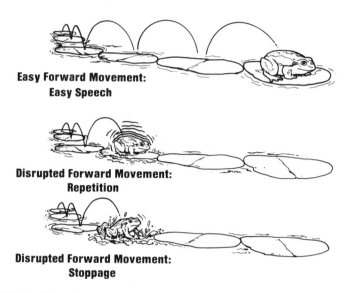

Easy Forward Movement:
Easy Speech

Disrupted Forward Movement:
Repetition

Disrupted Forward Movement:
Stoppage

FIGURE 3–9.   Forward versus disrupted sequencing of movement. Example 1: Frog jumping across lily pads analogy. For a frog to hop across a pond or stream on lily pads he would have to smoothly, easily, and *sequentially* hop from one pad to another. However, if he landed on one and repeatedly hopped up and down (repetition) or landed on one in a physically tense, fixed manner (stoppage) he would disrupt his forward movement across the pond. Likewise, speech requires physically easy, smooth, *sequential* behavior to make forward movement from beginning to the end of a sound, syllable, or word.

get across the stream easily, smoothly, and quickly if we land on one pad and stay there or jump up and down on it.

Essentially the same idea is conveyed by another analogy of a floating bridge, made of barrels tied to the each other with rope. Here, too, a barrel that is jumped on hard and stood on or repeatedly jumped up and down on will keep us from getting across the stream or from producing the word.

FOR OLDER CHILDREN: THUMB AND OPPOSING FINGERS ANALOGY

For older children, teenagers, and adults, who would naturally scorn or feel patronized by the perceived juvenile nature of the lily pad or barrel bridge analogies, we use one of our thumbs and its opposing four fingers in much the same way (Figure 3–10). Each finger is a letter or sound of a short word and our opposing thumb, the tongue, or speech system, is used to "produce" each letter or sound. Fluent speech, we tell the client (and his or

FORWARD VS. DISRUPTED SEQUENCE OF MOVEMENT: Example 2

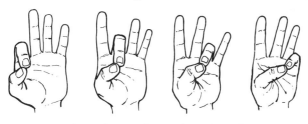

Smooth, easy forward movement

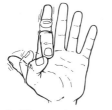

Disrupted forward movement: Repetition

Disrupted forward movement: Stoppage

FIGURE 3–10. Forward versus disrupted sequence of movement. Example 2: Sequential touching of fingers to thumb. To successfully touch each of the four fingers to the thumb, the person must smoothly, easily, and not too hurriedly move each finger to thumb in proper sequence. If thumb-to-one-finger contact is made repeatedly (repetition) or prolonged (stoppage), sequential, easy forward thumb to finger movement is disrupted. Likewise, with speech "forward" movement of vocal tract structures through the sound, syllable, or word requires physically easy, smooth, and sequential movement. Repetitions or cessations of vocal tract structural movement will disrupt forward movement through utterance.

her associates, if necessary), is something like having the thumb move smoothly, sequentially, and easily from one finger to the next. Conversely, we explain, stuttered speech is much like my pressing for too long with too much force between my thumb and any one of its opposing fingers (that is, a fixed articulatory posture or audible or inaudible sound prolongation) or repeatedly contacting the thumb and one particular finger (that is, a reiterative speech posture or sound/syllable repetition).

These analogies, of course, will not help anyone become fluent in and of themselves, but they serve as a common ground of understanding between client and clinician and provide essential insight for the young client into what he or she *does* that interferes with speech and what is necessary to change in order to speak more fluently.

Helping the child see, hear, and feel his stuttering   One of the fundamental problems with assisting young children do more and more things that normally fluent speakers do when they speak (Williams, 1971) is that the child cannot really see what it is that he or she is doing that is facilitatory or inhibitory to fluent speech. Furthermore, although the child can *hear* what he or she did that interfered or facilitated speech, audition is, by and large, an after-the-fact type of feedback. That is, although the child may have heard the stuttering, the speech behavior of interest has already taken place by the time the youngster has heard it.

Learning about speech and how to change it is different, therefore, than when the child is learning to hold a crayon or pencil for writing. When learning to write, the child can readily visualize—as they are happening—most of the correct hand postures, positions, and to some extent the necessary movements and coordinations of fingers, thumb, hand, wrist, and arm. Likewise, most sports that the child learns can be readily visualized and thus practiced and compared to the visual model (even though, of course, such visualization slows down actual production).

Many aspects of speech production, on the other hand, are for all intents and purposes invisible to the naked eye. Thus, you really cannot watch and, therefore, easily visualize (or draw a mental picture of) the necessary movements of the tongue, soft palate, pharyngeal musculature, and larynx for speech as you can, say the hand and arm movements used in tennis.

In a sense, our young clients are as baffled by the how and why of speech production and movement as we probably are by how and why our heart behaves the way it does. While we know the heart pumps blood and that it beats, few of us could really describe the physical movements, contractions, and configurations of our heart at work. (To get some idea of how naive most of us are regarding our heart, ask a few of your acquaintances to point to the location of their heart; many will point to the upper left side of their chest when in actuality the heart is located more centrally behind the sternum.) For most of us, speech and cardiac behavior are automatic events that we give little thought to: We simply speak and our heart simply beats. For children who stutter, however, some knowledge of how they speak and how they interfere with speaking is crucial in order for them to improve their speech fluency.

To counteract these difficulties, we have found that acoustic and videotape recordings are an excellent means toward helping the child see, visualize, and thus change his interfering (with fluency) speech behavior. Mirrors and clinician modeling or imitation are also useful in this regard. However, all such work must be done with caution and with a sensitivity toward the particular child's needs. We have observed that some children are excellent at discussing and demonstrating speech behavior and disfluency in the abstract, but become very emotional and resist or refuse to cooperate when their own actual speech behavior is touched, visualized, or heard. These children need the clinician's time and patience because they are not going to get over these feelings of fear, avoidance, and denial in a hurry.

We have also observed, in the P/C group, that children can, with clinician support and experience, readily identify their *own* speech behavior; however, we have also observed that inappropriate competitiveness and criticism between children starts to emerge if we require them to identify *each other's* speech behavior. Thus, experience has shown us, tasks that require a speaker's identification of his own behavior are very useful, but we have learned to be cautious when using tasks that require child speaker A to identify child speaker B's speaking behavior.

Sometimes actually showing children who stutter a model of the vocal tract or the larynx and allowing them to explore and ask questions about the model are helpful. They should be encouraged to ask questions about their own speech behavior and structures. Anything to mitigate the mystery and vagaries surrounding their speech behavior and the structures that produce it is desirable.

Of course, any approach with children must be used with an eye toward the child's level of understanding, experience, and ability to remember and assess complex concepts. And while there is a danger of being too intellectual with a young child who stutters, clinicians, particularly younger clinicians who have minimal experience with youngsters, must also guard against the opposite: oversimplification. An eight-year-old child in the third grade is not exactly receptive to approaches that would be used with a preschool stutterer. We should make every effort to interact with children at the level they present rather than the level we think they should present or that they sometimes present.

Helping the child understand "forward movement" in speech   Direct modification of the speaking behavior of youngsters who stutter (as with adults but using different methods) should focus on three factors: (1) the child's psychological and physiological evaluations and reaction *just before* he or she speaks (that is, what they do and how they get ready to initiate speech); (2) the child's speech production strategy used to *enter* or *go into* the production of the initial sound of the word, syllable, phrase, or sentence—the child's arresting gesture (McDonald, 1964); and (3) the child's speech production strategy used to *release from* or *move away* from this sound and on to the next sound. Like a stack of blocks, these three factors support and relate to one another. For example, the child's apparent difficulty with *releasing* from a particular sound and moving on to the next is probably an end-product of a behavioral chain that originated prior to the child's beginning to speak. (We hasten to add that the child should not be given the impression that the sound is like some sort of tar baby that once touched he or she can never let go of; instead, we want to emphasize that it is the child's behavior that needs modification and not the sound. If the child develops the idea that the problem is within the sound rather than within the speaker, the logical conclusion is for him or her to avoid the sound, an approach which would be as inhibitory to fluency as it is impractical to do.)

Therapy procedures like Van Riper's (1973) "pullout" or Williams's (1971) instruction to "move on" or our suggestion to "change" or "change and move forward" are among the many ways of assisting the child to make the necessary and appropriate releasing and transitional gestures on to the next sound. When helping the child learn to change or release speech production behavior for the sound(s) of interest and move forward, we want to make sure that we don't (1) simply have the child prolong the end of the stuttered sound or the sound after the stuttered sound, or (2) engage the child in long, didactic lectures about speech sound transitions and arresting/releasing gestures. As always with young clients, your demonstrations or examples of the model or target behavior are worth a thousand words. *Show* the child what you want him or her to do and try to minimize the *telling*.

CURSIVE WRITING AS AN ANALOGY
TO "FORWARD MOVEMENT" IN SPEECH

If the child has even a vague idea of what cursive writing looks like (as opposed to printed writing), the clinician can use the *transitional* gestures between cursive symbols as an analogy to transitions between speech movements. That is, the child can be shown that the connecting lines, curves, and so forth, between cursive letters are something like the transitional gestures known to occur during speech production. These connecting lines, the child is shown, need to be made in a smooth, easy, and continuously forward-moving fashion for the writer's cursive writing to appear "fluent." Carrying the analogy further, we ask the child to guess what would happen if the writer refused, was reluctant, afraid, or embarassed to, or could not make the necessary transitional lines between letters. We help the child understand that the writer would probably get stuck on or repeat the initial letter of the word. We use this analogy to help the child learn to appreciate and more readily produce a more appropriate rate and level of physical tension when (1) initiating speech and (2) when moving between speech sounds.

Sometimes having the child slowly and easily say his or her name in synchrony with the writing of it may help the child develop the idea of forward-flowing sound production and, in particular, the speech production gestures needed to move between sounds. Similarly, attempting to produce the word-initial sound too rapidly with too much physical force or tension will throw everything off. This too can be analogized through the use of writing. Indeed, the child can practice "hard" versus "easy" writing (with and without accompanying speech production) to get to the point where he or she must enter the word-initial sound with appropriate force and tension (neither too much nor too little, perhaps like Mama Bear's porridge!) and then concentrate on smooth, easy release and transition into the next speech sound. This approach can help the child learn what forward movement in a seriated motor task like speech is all about and also help the child understand what he or she is *doing* that interferes with smooth, forward movement. As mentioned above, we emphasize strategies, plans, programs, or rules rather than concentrate or focus on the child's so-called "problem" sounds, syllables, or words. We believe that the child needs help in understanding that he or she can use the same principle for many different sounds or sound combinations.

We want to help the child learn rules of speech production (both those that apply to initiation of speech as well as movement between sounds) that can apply to all sounds rather than learning one rule for /s/ and then another for /t/. In general, the rule can be stated as follows: *Use an appropriate rate and level of physical tension to begin or initiate speech production as well as move from the first sound into the following sound.*

Obviously, we don't explain this rule to the child using these words; furthermore, stating this rule is easier than actually following it. However, for the child to become more fluent, he or she will have to have help learning to change the time/tension domains of speech, particularly when initiating as well as moving between speech gestures, to initiate and continue speech at a rate and physical tension level that maximizes his or her chances for producing normally fluent speech.

All of this will require concentration and work (once again, we never said any of this would be easy); lasting behavioral change does take time and effort. It is also our job to encourage the child to expend the necessary time and effort without becoming overwhelmed and discouraged with the task.

TRYING NOT TO TURN OFF CHILD AND PARENTS TO SPEECH THERAPY

Sometimes in our sincere desire to help, our zeal for "improving" the child as fast as possible overcomes our abilities to consider long-term consequences. To paraphrase a song by Marlo Thomas, et al. (1972), there is some "kinda help" that is the "kinda help" these clients and their associates can do without. We really must try not to turn the child or his parents off speech therapy. Sometimes waiting until a child's and his/her parents' schedules are more conducive to therapy is preferable to forcing everybody to begin therapy when it requires the juggling skills of a circus clown just to get their feet in the clinic door.

Granted, a child can be *too* organized with tuba lessons on Monday, soccer on Tuesday, Boy Scouts on Wednesday, choir practice on Thursday, and so on; however, this frenetic schedule is the reality that the child and his parents live with and it is the wise clinician who doesn't insist that each and every one of these activities take a second or third priority to beginning speech therapy. Instead, the SLP should use gentle but firm terms to make it clear that the child needs therapy and that as soon as it can be done, some room in the child's busy schedule should be made to accommodate weekly therapy sessions. This "schedule adjustment" might take as long as three to six months to effect. Once this has been completed, however, on the initiative of the parent and child and not as a command performance because of clinician demands, this particular horse is going to be a lot more inclined to drink when brought to the water.

Maintaining a child's interest in therapy does not mean, however, that all therapy sessions have to be a rollicking good time or that children and their parents will not have to work hard during as well as outside therapy. Instead, we are simply trying to maintain, as much as possible, the child's enthusiasm for change in speech behavior and a belief that such change is possible. Speech-language pathologists can do harm by providing the child with such an aversive, nonrewarding experience at an early age that it may take many years before the child can forget this experience and be willing to resume therapy.

GIVING THE CHILD A BREAK BY CREATING A BREAK FROM THERAPY

Speech-language pathologists should be willing to give children a break from therapy when they or the child appear to become stale or bored with the process. However, the clinician should also, at the time of the break, tell the child, parents, classroom teachers, and other important adults in the children's environment about the break and explain why the clinician is instituting the break.

Moreover, it is helpful to let the child and related adults know the exact time and date when therapy will be resumed. Three to six weeks is a good break period, but individual clients' needs dictate the exact length and nature of such a break. Homework, if any, given during the break should be minimal; let the children alone, give them some time to reflect on whether or not they are interested enough and willing to make the necessary changes in their speech. It helps to tell the parents that they may call you any time they want during the break. It also helps to emphasize that they should not revert back to older, less appropriate ways of correcting the child's speech during the period of the break.

When the child and parent return after the break, try to greet them in as positive a tone as possible. Let them know that you are glad to see them once again and that you can now get down to the business of helping them speak more fluently.

MOTIVATING THE CHILD TO "THINK I CAN"

The power of suggestion, as Van Riper aptly points out (1973) and the field of medicine has long understood (Benson and McCallie, 1979), is tremendous, and the speech and language clinician should use it to help children (and their parents) believe in themselves, their ability to change, and their ability to work to the goal of improved fluency. Like the little train engine, the young child can be helped to believe, "I think I can"; conversely, the clinician certainly does not want to add to the young stutterer's all too common "I think I can't" philosophy. Undoubtedly, the speech-language pathologist, as Starbuck (1974) and Prins (1974) discuss, is a motivator as well as changer of behavior.

The clinician must routinely assess the child's degree of motivation and try to adjust clinician strategy to accommodate the natural rises and falls of client motivation. The SLP must not assume that the child's recognition of a problem is sufficient motivation to change because if mere recognition of a problem is all that is needed to improve, then people who know they are heavy would easily lose weight and people who know they smoke would easily quit. No, recognition of a problem may be necessary for motivation to change, but it is clearly not sufficient.

REFERRALS TO OTHER PROFESSIONALS

It has been said that the trouble with education is that everybody has a little of it. Unfortunately, SLPs suffer from a similar problem: Everybody uses speech and language, and therefore everybody understands it. Right? Wrong! Many readers of these pages devote their professional lives to understanding normal and disordered processes of speech, hearing, and language, and yet still may think that they have an inadequate understanding of these processes. This does not imply that our profession corners the market on information or knowledge regarding speech and language behavior, but it does imply that our professional education, training, and experience qualify us to assess and manage the myriad of communication problems that people present.

While it is important to know what we know, it is just as important to know what we don't know. (We hasten to add, that this is not only a problem for SLPs but for other professionals as well.) We need to realize that certain clients have problems and concerns that go beyond our scope of training and jurisdiction or have concomitant problems besides stuttering—problems and concerns that warrant attention from other professionals. With children, such professionals are most apt to be classroom teachers, special education teachers, reading specialists, family physicians, the child's pediatrician, child psychologists (and psychiatrists), social workers, audiologists, and otolaryngologists.

Academic and related matters are often detected *prior* to your entrance into the child's life; however, it is not uncommon for certain behaviors such as reading problems, difficulties with neuromotor development, psychosocial adjustment, and so forth, to be detected for the first time by the SLP during an initial speech and language evaluation. The parents should be told, in nonalarming tones, when such problems are apparent and that you will (with their permission) pass this information on to the appropriate school authorities.

Certain other problems, for example, a child who fails a hearing screening, or who appears to have abnormal reflexes, or who is extremely hyperactive, impulsive, and distractible, may require the SLP to consult with nonschool professionals. Once again, the SLP should try to explain to the parent, in clear nonalarming tones, his or her observations and recommendation that the child receive a *routine* or *standard* screening test or evaluation by the family physician or pediatrician to assess whether your observations warrant concern. Referrals, of course, are a two-way street. We are not physicians, nor are we psychologists or classroom teachers. Neither, we hasten to add, are these professionals speech and language pathologists.

Thus, while we refer to other professionals when needed, we also need to be prepared to receive referrals from other professionals. While a psychologist might observe and describe what to him or her is a speech problem, it is our purview as well as professional responsibility, after having the case referred to us by the psychologist, to administer a diagnostic evaluation and make, if needed, therapy recommendations regarding the child's speech and language function. When receiving such referrals, it is hoped the decisions we make and report regarding the child will be based on (as well as give the appearance of resulting from) a careful mixture of clinical intuition and objective data and avoid the appearance of being arbitrary and capricious.

Generally speaking, when making a referral, it is most appropriate to tell the parents of your observations and allow them to decide if they want further consultation with appropriate personnel. Certainly, you want to strongly encourage such referrals, particularly in those cases where you believe a referral is essential, but in the final analysis the decision to pursue the matter further rests in the hands of the parent. In a few cases, with parents of limited understanding, you may have to be more insistent and actually make some phone calls yourself, especially if the nature and degree of the problem (for example, a child who is physically acting out against other children or one who has threatened to harm himself or take his own life) require thorough and immediate attention from a professional other than a speech and language pathologist. It is our routine policy to tell the parents (after they have signed the appropriate parental consent and release form) that we will send to *their* family physician or pediatrician, or any other professional of *their* chosing, a copy of our report, findings, and recommendations, unless, of course, they would rather we did not. Although the SLP runs the risk of another professional's misinterpreting, misunderstanding, or ignoring his written report, it our belief and experience that more factual information is better than less and so we continue to forward reports routinely to the family's other attending professionals.

In the relatively few situations where the child has a psychosocial rather than stuttering problem, a referral to appropriate psychological or psychiatric agencies is in order. Many times, however, the parents and/or the child may resist such referral and insist that there is nothing wrong besides speech. If, on the other hand, you firmly believe, based on your clinical insights and objective data, that speech disfluency is not a significant problem or that it is secondary or even tertiary to some more chronic or serious psychosocial adjustment concern (our experience indicates that this is the case for approximately 5 percent to 10 percent of the child, teenage, and adult stutterers we encounter), then the parents should be told.

And if push comes to shove, and the parents disregard your recommendation, then you may have to decline speech therapy for the child (of course, providing the parents with the names of other SLPs who might be willing and able to handle the child) because you believe it inappropriate to administer speech therapy for a child whose real concerns lie elsewhere. Obviously, it is in your and your clients' best interest for you to develop and cultivate professional interactions with psychologists who work with children and their families. Such professionals can enter into such tough counseling situations and assist the parents in seeing that psychological services are warranted and most appropriate.

SOME PARTING THOUGHTS

We have viewed the remediation of stuttering in children in the context of dealing with the child's skills and abilities as well as the child's environment. Neither aspect—the child's abilities or environment—appears to be sufficient to cause stuttering, but both appear to be necessary for the problem to develop. Hence, the two aspects appear to interact in a complex way to make the whole greater than the sum of the parts. For the clinician, of course, working with both the child and the child's environment provides a sizable challenge, but it is a challenge that can be met with rewards that far outweigh any initial trepidations.

SUMMARY

Stuttering in childhood is highly variable with more than a few children resolving without formal therapy; however, we are still a long way from being able to accurately predict which children will become chronic, persistent stutterers. Severity of the problem is best determined by assessing the level of development of the particular child's stuttering, and this level of development may have little to do with the child's chronological age. Thus, a 3-year-old child could have a more severe and advanced stuttering problem than a 6-year-old child. The child's chronological age, however, may significantly influence the exact procedures used to remediate the child's problem, regardless of its level of development or severity.

Remediating stuttering in children may involve: (1) environmental modification (information sharing and counseling with parents regarding what they may or may not be doing to facilitate or inhibit their child's speech fluency as well as related aspects of development, for example, standards for "correctness" or perfection of behavior); (2) speech-language modification (indirectly and/or directly identifying and modifying those strategies and aspects of speech production that the child is using which cause the child to disrupt speech fluency, to either inappropriately cease, maintain, or reiterate a speaking gesture); or (3) both (1) and (2) together. The author is advocating, after appropriate diagnostic assessment, that most young children who stutter participate in a parent-child stuttering group; for those children who don't improve with group therapy, indirect or direct individual speech therapy is then advocated with the degree of "directness" being dictated by the nature of the child's problem, the child's level of development, and emotional/intellectual awareness of the problem.

Children and parents who seem most likely to profit from environmental modification may require some period of time before they show significant progress. Clinicians need to remember that they have the child for only a fraction of the child's waking hours while the parent spends most the remaining hours with the child. If environmental issues are apparently contributory to the child's stuttering, it seems reasonable that they be addressed for long-term improvement in speech fluency. However, this is not to say that the environment "causes" stuttering as much as it is to say that it may "perpetuate," "maintain," "aggravate," or exacerbate the problem. The skills and abilities of the child also are salient and those who would seem to most likely benefit from speech-language modification are children who are prolonging sounds (particularly if these prolongations are silent or inaudible in nature), and *frequently* blinking their eyelids and moving their eyeballs to the right or left during conversation, that is, avoiding eye contact with the listener. Directly identifying these youngsters' stuttering and modeling for them what they do and ways that they can change what they are doing appear appropriate. The third group, which comprises the bulk of young children who stutter, needs some environmental modification *and* speech-language modification. It would seem that these youngsters' skills, abilities, and environmental factors complexly interact to negatively influence the development of these childrens' speech fluency. The use of parent-child groups and/or indirect individual speech therapy is advocated for this third group as well as direct therapy for those whom the parent-child group and indirect approach only partially help.

FOUR
REMEDIATION: OLDER CHILDREN AND TEENAGERS WHO STUTTER

OLDER CHILDREN: BETWIXT THE CALM OF CHILDHOOD AND THE STEADY TRADEWINDS OF ADULTHOOD

As we move from the young child to the older child (although don't let any teenager hear you call him or her a child!), we are presented with a different sort of a challenge. Here the environment provided by the parents becomes less and less significant while the environment provided by peers assumes increased importance. The teenager finds him- or herself betwixt and between the role of the child that he or she seems so willing to discard and the brass ring of the adult role model they so eagerly seem to be reaching for.

Like a snake half in and half out of its shedded skin, the teenager clamors for the independent privileges of the adult, but is quite content to revert to the dependent ways of a child if the less than pleasant responsibilities of adulthood are thrust upon him or her. Onto this sea of adolescence physical, mental, social, psychological, and emotional disequilibrium we must sail if we are to deal effectively with stuttering in the teenager. Indeed, much more is going on than stuttering in teenagers who stutter.

While calm winds may be relaxing, they don't fill our sails and we can't make headway when becalmed. Likewise, hurricane-force winds filling our sails may rip our sails asunder and leave us at the mercy of the elements. It is the moderate to strong winds that test our sailing mettle, teach us how to sail, and make progress toward our destination. Between the relative calm of childhood and the hopefully steady tradewinds of adulthood blows the unpredictably strong winds of adolescence which rise and fall to test the mettle of teenager and parent alike but, hopefully, in the end, help develop independent sailors who no longer need parents or a skipper, navigators, and crew. Parents may not like the fact that their crew has taken to skippering another boat, but perhaps they can take some comfort in the fact that even though the young skipper may be sailing to other unknown ports, he or she now has the means to return home when needed, without the help of mom and dad.

OLDER CHILDREN ARE NOT JUST OLDER, THEY ARE DIFFERENT AS WELL

Older children (those about nine years and older) and teenagers who stutter differ in other ways besides age from those who are younger. Older children and teenagers have many times had some form of prior therapy experience. While some older children have had little formal therapy and thus, at least in theory, are eager for help, many others have several months to years of relatively unsuccessful formal speech therapy and are not as motivated and interested to receive more.

Besides stuttering, these older children present the typical preteen and adolescent concerns unique to their age group. Put another way, these youngsters are not only older but are somewhat different from the preschool or early elementary school child. For example, a fourteen-year-old girl who stutters, even one who noticeably and severely stutters, may balk at receiving help for her problem. She may complain that she does not want to seem different from her friends, leave school at unusual hours, or attend special classes not attended by her normally fluent peers. She may even tell you (as these youngsters have sometimes told me) that coming to your speech therapy sessions makes her feel like a "retard."

A third unique concern of these older children is the developing importance and influence of their peers relative to the diminishing importance and influence of their parents. While the influence of parents cannot be denied (indeed, some clinicians, for example, Mastrud, 1988, actively and extensively involve parents in the remediation of teenagers), neither can the tremendous influence of peers on the likes, dislikes, motivations, and so forth, of the older child. To manage the older child without understanding the influence of peers on the child's behavior, is to manage the child from a relatively incomplete perspective. Indeed, understanding the unique concerns of the older child and teenager who stutters is crucial for successful remediation.

Individuals with clinical experience attempting to remediate stuttering in teenagers (for example, Finkenstadt, 1988) report that few of these individuals appear free of some negative attitude about their speech and/or their abilities as speakers. These clinicians report that teenage stutterers' feelings of "being different" appear to be in opposition to their strong desire to look, act, and be like other teenagers, to conform, to fit in with their peers. What makes this situation even more challenging, clinicians report, is that often some of these teenagers' own attitudes about themselves as speakers appear far more negative than any feedback they seem to have received from their peers. (Teens, of course, are not the only people who may continually seek the cloud rather the silver lining in themselves. Some adults, nonstutterers and stutterers alike, may have a low self-esteem and opinion of themselves, regardless of environmental reactions to the contrary.)

While it is appropriate, in a society as complex as ours, to care about what others think of us, it is not conducive to our mental stability and self-esteem to be chronically and deeply concerned how others assess our every waking act. However, such continual concerns are exactly what some teenagers who stutter experience and this can lead to a "paralysis by analysis" whereby people, places, and things are avoided. Indeed for some teenagers, it is better not to act at all than to risk ridicule by their peers for their actions. As Finkenstadt (1988) reports, one of her initial goals is to help the teenage stutterer develop a "sense of freedom" from persistent and unnecessary concern about what others "think of you."

UNDERSTANDING THE PARENTS OF THE OLDER CHILD AND TEENAGER WHO STUTTERS

Parents of these children also have special concerns. First, some of these parents may have been trying for several years to get appropriate assistance for their child but have met with little success. Naturally, therefore, they may already be somewhat frustrated when an SLP, who has the training and experience necessary to significantly help them, meets them for the first time.

Second, some of these parents may have observed their child receive numerous hours of therapy and related services without much appreciable progress. These parents, therefore, may be quite skeptical or uncertain that yet another SLP can actually help their child.

Third, another group of parents—the ones we discussed in the previous chapter who were unconcerned about their child's problem—may have consciously decided to keep their child out of therapy. Perhaps they were previously denying the problem or hoping against hope that the child would "outgrow" it. They now seek services, but probably do so with a great deal of guilt or concern for the fact that their child should have previously received therapy. These same parents may now feel that their child's continued stuttering is their fault.

Fourth, many of these parents are also having the typical concerns that other parents of children of similar age experience with their rapidly maturing youngsters: concerns with schoolwork and academic achievement, responsibility for carrying-out household chores, willingness to listen and respond to parental requests and rules, dating and relations with the opposite sex, abilities to get along with peers inside and outside of school, driving their own or the family's car, (mis)use of drugs and alcohol, and future employment possibilities. Yes, no one ever said being a parent was easy but their job is not made any more so by professionals who fail to recognize the tremendous number and variety of issues these parents must deal with, on a daily basis, to raise and interact with their older children/teenagers properly.

We have mentioned before that the child who stutters and the parents of that child are children and parents first, respectively, and only secondarily involved with stuttering. Our belief that stuttering relates to a complex interaction between the stutterer and his or her environment suggests that stuttering neither develops nor operates in a hermetically sealed container but is interwoven with the fiber of human existence. We would encourage SLPs to gain understanding of the general human background against which the stuttering foreground exists.

Based on our understanding of this background, we have come to the belief that when managing the older child who stutters, we become less and less able to separate our own feelings of how things should be done because the child gets closer to our own age. I feel that this dilemma, which also is apparent when we try to remediate stutterings in adults, arises because we begin to observe with these children and their parents, more clearly than with younger children and their parents, problems that we ourselves have not successfully coped with in our own personal lives. These clients act as mirrors that reflect some of our own inadequacies. This is not something that makes us feel comfortable, but it is something we should clearly understand.

HOW OLDER CHILDREN DIFFER IN GENERAL FROM YOUNGER CHILDREN

It goes without saying that older children relate to adults in different ways than they did when they were younger. Whereas five-year-olds generally do what the clinician tells them to do because the SLP is an adult, the clinician finds that with the older child explicit rationale may have to be given for each and every request of the child.

Paradoxically, and this is important to remember, older children may want explanations for adult requests of them but be very much put off if the explanation is too detailed or stated in language they cannot understand! The SLP, to be successful with these children, must recognize the older child's growing independence (or need for it) as well as appropriate assertiveness which is not to be confused with inappropriate aggressiveness. (For an excellent discussion of the distinctions between aggression, assertion, and nonassertion, see Lange and Jakubowski, 1976, pp. 7–53.) In essence, the SLP must be prepared to interact with these children as they present themselves rather than as we might ideally like to see them behave.

Likewise, it is important to discuss with the older child's parents, school personnel, and others familiar with the child whether the child's social, emotional, psychological, physical, and academic development is on course. A child who is afraid to speak and is reluctant to use verbal expression during social and academic situations, is a child who may nonverbally act out to seek peer and adult attention, recognition, or approval.

The SLP must be sensitive to these signs and try to get parents and appropriate personnel to intervene to ensure that the child's acting out and other inappropriate behavior, inside and outside the classroom, does not become the child's standard operating procedure as he or she develops into his or her teen years. We have observed situations where stuttering becomes the least of a child's problems when that child keeps the classroom in a state of mild uproar and the police routinely visit the house because they suspect the child of the latest neighborhood vandalism. The SLP and other professionals should be sensitive to the child who, because he or she can't master the academic information and social rules of the typical classroom, tries to "master" his or her classmates by acts of physical and verbal aggression and interference. In our opinion, these children are crying out for help and should receive it as early as possible in the form of family or individual counseling, individualized academic instruction, and the like.

With the older child who stutters, but who exhibits minimal awareness, we like to continue the emphasis on parent-child activities. Any event that brings the family together is one that can potentially foster opportunities for positive emotional, intellectual, and communication sharing. Allowing the older child to spend week in and week out with minimal adult-child communication besides, "Clean up your room," "Don't talk that way to your mother," or "Be quiet, can't you see I'm talking," is counterproductive to successful remediation of the child's fluency problem. For example, a father who enjoys working with tools around the house could be encouraged to explain their use to his son or daughter; a mother who enjoys reading could explain her books to the child, in terms the child would understand.

Verbal sharing (which is to be differentiated from verbal lecturing) or quiet interactions between child and parent, regardless of what is discussed or the specific nature of the shared activity, should be encouraged by the SLP. Every opportunity can and should be used to encourage the child to keep talking, to praise him or her for his attempts to converse; that is, the child should not be allowed to become reluctant and afraid to verbally converse with his parents, other adults, and peers. Simply put, a child cannot practice speaking or attempt to modify inappropriate speaking behavior, if he or she does not talk except during therapy sessions.

HOW STUTTERING PROBLEMS OF OLDER CHILDREN
WHO STUTTER DIFFER FROM THOSE OF YOUNG STUTTERERS

It is somewhat obvious that stuttering in a 9-year-old child, who has been stuttering since he or she was 4, will be different from that of a 4-year-old child who has been stuttering since he was 3.5 years of age. However, it is not clear what these differences might be. In Chapter 1 we discussed some differences that might be observed as the problem develops. Similarly, Bloodstein (1987, pp. 40–44) discusses the "four phases in the development of stuttering" that are based on his assessment of the clinical case histories of 418 stutterers ranging in age from 2 to 16 years. Although Bloodstein provides broad ranges of age limits for each of these stages, he appears to believe, as do we, that chronological age is loosely related to routinely observed behavioral characteristics of stuttering.

What is needed is empirical research that investigates whether the older child and teenager who stutters is different, on dimensions other than frequency, duration, and severity of stuttering, from those children who, at an earlier age, with or without therapy, become normally fluent. If we had this information, we might be better able to predict, at earlier ages, which children are likely to recover and plan frequency and type of therapy accordingly. As mentioned in Chapter 2, Riley's (1981) Stuttering Prediction Instrument (SPI) represents an attempt to make such prediction; however, independent investigators need to assess empirically the SPI's ability to do what it is designed to do: predict chronicity of stuttering in young children who stutter.

Furthermore, we need to know whether the older child and teenager who stutter present a different or more complex problem than does the young stutterer who becomes fluent. Do older children who stutter exhibit more concomitant problems in speech and language, for example, delays in phonological development, than do younger children who stutter? Did these older children take longer to develop reading skills or fine motor control over speech musculature? Are there subtle differences in the home life of these older children that contributed to and perpetuated stuttering? Why are stutterers, between the ages of 12 to 14 years, sometimes so challenging in terms of achieving successful remediation? These questions and others must await empirical investigation for answers. For the present we must rely on insights and knowledge gained from clinical practice managing older children and teenagers who stutter which, we hope, has some general applicability to these clients in other clinical settings and locales.

The Age of the Client Is a Guide, Not an Imperative

Earlier we stated that the age of the client may be useful with the logistics and planning of therapy strategies, but that it is our experience that chronological age tells us little about the nature of the child's stuttering problem. What we are trying to point out is how important it is to consider each child in terms of his or her presenting situation rather than be locked in or rotely follow some a priori set rule that such and such an age child should be dealt with so and so.

Unfortunately, the problem with taking this approach—that age is less important for therapy planning than determining the nature of the problem—is that it does not readily lend itself to the confines of an organized book! Thus, for the sake of discussion, we have partitioned our clients who stutter into three age groups and assigned them each their own chapter: Chapter 3, children who stutter; Chapter 4, older children and teenagers who stutter; and Chapter 5, adults who stutter. This partitioning into separate chapters is not completely arbitrary since each age group does appear to have unique aspects and concerns; however, this does not mean that each and every client in a particular age group will present with similar problems or be treated in exactly the same way.

There are some common themes among older children and teenagers who stutter, but each of these clients presents his or her own unique variation on these themes. Our job, as SLPs, is to learn to recognize common themes but to be simultaneously cognizant of and prepared to deal with their numerous variations. Once again, it is silly to expect, for example, everybody to have an IQ of 100 just because that is what the mean for the population might be.

Variations among Older Children and Teenagers Who Stutter

Keeping in mind the above, we assume that older children and teenagers who stutter will vary a great deal among themselves. To make some sense of these variations we have divided these children into three different groups: (1) older children with little or no awareness of stuttering, (2) older children with definite awareness of stuttering, and (3) teenagers with definite awareness of stuttering. We have observed some teenage stutterers with minimal emotional and/or intellectual awareness of their stuttering, but we believe that these are probably the exception rather than the rule. Furthermore, we have observed a handful of individuals who began their stuttering in their teenage years (and even into adulthood), but this group is also probably the exception and not the rule. For the most part, we will be discussing older children and teenagers who have been stuttering for some time (two or more years at the least) whose problems are generally reported to have originated during preschool or early elementary school years. While some of these youngsters will have received previous therapy, some will have had little or no contact with SLPs, some of them seemingly only realizing they have a problem when they are in the latter stages of elementary school. To begin, therefore, let us consider older children with apparently little or no awareness of stuttering.

OLDER CHILDREN WITH MINIMAL OR LITTLE AWARENESS OF STUTTERING

To our knowledge, the Speech Foundation of America publication No. 21, edited by Fraser and Perkins (1987), is one of the few publications presently available that is specifically addressed to stuttering in teenagers. Another relevant publication (Ginott, 1969) deals with the unique relations between parents and their teenage children. Both of these publications deserve, in our opinion, consideration by any SLP interested in managing stuttering in older children and teenagers. Just as children are not little adults, teenagers are not big children but individuals with unique needs and concerns that should be understood, at least to some degree, by individuals who must professionally interact with them.

Awareness of Stuttering: What It Is, What It Means, and How to Deal with It Therapeutically

One of the first issues that SLPs encounter with the older child or teenager that is generally different from those observed in younger children is the level and type of "awareness" of stuttering. Awareness is a topic frequently discussed in clinical circles, but one whose outline and content are minimally understood, at best. In our opinion, awareness of an event takes at least two different forms: (1) general or (2) specific. The former is predominantly, for the sake of this discussion, an emotional-feeling level of awareness while the latter is a cognitive-intellectual (perhaps rational) level of awareness. Dichotomizing awareness in this manner is somewhat artificial because most of our awareness of ourselves, our actions, and interactions with the world around us involve both emotional and intellectual processes (Williams, 1978, makes a number of relevant remarks about stutterers' perceptions, evaluations, and thinking regarding their feelings and behavior). That is, our intellectual (relatively objective) and emotional (relatively subjective) selves are inextricably related to one another; however, for the purposes of this discussion, differences between the two can be discussed since although the two are related they do differ.

We have found, in the clinic, that it is useful to treat and discuss our clients' awareness of their behavior in terms of objective and subjective components. Many older children and teenagers will tell you, sometimes in a very emotional manner, that they stutter because they are stutterers (an interesting tautology), but when asked to show or describe what they do that they call stuttering, they will say, "I stutter." It is as if teenagers who stutter (and adults, for that matter) treat the word "stutter" or "stuttering" like a "you-understood" and that their use of the word is sufficient for you to understand what they *do* when they produce, as Young (1984) termed it, a "fluency departure." Along these same lines, Wingate (1976) has remarked that, "it is surprising how poorly most stutterers are acquainted with their own difficulty." We hasten to add, and with some certainty based on our clinical experience, that this acquaintance is not as poor on the emotional (or more subjective) level as it is on the intellectual level.

When we say that some stutterers are "unaware" or "lack awareness" of their stuttering, we seem to be actually saying that they are not concerned about or bothered by their speech. Such "unawareness" is, we believe, not really possible, at least on two levels—intellectual as well as emotional. In our opinion, even a young child, of reasonable emotional intactness and with any degree of intellectual ability, must be aware, on some level, of the fact that he or she talks differently from his or her parents, siblings, relatives, school-mates, or friends. And if in the beginning, at least, the child is not aware of his or her speaking difficulties, we can be reasonably sure that some other, less sensitive youngster will unsubtly remind the child of his or her differences and difficulties when talking. (For a fascinating, although horrifying, account of how individuals deal with and seem compelled to ridicule, shun, condemn and harm that which is different from themselves, read Kosinski's 1966 novel *The Painted Bird*.)

Perhaps, then, what we are saying when we say that a child is *unaware* is that the child shows no *overt* indications of being concerned, in any fashion, about his or her abilities to speak or speaking behavior. We submit, however, that not being concerned and not being aware are related but different issues. Intuitively, and ideally, we would like to see the child's speaking difficulties diminish prior to the child's becoming concerned about them, but we really cannot assume that the child is not aware at some level of his or her speaking difficulties.

Certainly, as speech-language clinicians, we try to do nothing to increase children's concern, worry or anxiety about themselves or their speaking abilities or behavior. Thus, for example, we would not hammer away at a young stutterer's occasional articulation errors, teaching him how hard or difficult these sounds are to produce and how much effort and physical tension he must use to try and correctly produce them. This approach has, in effect, the real potential for making the child aware as well as fearful of producing his or her "problem" or "error" sounds. It is not just the *degree* of awareness of a problem that is a problem but the *type* of awareness and whether the type of awareness experienced by the stutterer increases or generates concern on the part of the stutterer (and his or her friends, relatives, and family) that inhibits fluent speech production.

Matter-of-fact, Objective Approach
Helps Counteract Negative Aspects of Awareness

If the older child or teenager who stutters is clearly concerned and aware in an emotional, fairly negative way of his or her speaking abilities and behavior, then it helps if the SLP maintains an objective, matter-of-fact approach to the young client. Certainly, the SLP shouldn't get too philosophical or intellectual or totally ignore the child's obvious fear, anxiety, and worry about him- or herself, but neither should the SLP excessively dwell or focus on these concerns. What the SLP should do is recognize the reality of these concerns and acknowledge how these concerns may make the client feel when he or she experiences them but try to minimize the further development of these concerns.

Essentially, the SLP wants to arrest these concerns but this is, of course, harder than it sounds, and not all clients will react similarly to the SLP's attempts to do so. We have observed children with little apparent emotionality associated with their speech behavior refuse to listen to themselves on an audio tape recorder or watch themselves in a mirror as they spoke. These children are obviously concerned, at some relatively unobservable level, about their speech and these concerns or fears need to be dealt with if long-term improvement is to take place. We have also observed children with apparently high levels of emotionality associated with their speech appear to react objectively and positively to the clinician's description of their speaking problem.

Thus, the stutterer's level and type of awareness need not be observable to an external observer to be a problem; furthermore, the client can be "aware" of his or her speaking difficulties but as long as this does not engender fear or embarrassment, the client is unlikely to avoid examining his or her speech behavior.

Whatever the case, the client's type and level of awareness are difficult to judge in advance of therapy, and it is this difficulty that makes the thoughtful SLP hesitant to rush headlong into making assumptions about the child until further experience and testing of the child has taken place.

"Everybody Makes Mistakes" as Another Means
for Counteracting the Negative Aspects of Awareness

Older children and teenagers who present physically effortless repetitions are probably aware, on some level, of their speech disfluencies and that they may sometimes sound or look different from their peers when they talk. These children can often be helped through parental counseling, support, and encouragement to continue and enjoy talking. Their classroom teachers can also be enlisted to help them learn that talking can be pleasurable. At the least, the classroom teacher can be encouraged to (A) ask the child to talk on those days when the child seems particularly fluent and, conversely, (B) call on the child less on those days when he or she is particularly disfluent. These youngsters, we have found, can gain a great deal of perspective on their problem by considering their speech disfluencies as errors or mistakes that are not unlike those observed in other activities they are familiar with, for example, sports, walking, riding a bicycle, schoolwork, and so forth.

Williams's (1971) *hard* and *easy* speech concept may be used when discussing "mistakes," depending on the degree to which the client appears to be moving in the direction of producing more and more speech disfluencies. Fostering awareness of "mistakes," as in subsequently discussed procedures where we will actually be increasing the child's awareness of speaking behaviors, always begins with those events "far away" from the client; that is, those events that do not directly influence or are not produced by the child. For example, we would begin with a talk about how other people make mistakes when they are learning to print the alphabet, read aloud, write their name, or ride a bicycle, or how we, the SLP, are having trouble learning how to ski or use a computer. We suggest the use of audio or videotapes of *other* people making mistakes when they talk or walk or do anything.

Learning is not a smooth, error-free ride to skill mastery   We try to help the child begin to understand the concept that learning is not a smooth, error-free progression to mastery of a skill, but a process that is filled with mistakes, errors, and picking oneself up and trying again. We try to help the child develop an understanding for the gradualness of learning, so that she or he can develop an awareness of her or his own behavior based on reality, not some unattainable ideal of totally or completely fluent speech. The awareness we are trying to help the child develop is objective, as nonemotional as possible, and specific to speech behavior and disruptions; the SLP tries to foster this awareness by being nonjudgmental, objective, and rational in his or her examination of the child's and other people's speech and related behavior.

SLP concerns can be conveyed nonverbally as well as verbally   The SLP's noncritical but analytical assessment of the child's speech disfluencies will go a long way toward helping the child appreciate and come to deal with these behaviors in objective ways. One caution: the SLP, like the parents of stutterers, can convey concern, fear, anxiety, and worry through nonverbal as well as verbal means. In fact, as we discussed in the previous chapter, it is entirely possible that children, older ones and teenagers as well, may actually pay more attention to and learn more from your bodily/hand movements, head nods, eye contact, blinking and facial gestures, and prosody of speaking than any of the specific words you say and use. Our clinical observations suggest to us that many listeners, when they listen to a stutterer, tend to hold their breath, move their eyeballs to the left or right, close or blink their eyelids, turn their head, or immobilize their facial expression. Older as well as younger children, we believe, can pick up on and react to these nonverbal gestures. We believe it highly instructive for the SLP to have a mirror behind the client so the SLP can study his or her own nonverbal behaviors during the client's stutterings in order to learn how to identify and eventually change any untoward behaviors.

Use of "Awareness" as a Positive Influence on Changing Behavior

The above discussion of awareness calls attention to the ambiguities and uncertainties of dealing with awareness of stuttering, particularly with the older child or teenager. Objective awareness would appear to be a positive force for identifying and changing unwanted or inappropriate speech and related behavior. Subjective awareness, with its often attendant negative emotionality, feelings of frustration, embarrassment, and the like, is not viewed as a positive force and can contribute to a child's negative reaction to speech. The SLP should strive to understand the difference between the two types of awareness—objective and subjective—and how to change both if the need arises.

DESENSITIZATION

One procedure that we find assists with this type of child (and the younger child whose stuttering is clearly associated with various stimuli) is a desensitization approach (for example, Hall, 1966; Van Riper, 1973; Gregory and Hill, 1980). With this approach, the clinician attempts to assist the child/teenager develop more tolerance for events and stimuli that are associated with or seem to precipitate his or her stuttering.

In essence, the SLP, when attempting to *desensitize* the young client, tries to raise the youngster's tolerance level for those *fluency disrupters* for which the child seems to have a low threshold for reaction. Children are systematically presented with stimuli that have greater or lesser abilities to negatively influence or disrupt their speech fluency. Because the clinician never actually deals with the modification of speech and language behavior or concerns, desensitization is particularly useful when applied to children whose subjective awareness and concern regarding stuttering appear minimal. That is, the clinician can create and control the communication situation in such a way that the child's involvement is that of a spontaneous speaker rather than someone who is trying to modify his or her own speech behavior.

Beginning to "Desensitize" the Young Client

The SLP first tries to create a communication-emotional situation that is as free as possible from any pressures or frustrations (fluency disrupters) believed to precipitate the child's disfluency; for example, being an inattentive listener, talking at a rapid rate, interrupting the child, talking for the child, using very short or no turn-switching pauses, continually questioning the child, and so forth. The clinician gauges the success of this situational modification or control by monitoring the child's speech. When the child's speech is essentially fluent, when the child has reached what has been termed *a basal fluency* level (Hall, 1966), the clinician assumes that he or she has been able to minimize important fluency disrupters. The child's speech at this point should be normally disfluent, not perfectly or abnormally fluent, and the child should appear to communicate reasonably freely and with apparent comfort.

The clinician should carefully observe—audio and/or video recording help with retrospective study—the number and nature of salient aspects of the situations in which the child exhibits basal fluency. This is because during therapy the child may have to be repeatedly brought back to basal fluency and the clinician needs to clearly understand what variables are most highly related to the child's basal fluency. Once basal fluency can be reliably and predictably obtained and maintained for appropriate periods of time relative to the child's severity of problem and stage of therapy, the SLP can begin to introduce fluency disrupters or *barbs* or *probes.*

Before we proceed any further, let us make it clear that this form of therapy, as with many other forms, relies heavily on the SLP's ability to "read" or discern accurately and quickly those stimuli and events that facilitate versus those that inhibit the client's speech fluency. The clinician's observational skills are every bit as important as his or her manipulation of environmental events to the success of desensitization. The SLP should observe and manipulate the fluency disrupters that *actually* seem to influence the child rather than those the SLP *assumes* to be of influence or is familiar with. In our experience, many therapies achieve little success in the clinic, not because they are fundamentally unsound forms of remediation, but because the therapies are poorly applied or understood.

In all fairness, of course, some therapies are poorly conceived as well as stated and thus lead to less than ideal results when put into practice. With desensitization, the SLP must spend some time assessing and testing which events are fluency inhibitors and which are fluency facilitators for which children, and when. This continual assessment and experimentation, at least in the initial stages of therapy, is no small task and are just another reason for considering remediation as ongoing diagnosis.

Introducing "Barbs" or Fluency Inhibitors

The "barbs" or fluency disrupters or inhibitors introduced into the speaking situation are used to toughen, strengthen, or increase young stutterers' resistance to fluency disrupting influences. Barbs should be selected from those events the child is likely to encounter in his or her daily, outside-the-clinic environment and should be based, as much as possible, on clinician observation of the child's speaking while in the presence of these events.

We have used the following events as fluency disrupters or barbs: answering children's questions with questions; asking questions that involve rather large, abstract responses from children; changing the topic of conversation with children; looking away while children talk; interrupting children while they talk; asking children to repeat themselves; asking children to hurry up their responses; asking the child a question and then answering our own question without giving the child a chance to respond; talking very rapidly ourselves; providing minimal or no turn-taking or turn-switching pause between the end of the child's response and the beginning of our reply. This list is, of course, only partial and is presented solely for the purpose of providing some examples of fluency inhibitors or barbs. The list is not meant to be all inclusive and in no way should inhibit or preclude readers from adding or developing their own "barbs."

At first glance, the reader may think that the listed fluency disrupters are "cruel and unusual punishment," but under the right circumstances, done in the right manner (mildly stressing the child's resistance to fluency disrupters without ever provoking the child's stuttering), they can be used to positively influence the child's fluency and strengthen the child's tolerance for such fluency disrupters. At no time should these barbs be used by the SLP or other interlocutors to "get back at" or punish the child or to show SLP disapproval for client behavior judged to be inappropriate or undesirable by the SLP.

It seems reasonable to assume that many children experience fluency disrupters in their everyday communication situations. Therefore, it seems both commonsensical as well as prudent to help these children learn how to deal effectively with these disrupters if they are demonstrating that they are having difficulty. Each disrupter, or barb, is presented into the speaking situation only *until* the child shows that he or she is about to become disfluent. The SLP removes the disrupter(s) *before* the child begins to stutter, not *after.* This is much like the allergist I see for treatment of allergies. The allergen dosage, for example, the miniscule amount of ragweed pollen in the desensitization injections I receive, is slowly increased but leveled off if I exhibit any signs that the desensitization shot is precipitating an allergic reaction (sneezing, wheezing, itching, or watery eyes). If need be, the allergist may even decrease the level of my allergen dosage, say from 0.3 cc to 0.2 cc, if the higher level causes too many problems. Likewise, the SLP is not trying to elicit or precipitate stuttering but to slowly and systematically increase the child's ability to react fluently to communicative situations that are increasingly stressful.

Inattentive Listeners: A Potent but Difficult to Discern Fluency Disrupter

One relatively subtle but potent fluency disrupter that some parents and other listeners unwittingly expose their child to is ignoring the child when he or she talks to them. For example, this may be seen when the parent and another adult are conversing and the parent's child *continually* tries to interrupt to ask the parent something or to get the parent's attention. The child may repeat "Dad" ten to 15 times (I've actually counted!) before the father will respond to the child; sometimes the father never responds but continues to converse with the other adult, seemingly oblivious to the child's presence or attempts to communicate. Instead of the father's stopping the adult conversation momentarily and explaining to the child that it is impolite to interrupt or telling the child to wait his turn, the parent essentially ignores the child. (Of course, feeling "ignored" is somewhat in the eye of the beholder. As we will subsequently discuss, a parent cannot and should not be expected to make eye contact with a child while the parent is driving a car or cutting vegetables with a sharp knife. Instead, the child should be told that the parent is listening but can't look away at the moment.)

To my mind, the only thing worse than continually and destructively criticizing someone is not paying any attention at all to that person. When children are *frequently* ignored by their parents, some youngsters seem to figure that any attention is better than none at all and do things that their parents simply can't ignore, for example, throw a match into the paper in the kitchen waste basket, punch or verbally abuse or tease the younger brother or sister, play the stereo at a window-rattling volume level, and so forth. Children who must constantly repeat and lobby for their parents' attention experience far more than their fair share of fluency disrupters. (Besides desensitizing the child to these disrupters, we should also try to mitigate their excessive occurrence.)

Being a parent is very rewarding, but as in any other endeavor, these rewards are earned through a lot of hard work. Perhaps it is fair to say that a parent's work is never done and although exasperating, especially after a long day of work (either inside or outside the home), the parent needs to let the child know that he or she was heard, but that his mother or father is busy and tired right now and, after such and such is done, the child will be listened or talked to, interacted or played with.

Another example of this type of situation is the mother's busily preparing dinner over the kitchen counter when her child comes up behind her and starts excitedly explaining how he just scored the winning goal in a neighborhood soccer game. The mother, as she slices the carrots, and scurries around the kitchen looking for the cookbook containing the recipe for tonight's main course, says such things as, "Hmmmm," or "Oh, yeah," or "That's nice," while the child rattles on about this most recent example of his athletic prowess (perhaps she thinks her youngster's soliloquy is only too similar to her husband's reminiscences about the halcyon days when he was a star high school basketball player). Sometimes the mother may not even say anything to the child but silently nod her head and silently prepare dinner. The child, who begins to feel that he or she is losing his or her listening audience (if there ever really was one), may get frustrated, nervous, and upset over the parent's apparent lack of interest or willingness to communicate and may begin to repeat sounds, syllables, or whole words. Interestingly, *now* the mother turns and reacts either overtly or covertly to this new form of the child's verbal expression. Perhaps the message the child is getting is: When you begin to lose your audience, when your audience pays you little or no attention, when your audience seems unwilling to communicate, start to repeat and prolong; it gets their attention every time! The mother's disregard for the content of the child's communication but attention to its manner acts as a differential reinforcement that may actually lead to more of the very speech behavior by the child that she actually doesn't like (cf. Shames and Sherrick, 1963; Ryan, 1980).

Helping parents recognize (and reduce) and the child resist such fluency disrupters is one of the tasks of the speech-language pathologists. While this desensitization procedure has seen much use with younger children who stutter (Hall, 1966), its use with older children is also quite appropriate. One cannot claim that the child will successfully deal with all fluency disrupters and frustrations as a result of this form of therapy or that parents will cease and desist each and every instance of fluency disruption. However, this approach is a good beginning, a good way as Van Riper (1973) suggests, to "toughen up" the child.

Evaluating Successfulness of Desensitization Approach

In truth, there are no firm guidelines that the SLP can follow to evaluate the success of desensitization approaches with children who stutter. Success with this procedure will be relative to the nature of the individual child and the type and severity of stuttering that individual child presents. For example, "fluency" during the introduction of fluency disrupters or barbs for one child may contain as much as 5 percent disfluency whereas for another child it may contain 1 percent or less. The clinician is using this procedure in attempts to help the child successfully resist the types of fluency disrupters that will be encountered during speaking situations.

Desensitization may or may not be employed when the SLP is *directly* helping the child learn to identify and modify specific instances of disfluency (its use being determined by the clinician's judgment about its compatibility with these procedures). The emphasis with this desensitization therapy is on the situations that evoke disfluency and the child's ability to respond fluently to these situations. With desensitization, it is the child's *tolerance level for fluency disrupters* and *not the disfluencies themselves* that the SLP is trying to influence directly. In this case, the speech disfluencies are used by the clinician to determine the relative success with which the child is coping with the pressures.

It is also helpful, when employing desensitization, to meet with the child's parents and discuss some of the fluency disrupters they may knowingly or unknowingly be exposing their child to (for example, "When your child is stuttering a great deal, what is typically going on in the home? What are you typically talking about or doing?"). Along these lines, Zwitman (1978) explicitly describes some parental reactions to child's speech which *do* (for example, pay attention to *what* the child says) and *do not* (for example, appear angry or impatient) facilitate fluency. The keys to uncovering fluency disrupters that seem to be highly related to the child's stuttering are observing their frequency and consistency of occurrence since it should be realized that all parents, indeed all listeners, exhibit fluency disrupters when they are talking with other people.

ENCOURAGING THE CHILD TO INTERACT (NON)VERBALLY WITH PEERS

We like to spend some time discussing with parents and encouraging them to see what hobbies, sports, or extracurricular activities their older child or teenager might like to become involved in or would benefit from participating in. It is not uncommon for these older children to come home every day after school and go into their room by themselves or turn on the television. Certainly these children, like all children, need some time to themselves, but *routine* isolation from peer interaction makes it difficult to develop interpersonal skills (and, after all, it is their peers and not their parents with whom these children will be spending their school years and later life). Furthermore, watching television three or more hours *every* afternoon provides the child with little opportunity to communicate verbally with others. Winn (1977) likens the experience of watching television to that of staring into a fireplace relative to the amount of intellectual stimulation that takes place.

These children should be encouraged to develop the friendship of other children their age. Perhaps this will mean, initially, inviting other children over to play. It is certainly all right to have some friends markedly younger or older than themselves, but when this is the rule gentle, parental encouragement to form friendships with their age peers should take place.

Alternatively, an organized team sport like baseball, soccer, basketball, or football, or more individualized activities or sports like chess, tennis, archery, fencing, wrestling, bowling, swimming, gymnastics, golf, or track might be good ways for the older child or teen to develop friends and learn appropriate verbal and social interactions. Perhaps courses at a local school or community center on how to: play the guitar, take photographs, raise tropical fish, learn juggling, train the family dog, learn about computers, magic tricks, crochet, painting with oil colors, first aid, or the use of woodworking tools may help the child get out of the house and interact with new and different people. Needless to say, if mom or dad get involved in these extra activities, the greater the likelihood that parent and child will socially and communicatively share common experiences or skills to be learned, and, once learned, mutually enjoyed. If these children learn some skill, sport, or acquire special information (for example, knowing detailed information about Civil War battle sites or United States stamps since World War II) in which they can take pride and gain the respect of others, so much the better. These skills, sports, hobbies, or expertise can only serve to build the children's positive regard for themselves. Furthermore, there is no better place for a parent to see how typical their child is than by regularly watching the child perform, play, or interact with other children of the same age.

The Gradual Process of Learning

Some parents need to learn about learning Some parents, like their children, do not understand the gradual process of learning, in general, and the gradual process of learning to change behavior, in specific. That is, these parents give the impression that all one must do to master a particular skill, event, activity, or sport is have will power and positive thinking ("All is mind"). They seem quite reluctant to accept the fact that complex skills, for example, catching baseballs, reading, using a hammer and nails, take months and years to develop and that the first time you sit down at the piano you do not play like Chopin. This attitude on the part of some parents is most unfortunate because their children, due to their immaturity, are already impatient with learning. Thus, instead of helping the older child or teen learn patience and how to concentrate on small signs of positive improvement, some parents become impatient, discouraged, "shop around" for "quicker cures," or push their children to use skills they are simply not ready for or have had insufficient opportunity to develop. Once again, time urgency, this time on the part of the parents, or the inappropriate attempt to "speed things up," interferes with the therapy process.

In these cases, the SLP must be patient and continually encourage the parents to accentuate the positive in their child; the SLP should try to support the parents' positive intervention in their child's development and help them change or mitigate their more negative forms of intervention. Our experience suggests that parental impatience with or intolerance for their child's overall development are two of the main reasons that they express impatience with their child's progress in speech therapy. When the SLP recognizes the existence of such impatience, the SLP must clearly tell the parents the short- and long-term goals of therapy and approximately how long, in weeks, or years, he plans active speech therapy. If a period of "maintenance" therapy or a "transfer" period is to follow active speech therapy, the parents should be so instructed with the time line explicated as clearly as possible. Parents need and want such time lines and while it may not decrease their impatience for the relatively slow process of human change, it certainly makes things less ambiguous for them.

OLDER CHILDREN WITH DEFINITE AWARENESS OF STUTTERING

It is difficult to provide a precise age range for these individuals. They could be as young as seven or eight but are probably at least nine or ten, with a ceiling somewhere around twelve years of age. Once the child gets much beyond twelve, adolescent concerns begin to enter the picture and considerably change the course of remediation and prognosis for improvement.

Older children with cognitive and/or emotional awareness of stuttering are probably producing both sound prolongations and sound/syllable repetitions. Glottal fry and/or breathy voice quality may be associated with either or both disfluency types. Some indications of physical tension may be associated with these youngsters' stutterings, particularly on the cessation-type of speech disfluency. Eye contact with listeners, as noted in Ainsworth and Fraser (1988), may be poor, particularly during instances of the child's speech disfluencies. The child may give verbal as well as nonverbal indications that he or she is psychologically and physically tense prior to or during speaking. Many people, even casual observers, in the child's environment will recognize that this child is stuttering, and the parents and the school system will often express a good deal of concern.

Within the context of Bloodstein's (1960a, 1960b, 1961) description of the four phases in the development of stuttering he would probably characterize these children as phase three stutterers, that is, chronic with certain situations, words, and sounds more apt to be associated with stuttering; word substitutions and/or circumlocutions, but with little or no clear evidence of fear, embarrassment, or avoidance of speaking. While, as Bloodstein (1987) notes, these four phases represent an attempt to describe the typical (or "average") stutterer of a particular age-development level, they may inadequately describe any one individual stutterer. Furthermore, any attempt to use categorical "phases" to describe what appears to be a continuous process (that is, the development of stuttering) is problematic. This is because the variables being categorized are dynamic and ever changing and are resistant to being "pigeon-holed" into static or relatively fixed slots or groupings. However, such categorical schemas certainly provide one reasonable means to organize and discuss the multidimensional nature of stuttering, but they should be taken as conventions for the improvement of our thinking and communication about stuttering rather than inviolate laws of nature.

The emotional concern exhibited by these children is clearly unclear. It may be, as Bloodstein suggests, *irritation*, but it can be concern that is more aptly described as *emotional discomfort*. We do not think that it has yet developed to the point where terms like *anxiety* or *fear* could be applied, at least not in the sense that these relatively strong concerns are chronic. Once again, we are talking about the rule rather than the exception, the group rather than a specific individual. And, as mentioned above, it is always difficult to categorically label behavior and events that are continuous as well as multidimensional in nature. We can say, however, that it is apparent that these youngsters "know" and are "concerned" at some level that they stutter, although the nature and degree of their knowledge and concern are probably dissimilar from those of older teenagers and adults who stutter.

Motivation

One of the first and most important, but probably most challenging, things to ascertain when remediating any client (especially these clients) is the nature and depth of motivation for seeking therapeutic services. The essence of this investigation can be summarized in the following modified analogy: Is the horse being led or is he coming of his own free will and desire to water? Obviously, not too many ten-year-olds will actively seek help (for example, pick up a telephone and call a professional agency), but many of them will at least tell their parents (or some other adult they trust) that they are concerned about their speech or wish their parents would take them to someone who can help with their speech. Another group of children will say nothing as direct but indicate indirectly that they are concerned, irritated, or frustrated regarding their speech. Still yet another group will express very little, either explicitly or implicitly, that indicates concern. Parents may be the motivating force behind this latter group's coming in for therapy services; sometimes it is a concerned physician, social worker, or teacher who makes the referral.

Unfortunately, no matter how severe, frequent, or noticeable the stuttering, children with a passive or blasé attitude toward their own speech will be children whom the SLP will find it difficult to help. The child has to care somewhat about changing his or her speech. No matter how badly the parents or teacher desire fluency for the child, if the child is minimally desirous of expending the necessary effort to change behavior, then prognosis for change is poor. Starbuck (1974) and Prins (1974) discuss these problems and make a number of suggestions for dealing with them.

Identification

Although a variety of situations impact these children's stuttering, we do not always attempt to modify the association between situation and stuttering. For a more complete description of situations associated with stuttering, developing situational hierarchies, and systematic desensitization, one may read Brutten and Shoemaker (1967). These authors present rationale and therapy for dealing with situational fears and concerns that may be adversely influencing a person's speech fluency. Instead, when possible, we have the child's parents provide us with a general situational hierarchy—those situations where the client exhibits the most to the least number of speech disfluencies—in order to gain some perspective on those events and stimuli associated with the child's stuttering.

Working on problem sounds   We believe that concentrating on the child's "problem" sounds, syllables, or words is therapy time misspent. In our experience, this procedure all too often leads the child to develop more, rather than less, concerns, fears, and avoidances regarding specific sounds, syllables, or words. It is almost like telling someone driving a car to be especially careful and on-guard anytime he crosses a bridge. If these instructions are persistent enough and the driver listens and takes them to heart, it would not be surprising to see this same driver quite physically and mentally tense when driving over bridges, to the extent that he or she may go out of his or her way to avoid bridges or get someone else to do all the "bridge driving."

Instead, we like to have children and teenagers (and adults for that matter) deal with their speech behavior and disruptions by using a more general, problem-solving approach where the emphasis is on changes in their overall strategies to initiate and continue speech rather than to watch for and modify their behavior when certain speech "hurdles" must be jumped. The emphasis is on them and the way they act when speaking (an active approach) rather than on the way various sounds, syllables, and words act upon them (a passive approach).

The use of analogies   To begin, we use the previously described garden hose analogy and others like it to help these older children learn something about their speech mechanism and the various ways they can *use* it. This approach helps them come to grips with what they do that is *facilitating* versus *inhibiting* their speech fluency; however, it does this in a rather down-to-earth, understandable fashion (one that these youngsters can relate to). Once again, rather than concentrate on certain sounds or words, we concentrate on *strategies* the child appears to use that interfere with the smooth, fluid flow of ongoing speech (for example, "stopping the air from flowing at the nozzle" or "making sounds hard with the faucet").

We believe it is extremely important to get these older children to *physically feel* what they do when they produce speech, both the disfluent and fluent aspects. Hearing and seeing what takes place during stuttering supports the changes in client speech behavior that must take place; however, audition and vision are generally *after*, rather than *before* or even *during*, the act of stuttering. Often by the time the client hears and sees the stuttering, it has already begun. While we want them to change once they have begun, we also want them to change prior to or at the very beginning of speech production. To do this they must physically feel what they are *doing*.

This age client can come to feel and recognize what she or he does that interferes with speech and contrast this with what is done that facilitates speech, that is, what produces fluency. In our opinion, identifying and recognizing inappropriate strategies used to produce speech are crucial, for the child to learn how to modify speech and once such modification is learned, to recognize those situations where they are reverting back to inappropriate behavior or strategies so that change can be made. Long-term recovery, we think, requires these clients to understand that they can physically feel and closely imitate these inappropriate strategies and that these strategies can be changed in ways that they can physically feel to facilitate their fluent speech production.

Imitation is not the same as mocking   One problem with identifying and recognizing speech disfluencies is clinician imitation of the child's disfluencies. Imitation, in and of itself, is not inherently bad, but some clinicians may do it, albeit unconsciously, in such a fashion that the child may feel mocked or "put down." This is not a common problem, and many times it is the child's hypersensitivity toward imitation, rather than the nature of the clinician's imitation, that engenders a problem. However, the sensitive as well as sensible clinician should be aware of such events and head them off before they happen (in some cases, the child will have to be specifically desensitized to observing his or her own stuttering). The clinician should realize that, even for children, there may be relatively strong fears associated with stuttering and that showing the child, no matter how innocuously, what his or her stuttering sounds or looks like may be a fairly unpleasant experience, at least at first, for some of these children.

Unnecessary emphasis of nonspeech behavior during imitated disfluencies Another problem with the SLP's imitation of the youngster's disfluencies, and one that seems quite common in our experience, is the clinician's inappropriate, unnecessary emphasis of nonspeech behavior during imitated disfluencies. Here, for example, we may see a clinician showing a child a sound prolongation on the /b/ in the word *boy* by pursing her lips and then quickly and tensely jerking her head forward as she releases the /b/ and moves through the word.

This clinician is teaching something in addition to the nature and feel of the speech disfluency and its locus within the speech production mechanism. She is also teaching the child inappropriate associated behavior. These more molar or "grosser" nonverbal behaviors are readily perceived and picked up by the child and can easily become part of the child's disfluency. Clinicians should try to avoid producing such unnecessary head and body movements and only imitate that which is necessary to produce the actual speech disfluency. If the clinician feels the need for emphasis, large magnifying glasses, small high-intensity lamps, and the like can help the child focus in on the area and speech behavior of import.

The older child's desire for a "passive" cure   Of course, these children, not unlike many of us, wish for a pill or some passive device to take away their stuttering. This wish is only natural since humans, like electricity, tend to take the path of least resistance. The SLP needs to help children use their mind and sensing powers to intercede between the communication environment and their speech reaction in the presence of that environment. Such intercession obviously takes some work and patience on the part of the child and the SLP. Change, long-term change, can only come about if the young client takes more of an active role in the process of changing his or her behavior.

Some clients and their associates seem to hope against hope for divine intervention, a miracle drug, or passive, osmotic assimilation of the SLP's admonishments to change. These hopes of finding the "silver bullet" to eradicate the problem are about as productive as staying up all night to catch the tooth fairy. What a shock when we realize that the magical appearance of money under our pillow comes from good old mom and dad; likewise, it is an equal shock to learn that the seemingly magical change in our speech must come from our own acts, thoughts, and efforts. To hope for and believe in tooth fairies and miracle cures may be human, but it also reflects an inability or unwillingness to face reality as we now know it.

Getting off the identification dime   We, as SLPs, sometimes make the process of change unnecessarily difficult for our clients when we get so involved with identifying and recognizing the child's behavior that we fail to make the adjustments necessary to move into the next phase: modification. That is, the SLP carries on the identification phase of therapy long after it has achieved its desired goals. Moving toward modification is something the SLP must be doing, at least in small steps, from the initial evaluation onward. Nothing is as motivating as change, even if it is slight and temporary; it signals to the client that things can get better. Indeed, the clinician must constantly assess the client's ability and willingness to change as well as demonstrate to the client that change is possible—that there is hope for the future.

Modification

Modifying a child's speech assumes that the SLP knows what changes in speech signify movement in the right direction, in the direction of "doing more and more things like normally fluent speakers do" (Williams, 1978). That is, the SLP must be able to recognize and reward small positive changes in the child's speech if he or she is to systematically reinforce and shape that child's speech (cf. Shames and Egolf, 1976). It is not too difficult to recognize that a decrease in the frequency of a particular within-word disfluency is indicative of positive change. Likewise, it is fairly easy to see that diminution of inappropriate facial gestures or bodily movements during stuttering indicates positive change. However, in the beginning of therapy, when changes are less noticeable and more subtle in nature, what can we use to indicate to our clients (and ourselves) that they are changing? That is, before the client produces noticeable changes what can we use to indicate improvement?

We can count behavior but do we know what behavior to count? In the beginning of therapy, before dramatic change takes place, what changes indicate that positive change is occurring? Here, unfortunately, we come up against a blank wall. In the past 20 to 25 years, our rush to be clinically quantitative, to count and assess behavior within this or that behavioral theory framework, has, to some degree, led us to lose sight of the *content* of our client's behavior. While we can easily design charts to depict behavior change over time, we cannot as easily explain to ourselves and others *what* behavior *needs* to be charted.

Fortunately, information is beginning to accumulate that objectively describes those speech production behaviors associated with those speech behaviors we perceptually evaluate as stuttering (for example, Hutchinson, 1974; Guitar, 1975; Conture, McCall and Brewer, 1977; Freeman and Ushijima, 1978; Zimmerman, 1980b; Shapiro, 1980; Conture, Schwartz and Brewer, 1985; Caruso, Conture and Colton, 1988; Kelly and Conture, 1988). These studies make it abundantly clear that the number and nature of these speech production behaviors vary as much as the labels, for example, broken words, sound prolongations we use to describe our perception of them. Along these lines, it will be recalled that Van Riper (1971) posited that during instances of stuttering vowels sound more like the schwa /ə/ than the intended vowel; however, it has been shown that the intended vowel quality during stuttering remained but listeners did not perceive this because vowels during stuttering have lower amplitude and shorter duration (Howell and Vause, 1986; Howell, Williams and Vause, 1987). Further, as Howell, Hamilton and Kriacoupoulos (1984) have shown with their attempt to identify stutterings automatically through the use of computer algorithms, no single algorithm can capture or identify all instances of stuttering. Therefore, as much as we find the counting of behavior attractive and understandable, it may not adequately circumscribe all aspects of stuttered speech. Indeed, it may overlook very salient behaviors.

Improvement in the beginning: changes in duration, number of sound prolongations, and physical tension   Our clinical observations indicate that in the beginning of therapy, three of the first things that signify positive change in stuttering are (1) decreases in the duration of within-word disfluencies; (2) a change in the ratio of sound prolongations ("cessation" type of disfluencies) to sound/syllable repetitions ("reiteration" type of disfluencies)—fewer sound prolongations and more sound/syllable repetitions; and (3) subjective listener impressions that instances of stuttering are being produced with less physical tension (they sound more physically "easy" or "relaxed"). These changes may occur even while the child continues to stutter at about the same frequency. In essence, as some have suggested (Cooper, 1986, 1987), we need to look beyond the frequency count of instances of stuttering. Instead, we need to examine more closely the time course and relative predominance of certain other behaviors, some of which may be less quantifiable than frequency of stuttering but just as relevant to understanding and remediating the problem.

For example, it has been our observation that duration of instances of stuttering will start to change as children become more and more objectively aware of where and when in the speech utterance they begin to stutter. As they learn more and more about the *where* as well as *when* of their own behavior, they seem to begin to learn more and more about *what* they do that interferes with speech. This level of objective awareness appears to help many children and adults shorten or truncate the duration of their disfluencies. It is my hunch that longer disfluencies are associated with higher levels of muscle activity or physical tension (particularly if they are the cessation kind of speech disfluency earlier mentioned) than shorter disfluencies. Objective awareness of these disfluencies seems to assist children, in the early stages of therapy, to begin decreasing the amount or level of physical tension associated with their speech disfluencies.

Helping children change physical tension levels   Helping children *directly* decrease the duration of their disfluencies is hard but not impossible. First, the child needs to understand something about the difference between physically tense versus relaxed muscles *and* the gradations of physical tension in between these two states of muscle tonus. This is, of course, a difficult concept for even older children to grasp because the vocabulary used to describe physical tension is generally beyond the comprehension of most youngsters. Besides, even adults, in our experience, have trouble sensing physical tension in their muscles. Perhaps, biofeedback may be of some assistance in this regard; for a critical review of the use of biofeedback with school-age children, see the comments of Guitar, Adams and Conture (1979). (Readers may get some perspective on the difficulty of recognizing the sites and amounts of bodily tension by trying to figure out, without palpitating or touching with fingers or hands, whether the muscles of their forearms and shoulders/neck region are physically tense and, if they both are, which one is more tense!)

As shown in Figure 3–2, on page 116, we try to help children understand, at a level they can relate to, the concept of physical tension by using the Scarecrow and Tinwoodsman in the *Wizard of Oz* as analogies, with the bendable, rubber stick figure as mid-way point between the excessive floppiness of the scarecrow and the excessive tension or stiffness of the tinwoodsman. Most children have seen or read the *Wizard of Oz* (and seen such rubber stick figures) and can readily identify and imitate the floppy, relaxed scarecrow and the creaky, stiff tinwoodsman. It is, however, very instructive to see them imitate how the rubber stick figure might talk, walk, or run since this gives the clinician some idea how they view the more in-between state of physical tension.

We explain through word and deed that speech takes some degree of muscle tension—not as much as the tinwoodsman or as little as the scarecrow but more like the rubber stick figure. We have children throw balls, walk, skip, run, sing, write, or clap their hands with tinwoodsman, scarecrow, or rubber-stick-figure-like muscles or movements. In these ways the idea of (in)appropriate degrees of muscle tonus are imparted, to greater or lesser extents, to the children.

Changing tension during speech production   Assuming the children understand muscle tension in terms that are clear to them that they can relate to us and show us by example, we show them how they can apply these ideas to speech. In essence, we want them to understand that they can decrease as well as increase muscle tension throughout their vocal tract and that it is clearly within their power to make changes in muscle tension during speech production. We employ the garden hose analogy to help the child more readily identify and sense the various locations within the vocal tract where physical tension can be felt and changed. With mirrors and face-to-face observation, the clinician makes speech production physically tense ("hard") at the level of the faucet (larynx) or nozzle (lips), and then has the child do the same. As mentioned previously, using magnifying glasses and small high-intensity lamps helps emphasize the areas that the clinician wants the child to attend to. We repeatedly demonstrate to children through both word and deed that they can tense and relax various aspects of their speech mechanism and that these states of muscle tension are within their control and that they can govern the tension level of their muscles.

The child is then given practice in physically tensing on sounds and relaxing on the same sounds. In the beginning, the use of bi-labial sounds like /b,p,m/ helps the child more readily visualize what is going on; however, the specific sounds are not as important as the child's recognition and sensing the difference between muscles that are physically tense versus relaxed and the states in-between. We are not talking about an understanding of the level of a speech physiologist, but rather an objective awareness that is sufficient to serve the child as a basis for subsequent modification.

Changes in time and tension: The essence of modification of stuttering At this point, other therapy procedures may be employed; for example, Van Riper's (1973) well-known cancellation, pull-out, and preparatory set sequence, Webster's (1978) precision fluency shaping, or Williams's "hard"/"easy" speaking approach. Although the names of various therapies change and philosophies differ in whole or in part, one common element seems to stand out: The modification of stuttering involves, to greater or lesser degrees, *changes* in the *time* and *tension* domains of speech production. Whether, as with precision fluency shaping, it involves a systematic change in the initiation of vocal sound pressure level ("vocal loudness" or "volume") over time (neither too gradual nor too sudden a change) or, as with the pull-out procedure, a gradual stretching or elongation in time of the articulatory contact for the sound following the word-initial stuttering or, as with the hard/easy procedure, starting or "going into" the sound in an "easy" (less physically tense) manner, all modification procedures for stuttering appear to involve, in one way or another, manipulation of the time and tension factors of speech production. In essence, the person who stutters is encouraged to begin and continue speaking in a less rushed, more physically relaxed fashion—a goal that is easier said than done. This is the essence of *all* stuttering therapies.

It is appropriate for therapies to focus on changes in the time/tension domain of speech production since an instance of stuttering takes more time per sound or syllable than it ordinarily should and is probably produced with inappropriate levels of muscle tension with the speech and related musculature. Therefore, an unspoken goal of therapy is to help stutterers normalize the time course and physical tension level of those sounds/syllables/words they stutter on or at least bring the temporal/tension aspects closer to typical values for producing these speech events. Interestingly, some stuttering therapies appear to change stutterers' stutterings by *lengthening* the duration of their sounds and syllables (see Metz, Onufrak and Ogburn, 1979). It is my hunch that therapies that require stutterers to *volitionally* increase the duration of sounds and syllables in order to bring about a change in stuttering probably do so by bringing about a concomitant *decrease* in physical tension levels, when compared to instances of stuttering.

Time and tension are different but related aspects of speech production and it is by no means clear which of these two aspects of speech production should be "worked on" first in therapy. It is our guess, however, that therapies that concentrate first on tension and then time result in speech that contains more disfluencies but sounds more natural. Conversely, therapies that concentrate first on time and then tension result in speech that contains fewer disfluencies but sounds less natural. These are, of course, empirical issues that must await careful, objective research studies.

We are partial to Williams's hard/easy approach and try to help children learn to quickly recognize what they are doing—in terms of temporal as well as tension disruptions—to interfere with their speech fluency and then learn to change it. At this point in therapy we continually instruct the child to "move on to the next sound," "move on," "change" (reduce the physical tension level associated with speech production and move on to the next sound), "make the sound easy," or "easy." Such instructions must obviously be repeated, and praise should be offered for *small* as well as large changes in the child's demonstrated ability to follow such instructions and make appropriate change successfully.

Once again, we hasten to add that these instructions *should not* become an old-wine-in-new-bottles situation: Changing the name ("stuttering" changed to "hard") but keeping the game the same (instead of criticizing for stuttering the listener would now merely criticize for "hard" speech or even telling the child to "stop that hard speech!"). If the child appears discouraged or confused, or is having a great deal of trouble, the therapy task should be changed, and this direct work discontinued until later in the session or the next session. We firmly believe that lasting change requires lasting long-term therapy. We may have to prolong this challenging stage of therapy for some time until the child demonstrates that he or she is ready to make these changes consistently.

Older children who stutter do almost anything to "get unstuck" Not being able to move on from one speech posture to another, feeling stuck on a particular sound, syllable, or word, and being unable to move forward is a frustrating, frightening feeling for a young or even more mature speaker. It is indeed a sense of helplessness (in Chapter 6 we discuss the concept of "learned helplessness"), of being out of control, or being unable to control one's acts. For some older children, some of the time, the feelings surrounding these events can be strong enough to create a temporary *white-out* from reality or tuning out of one's surrounds and behavior. Physical pressures are felt in the chest, neck, vocal tract, and stomach regions (we've had a few adults who stutter also tell us that they felt that their head was "under pressure" or "about to explode"). During these sensations, the child who stutters is solely occupied with getting the sound, syllable, or word out, and will use any means at his or her disposal to do so. It seems that the ends (getting the word out) justify the means (any speech or nonspeech strategy that completes the word).

Coming to grips with the emotional aspects of stuttering It is, therefore, unfortunate that at the very moment when it is most important for children to make a change, they are the least aware or objective regarding what they are doing that interferes with talking. Perhaps we can equate these feelings to those we have when we almost fall off a high ledge but pull ourselves back from the edge in the nick of time. We feel momentarily panicked, frightened, and do something, anything that we can, to keep from falling. If I then ask you, "Tell me what you did when you almost fell off the ledge," it is almost certain that you will have some difficulty. Even some time later, when trying to recall the events surrounding your near-fall, you may become emotionally uncomfortable and draw a blank or be very hazy on details. Indeed, you'll probably remember the emotion far better than the specific acts involved in righting yourself. You will probably be even less clear if I say, "What did you do to get yourself in such a situation in the first place?" The antecedents to, as well as the events of, the near-fall are most likely lost in a haze of emotion.

The point of this analogy is that youngsters who are trying to make changes in their speech fluency are being trained to attend quickly and objectively to specific physical aspects of their speech production at the very moment in time when they are the least objective regarding their own behavior (see Williams, 1978, for elaboration on this point). Thus, the emotionality associated with the child's instances of stuttering must be brought within some reasonable limits if children are to make the necessary change. The good news is that we find that success with making changes in speech—no matter how small the change—leads to an increased willingness to make changes and a diminution of emotionality. Once children have demonstrated an ability to make the type of change necessary (physically moving their speech structures onto the next posture from the posture they were holding or repeating), you may then engage them in spontaneous conversation. Beginning with the more noticeable, longer instances of stuttering, the clinician instructs the child—near the beginning or at least in the middle of the stuttering—to change. We often do this by saying gently but clearly to the child, "Change," or "Now," or "Easy," in association with a head nod, motioning, or pointing. We clearly and emphatically reward ("Good!") the child's attempts at changing speech behavior, whether it was a partial or clearly apparent change. We believe that our verbal instruction, hand gesture, and/or head nod help the child focus on the specifics necessary and, we think, break through the sometimes inappropriate levels of emotionality associated with the instance of stuttering.

Handling a child's inability to make change If the child does not seem to make an attempt at changing upon our instructions, we immediately back up and halt the forward flow of our own therapy. Does the child know or understand what we mean by change? Is the level of the child's emotionality surrounding his or her instances of stuttering still so high as to preclude objective appraisal and change of behavior? Can the child *show* you an easy change on an isolated syllable or word? Can the child imitate an instance of stuttering and then, with your help, change it? We clearly do not want the child to spend the entire session, or large portions thereof, being frustrated, discouraged and embarrassed by an inability to make change. We try to assess right then why change is not taking place. We cannot overemphasize the clinician's sensitivity to the client's behaviors and feelings. In our opinion, one of the hallmarks of effective clinicians is that they are sensitive individuals who constantly monitor their client's activities and make changes in their procedures, on the spot, as the client's behaviors dictate.

Model the type of change you want the child to produce. Have the child try to copy your model. Then have the child shadow your modeled change immediately after you. The perceptual reality of the change—moving forward onto the next speech posture—is that it sounds a bit like a fluent pull-out. That is, the child is moving from the cessation of forward speech flow on a sound (that is, the stuttering typified by a fixation of speech postures) by making the correct speech production gestures or transitions for the next sound.

At first, these transitions might appear longer and more gradual in nature than they would ordinarily, but as the child more quickly and precisely recognizes and changes the original nonmoving-on posture, he or she will shorten these articulatory transitions. We do *not* want the child to end up with speech that sounds like the ends and beginnings of adjacent sounds that were elongated like stretched taffy. Rather our goal is to help the client produce speech that sounds reasonably fluent and natural.

Of course, on a particular day, in a particular speaking situation, for a specific sound or word, a deliberately longer moving-on posture might be appropriate because it handles, in the best way possible, a particularly difficult to change disfluent production. In the main, however, the child will, with time, learn to make more and more of the movements that are necessary to produce the sound within a reasonable time frame and within reasonable limits of physical tension.

Changing rather than pushing or pulling on speech postures We try to emphasize to children that pushing or pulling on the speech posture of the sound they are stuttering on is only causing them to hesitate or stutter even more. For emphasis, we might tell children that it is as if they were the Three Stooges or Laurel and Hardy (or some other silly cartoon or comic figure they know) who keep running into a closed door, each time with a little more force and with a longer start. Instead, we say, they need to open the door and move on to the next room (or speech posture). "Opening and moving on or through" is one more relatively graphic way we have of explaining to children what they do when they fail to move on to the next posture and exhibit inappropriate levels of physical tension. We tell them they can repeatedly kick at the door, each time with a harder and harder kick, or they can push on it with all their physical might, but they will not go on to the next speech posture (or into the next room) until they open up (the door) and move on. Most children seem to comprehend such descriptions and act, to greater or lesser degrees, on these recommendations.

Children must speak before they can change their speech   Children who stutter must be encouraged to communicate and be supported in their efforts to do so. We firmly believe than an important adjunct to therapy with this age group, indeed any age group, is to keep the clients talking and foster their attempts to communicate (cf. Johnson, 1961). Talking should be encouraged at home, at school, at play, in therapy, and any situation where verbal communication is appropriate. One of the tragedies of stuttering, when the problem goes unchanged and worsens, is that the stutterer begins to talk less and less and society begins to lose the stutterer's potentially beneficial, worthwhile, and interesting contributions.

The well-known clinical practice of having stutterers accompany their clinicians on visits to stores and shops has, as one of its goals, the maintenance and reinforcement of talking. It seems logical to assume that if the child *only* talks and practices changing their talking during the therapy session, the child has less than a favorable prognosis for improvement in speech fluency. It is much like practicing to drive only in the driver education class and in the school parking lot. (Conversely, we shouldn't practice only during the Indianapolis 500 race!) Classroom or in-therapy practice is important, but nothing can take the place of actually using the skilled behavior in the forum or situation in which it must be displayed. "Learning by doing" is at least as important to remediation of stuttering as all of our skillful and supportive in-clinic therapy procedures.

One suggestion to encourage talking in older children who stutter was made by Johnson (1961). He encouraged children to read aloud, at first to themselves, then to their mother, father, or friend. His suggestion, which I use with this age group, helps the child practice talking. The parents, after instruction, are encouraged to listen to the child and be uncritical of the child's speech fluency during the reading. The parents are to attend to the content of the child's reading; children are encouraged to read something they find interesting that can be read in three-to-five page blocks. This activity is not to take a half hour of the parent's or child's time but more like five to ten minutes every day, or at least every other day.

What the clinician, parent, or teacher want to encourage is the act of talking aloud, the physical feeling of speaking, the joy of conveying a message to attentive listeners. Fully realizing the relative intolerance of some adults for listening to oral reading, this activity is not to be undertaken by every child and his or her parents. When it is used, the clinician needs to clearly, and sometimes repeatedly, describe the purpose and procedure of this task and to maintain weekly monitoring of its progress. The clinician should not hesitate to discontinue such an assignment if it appears to be more of a hindrance than a help.

Practice

Getting children to practice outside of therapy what they demonstrate they can do during therapy is a major task for the SLP. First, the SLP must make the practice exercise or assignment something that can be done within a short period of time each day between therapy sessions. Second, the child must be helped to see or understand some reason why the homework assignment is given—busywork will seldom get done. Third, whenever possible, we should explain to parents the nature of the practice exercise and its rationale. As mentioned above, parents need to be given positive ways of responding to changes they notice in their child's speech. Fourth, partial or totally uncompleted practice assignments need to be dealt with as they occur and not allowed to become a routine occurrence. Why wasn't the assignment done? Was it too hard? easy? silly? unclear? irrelevant? Does the child have a particular place/listener, specific time each day to practice? Is the child sufficiently motivated to change? Are you a sufficient motivator (a necessary if challenging role for the SLP)? We want to make clear that allowing "homework" assignments to go undone from week to week is poor therapy and sets a poor precedent (better almost to give no "homework" than to assign exercises that are never completed, handed-in, or checked-up on). Make it clear to the child and parents that change in speech will come, but not without time and effort on their part *outside* the confines of the therapy session.

I forgot to practice One of the big problems with practice assignments is that they are handed in at the beginning of each therapy session. What more discouraging way—at least for the clinician—to start a therapy session than with the child's report, in deed or in words, that he or she forgot, was not interested in, or did want to do the assignment? Your post hoc scolding generally accomplishes very little. Conversely, neither will ignoring the situation accomplish much. Some sort of talk is in order, where you ask questions and listen to the child's answers. Try to impress upon the child the need for practice and its importance to you and the therapy program. Show that you care about the assignments' being done, but that you aren't disappointed in the child as a person. Request the child's help in carrying out the assignment. Let children know that you trust them to do the right thing, and encourage them to ask questions and raise their concerns when they feel your homework assignments are unclear, unfair, too hard, or simply meaningless to them.

Show children—actually demonstrate the assignment—before they leave therapy. Tell them the assignment requires so many minutes each and every day (a brief period every day is, in our opinion, worth much more than a long period only one day per week). Help them develop a chart they can hang up at home that allows them to check off the days and times when they did their homework. Praise them for successfully completed practice assignments; try not to accept the assignments as if it is a "you-understood" that they get completed. Show them you are pleased with their completion. Let the clients know you are proud of them and that it is important to you that they have done their assignments successfully and on time.

We really shouldn't expect sudden or dramatic change with such a complex human problem as stuttering; however, we should make every attempt to reward successive approximations to the final goal: regular successful completion of reasonable practice assignments.

Parent's Role in Modification

Sometimes, when parents observe you directly trying to modify or change their child's speech, they may ask what they can do at home to help. This is not a situation to be feared, but it is one to be dealt with in a thoughtful manner. Once again, some kind of help is the kind of help these kids can do without. For example, parents may observe our *neutral tone* suggestion to their child to change speech behavior, but attend only to the word "change" and ignore our neutral affect. Thus, parents' use of the word "change" with the child becomes nothing more than "stop that stuttering" if said by the parents (or us!) with the wrong inflection or as a means to "get at" or "pick at" the child for unwanted behavior.

We caution against parents using the same instructions we use, at least in the beginning of therapy, because we have so little control over how some of the parents will use these instructions. Our tentativeness in this area reflects the fact that we have been hampered by parents who inappropriately use our instructions, outside the clinic, to the point that when we employ them in therapy, they negatively influence the child.

Instead, we like to encourage parents to keep their child talking, to ensure that the parents try to listen to the content of the child's speech, that they not request too much speech from the child on a day when the child is obviously disfluent, and that they reinforce any and all positive *changes* in their child's speech.

The last suggestion—reinforcing changes in the child's speech—is difficult for parents to implement because it requires them to be able to detect changes, just like you, the SLP. This, of course, means training the parents to be more observant of their child's behavior and this of course means more work. It also means that parents must learn what differences in their child's speech and related behaviors make a difference in terms of long-term recovery from the problem. For example, in the beginning of therapy, this may mean helping parents observe that even though their child's frequency of stuttering remains the same, the duration of each instance of stuttering is shortening, suggesting that the child is beginning to make progress toward becoming more normally disfluent.

In a public school situation, of course, parental involvement is often very difficult because of facilities, time factors, and school policy, but in a clinic, involvement of parents is not as problematic. Perhaps this suggests that schools and local clinics could cooperate in such a way that in the beginning, when parent concerns, information sharing, and the like are most acute, the child could be managed by the clinic, but as the child progresses and parents become more facilating and less of an issue, the public school SLP could take over management of the child.

As a matter of course in our clinic, *all* parents of children who stutter must be present and observe a significant proportion of their child's therapy sessions (this is particularly true for our P/C groups). Parents, unless there is an extremely pressing reason, cannot routinely drop off their child at the clinic—like a pair of pants at the dry cleaners—go shopping, and then come back in an hour. We explain this policy kindly, clearly, but emphatically to parents *prior* to the beginning of therapy. If they decline to become so involved we give them names, addresses, and phone numbers of other agencies that they can consider. We are very desirous of having the parents know what is going on, and we want the parents to be a part of their child's remediation program. We show the parent what we mean by change in their child's speech; we have them observe the child in therapy and point out to them changes their child makes. We tell the parent that spontaneous examples of these changes at home or elsewhere outside the clinic should be praised by the parent: "Boy, Johnny that was a nice change you made there."

How to Handle Parental Observation of Therapy

It should be noted that parental observation of therapy, not unlike student-clinician observation of therapy, must be *guided* to be of any real value. If the clinician does not guide the parents' observation, tell them what behaviors and events to attend to and why, the parents may gain little real understanding from the observations other than fatigue. This procedure may require two clinicians, one managing the child and the other the parent, pointing out the therapy's strategy, procedure, and rationale, changes in clinician behavior that appear to influence changes in child behavior, and progress (or lack thereof). Two SLPs are obviously not a luxury every clinic or school system can afford. One way around this, if the parent can observe without the child being aware, is for the SLP to arrange with parents in advance certain nonverbal signals or verbal cues or codes that the parent is to listen and watch for and then attend to this or that aspect of the child's behavior.

At least in the beginning, the parent should not discuss with the child what the parent has observed in therapy. In fact, in the beginning, the parent should not tell the child that he or she is observing therapy. If the child directly asks the parents if they are watching therapy, they can say that the clinician discusses what is going on in therapy with them. With time and positive change on the part of the child, the child will probably come to realize that mom and/or dad occasionally watch therapy but this will concern them less and less. In fact, we have noticed that this lack of concern seems to closely parallel positive change in the child's speaking difficulties.

(Dis)continuing Therapy

When children do not change their speaking behavior, no matter how hard the clinician works, several things must be considered: (1) Do the individual children really understand how they are interfering with or disturbing their speech production and how, when, and where they can change these interfering behaviors? (2) Is the environment counterproductive to the child's making significant (or any) change in his or her speech disfluencies? We have had parents complain, once a child becomes significantly more fluent, that the child is talking too much and they do not like this. Some of these children may revert back to their earlier forms and frequencies of stuttering. (3) Does the child practice outside the clinic, to a sufficient degree, what you and the child do during the therapy sessions? (4) Is the child and his or her family ready, willing, and able to put in the time, effort, and energy to make the necessary changes that will facilitate the child's speech fluency? and (5) Have you adequately assessed the child's problem and sufficiently geared your therapy to the child's particular needs? These and many more questions arise when change does not occur or when change plateaus and levels off.

Perhaps this is the time for a break from therapy with all the precautions previously mentioned duly taken into consideration (Chapter 3). It may also be the time for you to reassess the client's intellectual and social skills; perhaps you have been overestimating his or her ability to quickly and clearly follow your therapy plan. It is also possible that the child's social maturity is still not at a level where he or she can independently carry out assignments at home. Perhaps these children understand the idea of change in the abstract, but when applied to their own behavior during an instance of stuttering when many things are happening rapidly and they are the least objective, they cannot apply what they actually know, feel, and can do. Perhaps, they know those behaviors that will facilitate their speech fluency but will not do them because they feel, "It won't sound like me," or "It doesn't sound or feel right." Sometimes lack of change simply comes down to the fact that it takes too much work, too often for the child to maintain or increase his or her speech fluency. In effect, the child finds it easier to stutter and/or that the costs of improved fluency outweigh the benefits. As much as we want to try to help, we must recognize that in order for anyone to be helped she or he must be capable of being helped.

We continue to encourage and support those children who do seem to be able to change. We have already mentioned the *placebo effect* in therapy; however, rather than reject this out of hand, I think that we should recognize a powerful therapeutic adjunct when we see one. Better, in my opinion, that we recognize its presence and use it for our clients' benefit than deny its existence like an ostrich with our collective clinical necks in the sand.

Nothing is to be gained by being reluctant to tell parents and child that they are doing a good job, that you see signs of positive progress, or that this was a good session, even when things are not exactly ideal. We realize that unwarranted touting and praising of a particular therapy approach has given the placebo effect a bad name (and deservedly so), but we also recognize that every clinician, either consciously or unconsciously, is involved with the components of the placebo effect in his or her therapy: (1) the beliefs and expectations of the client, (2) the beliefs and expectations of the clinician, and (3) the client and clinician relation (Beecher, 1955; Shapiro, 1964; Benson and Epstein, 1975; Benson and McCallie, 1979). We can reinforce and raise children's expectations for change by encouraging and supporting them. Likewise, the parents' feelings that change has taken place can be reinforced and supported; this in turn should help the parents try even harder to change and maintain change in themselves and their child. Nothing succeeds like success, and we can gain much by telling our clients and their parents in positive tones when they are making change, and when their efforts appear to be paying off in improved performance.

TWELVE- TO FOURTEEN-YEAR-OLD STUTTERERS: TURNING THE CORNER INTO ADOLESCENCE

The General Lay of the Land

Along the road to becoming a reasonably organized, stable adult, we all go through a period of relative disorganization and instability called adolescence. This period of personal development begins for some by 11 to 12 years of age and for most, by 14 years of age. During this period, young people find themselves in the throes of physical, social, emotional, and psychological forces and changes over which they have little control. Emotions are readily expressed and keenly felt. The strong urge to be like and to be liked by their peers many times replaces their better judgment. The here and now becomes paramount. Parents discuss the future, for example, plans for college, while the furthest into the future the teenager is thinking about is this weekend and whether the girl in third period math class will go with him to a party.

Sometimes one of the last things members of this age group may want to hear and attend to is speech therapy. The mood swings of this period make speech therapy less than a steady course of action. The young person's struggle with independence from parents reminds one of the approach-avoidance conflict previously discussed by Miller (1944) and Sheehan (1958, 1975). One minute teenagers want freedom and disassociation from parents, and the next they are asking for parental advice and support. While they clamor for the privileges of adulthood, for example, staying out late, driving a car, and drinking alcohol, they may simultaneously refuse adult responsibilities, such as taking out the trash, daily working toward a future goal, saving for the future, cutting the grass, or taking care of their rooms and their health.

Into this whirlpool of human change and disequilibrium enters the speech-language pathologist trying to help teenagers become more fluent. These clients present us with a unique challenge in terms of remediation. To begin understanding this age group, one might want to read Ginott's (1969) common-sense approach to interactions between teenagers and adults. Ginott covers many of the feelings, actions, and issues involved with being a teenager, and for this reason alone his book is worth reading.

We firmly believe that SLPs must be well grounded in the totality of the children and adults we remediate. Shames and Egolf (1976) put it better when they said, "Stuttering neither develops nor exists in a vacuum. Stuttering is a behavioral response of a living, feeling, reacting individual who is operating in some form of socially interactive system with other people." With teenagers, young teens in particular, it is crucial that the speech and language pathologist know the general bounds of that system so that he or she can successfully navigate through its pathways. Such knowledge can also be enhanced by Fraser and Perkins's (1987) booklet that is especially directed to the teenager who stutters; the teenage stutterer, his parents, and the SLP can all benefit from this booklet.

Teenagers' Interest in and Cooperation with Therapy

We have observed that sometimes adolescents do not appear particularly interested in speech therapy. Paradoxically, this disinterest in therapy may relate to the fact that teenagers are becoming acutely aware of their stuttering and themselves as speakers, and that this awareness is beginning to become increasingly emotional in nature (which is completely in keeping with teenagers' general modus operandi). They may be starting to develop real fear and avoidance of speech and speaking. Their speaking may be making an already challenging age period even more so because they may be reluctant to be outgoing and speak because of the embarrassment it will cause them. Just when they might want to become one of the gang and impress their friends (particularly those of the opposite sex), they may become shy, withdrawn, and reticent because of fears and concerns regarding their speech.

Once again, paradoxically, the last thing they may want to do is touch, see, feel, and discuss (with an SLP, or anyone else for that matter) what is bothering them the most: their speech. Of course, this is exactly what the speech and language pathologist wants them to do—confront the very thing (speech) that the teenage stutterer fears the most. Some of these clients give the impression that they will change the problem as long as (1) none of their friends know they are receiving speech therapy and (2) the therapy process involves them as passive recipients of the clinician's administrations.

Along with these concerns goes the fact that so many things are changing for adolescents. They must attend to so many different things that they may feel they have little time left over for attending to or changing their speech behavior. Perhaps, teenagers may be likened to a beginning juggler with too many clubs to juggle; some of them are going to be dropped and only picked up later when the juggler becomes more proficient at balancing many things at once.

Teenagers need adults who will be patient with them and provide them with support, yet as adults we often feel inclined to direct and scold teenagers. We find it too easy to lose our patience with teenagers' apparently flip dismissal of what we consider well thought out therapy plans or suggestions for change. Sometimes the best course of action when we face the challenge of remediating adolescents is a break from therapy where client and clinician can separate, regroup forces, and wait for a more advantageous time to resume therapy. The SLP must make it clear to teenagers, however, that therapy will resume after a period of time when *they* can apply more time, effort, and thought.

Discontinuation does not mean disregard; that is, the SLP's discontinuation of therapy should not be taken by the teen to mean that the SLP is disregarding the teen's speech problem, but that the SLP is calling time out from formal active therapeutic intervention. The SLP's decision to discontinue therapy may not be agreed to by the client and his or her parents, but periods of plateau, stabilization, or lack of forward progress in behavioral change and/or relative uncooperativeness in therapy dictate that something should be done. It is not fair to the teen nor is it good therapy practice to prolong the agony of unsuccessful treatment when a break would be a better long-range solution even though the short-term security of weekly therapy ("At least I'm doing something about my speech") is missing.

Using Other People to Assist with the Teenager's Therapy Program

Specific procedures for speech modification used with this age group are not unlike those used with clients slightly younger or older; however, with the twelve- to fourteen-year-old client, we must proceed in somewhat different ways. We need to enlist, if we can, people in the client's environment whom the client can relate to, for example, a friendly school guidance counselor, a kindly piano teacher, or a supportive mother or father. These people can be asked by the SLP to reinforce change outside the confines of therapy, to praise the client's increased amount of talking, and so on. When sufficiently informed regarding the client's problem and therapy plan, they can help monitor the client's outside-of-clinic progress. Naturally, the SLP should also ask the teenage client if the SLP may discuss with the outside person the client's speech problem, therapy plan, and progress. We have found that clients' discussion and responses in these matters are very instructive regarding their desires to conceal, cover up, or hide their problem from friends and relations (for discussion of the *interiorizing* of stuttering, see Douglass and Quarrington, 1952); the degree to which they are willing to share personal information with friends; and the degree to which discussing stuttering with anyone is a fearful, shameful or embarrassing topic.

Some teenage clients may balk at your suggestions and others will readily agree; however, it is prudent, as well as good therapy, to obey your client's desires concerning the discussion of personal matters with outside-of-clinic friends. Besides, given some time to think about it as well as the SLP's encouragement and support, many clients eventually come around to the point where they will accept the involvement of outside-of-clinic friends, particularly as they become more fluent and begin to receive the spontaneous praise of their friends for their improved speaking abilities.

Differences between Young Teenagers and Younger Children Who Stutter

As mentioned previously, a 12- to 14-year-old person who has been stuttering since say, 4 or 5 years of age, probably has a more habituated speech problem than the six-year-old who has been stuttering for only 6 to 12 months. This habituation plus the young teen's fundamental flux in development make it a challenge to change speech behavior. Lasting change, I believe, involves engaging more of the client's intellectual cooperation than his or her emotions in the change process (this is a relative increase in cognition since teenagers' emotions are something that even they find hard to dampen). Interestingly, as Ginott (1969) points out, this comes about by talking to the teenage client in a manner that conveys your understanding of some of the emotional changes and concerns the client is experiencing. It does not mean that the SLP becomes a psychoanalyst or psychotherapist, but as a professional, the SLP should have sufficient sensitivity to recognize the adolescent client's particular needs and concerns.

While the SLP is not directly involved in influencing the teenager's psychosocial-emotional behavior, the SLP should make it clear to the client that he or she appreciates the client's feelings. Perhaps it is obvious, but understanding the young teen's feelings provides the SLP with a broader perspective from which to view his or her stuttering problem. Furthermore, the SLP must search, largely through trial and error and the use of common sense, for a middle-ground of expression whereby the teenager feels neither patronized by the apparent immaturity or child-like manner of the clinician's expression nor overwhelmed and confused by high-level, sophisticated, and adult-like vocabulary and manner of clinician expression.

Some Demographics about Teenagers Who Stutter

Interestingly, little published information exists on the specific nature of the teenage stutterer's speech problem; therefore, we decided to remedy this in part by studying the characteristics of a small but representative group from our clinical population. Table 4–1 presents information for 15 stutterers in the 12- to 14-year-old age range (as usual, most of these clients are boys). Approximately two-thirds of these clients report or have clinically demonstrated speech sound articulation/phonological difficulties. A similar proportion were significantly consistent (values of 1.0 or greater; cf. Johnson, Darley, and Spriestersbach, 1963, pp. 272–76, 292) in the loci of their instances of stuttering, which suggests that there is a fairly well-established relation between certain speech-related stimuli and their instances of stuttering. Eight out of the fifteen clients produced sound/syllable repetitions as their most frequent disfluency type.

While these facts suggest that persons who are still stuttering at ages 12 to 14 are in some ways similar to those who resolve their stuttering with or without therapy before 12, these facts also suggest that their stuttering has become more consistent and that more of these teenage clients appear to have had (or still have) concomitant speech/language problems than younger stutterers. Whether this rather small sample ($N = 15$) is representative of teenage stutterers as a whole remains a question that must await future research; however, we need to keep these facts in mind as we plan our remediation programs and realize that teenage stutterers may not be merely older versions of younger stutterers.

Planning Therapy: Factors to Consider

As the data in Table 4–1 suggest, the SLP should try to determine whether concomitant language, articulation, cognition, or social concerns are evidenced by the teenager. Far too often significant problems in other areas are overlooked or overshadowed by the SLP's focus on the client's stuttering (we'll give an actual example of this in Chapter 6). A significant problem in any of these related areas may dictate that the concomitant problem, and not stuttering, should be evaluated in greater detail and, if appropriate, remediated initially.

TABLE 4–1.   Descriptive information regarding a sample of older children and teenagers who stutter (N = 15). Clients were selected because of their representativeness of this age group of stutterers whom the current author has evaluated and remediated. Significantly consistent stuttering determinations were based on the Iowa Measure of Stuttering Consistency (Johnson and others, 1963). Presence of speech articulatory disorder resulted from either reported histories of three or more sounds in error or actual observation by the present writer of such a disorder; these data relative to articulatory problems are, therefore, considered preliminary and in need of further, more refined and controlled analysis.

Stutterings per 100 words spoken
Mean   16.5
Range   1.0 to 43.0

Stuttering Severity Level
Mean   3.5
Range   1.0 to 6.0

Disfluency Type
Most Frequently Produced by Most Clients: Part-word repetitions (8 of 15 clients)
Least Frequently Produced by Most Clients: Part-word repetitions (7 of 15 clients)

Child's Age at Time of Initial Evaluation
Mean   13.6 years
Range   12.2 to 14.8 years

Sex of Child
Male   14
Female   1

Child's Position in Family
First   7/15
Second   3/15
Third   3/15
Fourth   2/15

Presence of Speech Articulation Disorder
10/15

Significantly Consistent Stuttering
10/15

Source: Iowa Scale for Rating Severity of Stuttering (Johnson and others, 1963).

Assessing the teen client's past therapy record   The SLP should make every attempt to assess the teenage client's past record in terms of speech therapy. For example, did he or she already receive three years of public school therapy to no apparent avail? Why does the teenager think or feel that this therapy was of little help? Why do you think previous therapy was unsuccessful? Likewise, has this person received two years of articulation therapy only now to be referred to you for a "stuttering problem"? What was the nature of this former articulation therapy? Are the "problem sounds" (that is, sounds in error) that were concentrated on in the articulation therapy the sounds the teenager now stutters upon? What role did the parents have in changing clinicians or therapy agencies? Do the client and/or parents blame previous therapy and therapists for the client's lack of progress?

Clinicians who ignore history are bound to repeat it We sometimes think that a client's past failure or relative failure was due to poor therapy else-where or a misevaluated case. However, many times these failures are just as much due to the client, his or her particular problem, relatives and/or associ-ates, or some combination of all three. Thus, a client of this age group who is referred to you for evaluation and assistance should be carefully assessed by *you*, and all such background questions should be asked. If the client's atten-dance record was poor and you know this for a fact, you should discuss it directly with the client and the parents *before* you begin therapy. At the risk of redundancy, we cannot help repeating (and slightly changing) Santayana's famous remark that those who ignore history (or a client's history of thera-peutic progress) are destined to repeat it themselves (see Van Riper, 1970, and Rieber, 1977, for an overview of historical perspectives on stuttering therapy).

Attempting to discern typical from atypical problems It will help if you try to decide whether the teenager's presenting problems, for example, withdrawal from social events, reluctance to use the phone, or meet new friends, are more related to teenagers' typical "disorganization" or to his or her stuttering. Realistically, we seldom can make such fine distinctions, but by trying to do so we give the client every benefit of the doubt so that we are less eager and willing to label each and every one of his or her problems as those *typical* of a stutterer. Simply put, some of the teenage stutterer's problem will have little to do with stuttering but everything to do with his or her unique personal characteristics as well as being a teenager. Our knowledge of typical teenage mood and personality swings and quirks should also help us explain the client to his or her parents (conversely, the SLP's knowledge of parent-child interaction should help in translating "parentalese" to the teenager). Particu-larly today, with the dissolution of the extended family, when grandmothers and grandfathers do not live at home and are not available to routinely provide parents with perspective, parents tend to think that they and their child are the only ones with these problems. You can help if you strive to deepen your understanding of typical teen concerns so that you can begin to explain them to parents, if the need arises. Obviously, you do not want to be too optimistic about this and will want to identify any real problems relating to the teen's stuttering that need your attention.

Teens need adult support not adults posing as peers, or, understanding where teens are coming from does not mean you have to come from the same place yourself Try not to fall into the trap of becoming a buddy, compatriot, groovy or cool friend, or the like. Teenagers need and want adult guidance, help, and counsel. They learn as much from your model as from all your words (Bettelheim, 1985). This, as in most things, requires moderation. While you do not want to be too authoritative like a Marine Corps drill instructor who coldly and loudly barks out orders and assignments, neither do you want to be too chummy and essentially deny your adult experience, dignity, and maturity as well as professional training in a mad rush to relate like a teenager to the teenager who stutters. The posture of a chum or teenage-like buddy is easier for older, more experienced clinicians to avoid than those in their twenties who most vividly remember their teens; however, it is not unusual to see forty-year-olds act like teenagers themselves in order to relate better to their teenage clients. Understanding where your teenage clients are coming from is not the same thing as trying to come from the same place yourself.

The SLP does the guiding, the client does the walking   Most importantly, make it as clear as you can to the teenager that you are the *guide* and he or she is the person who must do the *walking* (that is, work). Promises of quick cures and fantastic overnight changes are what everybody, particularly the uncertain teen, appears to want, but nothing in the long run is more debilitating to the client than the subsequent reality that they were misled. Sad, but true, instant fluency, like Cinderella's coach and gown, frequently disappears at the stroke of midnight. Easy come, in this case, will all too often be easy go.

I realize that stutterers and their families are not going to like what I have to say. However, they must realize their definite role in fostering therapies that claim quick cures. While charlatans may know in advance that their fast fluency therapies produce only temporary, albeit dramatic, changes in stuttering, all too often the lay public seems far too eager to believe and shell out their hard-earned money. Obviously, these charlatans are telling the public what the public wants to hear because if they weren't, these charlatans would quickly go out of business. Professional groups should certainly be taking a leadership role in eradicating the therapies of the charlatans and mountebanks; however, professional organizations can't do it all themselves. As long as the public continues to patronize these therapies in hopes of receiving the silver bullet to "cure" their stuttering *without* any real or active attempts on their part to make long-term changes in behavior, these fast fluency therapies will be encouraged to develop and multiply. Our only hope is developing a more educated, knowledgeable, and sophisticated public who will, *before beginning therapy,* ask themselves questions, as well as question the so-called authority about his or her claims. This same public especially needs to scrutinize claims that the changes resulting from fast fluency therapies will last longer than a week or two.

Contrary to the fast fluency, silver bullet forms of therapy, we try to help the teenager understand his or her *active* role in changing his or her own speech. We try to explain to our teenagers (and adult clients) and their parents that we are a bit like a person guiding a tour on which the clients and their parents are about to embark. We say that we will facilitate their trip and point out salient aspects for their consideration along the way, but they are the ones who must do the considering, walking, and touring. It is they who must pay attention to the landmarks we point out and think about what they mean to them. We tell them that we cannot and will not carry them on our backs but will, on occasion, let them lean on us for support. If they refuse to go down trails we think are important, we cannot (and will not) force them. We are guides not magicians: We point out ways and means for them to change, but we cannot make their problems disappear into thin air. We are not behavioral alchemists brewing up potions to turn their stuttering into Walter Cronkite fluency without any effort on their part.

Obviously, the concept of being a guide versus magician is not one that makes the client and parent particularly comfortable because it will undoubtedly mean more work on their part. However, we must say it in as honest and straightforward fashion as we can muster. I think that it is this honesty and directness that convinces and motivates people to try to help themselves. We try to show that we believe that the teen, with sufficient guidance, can and will change and that we trust him or her to put out the necessary effort and spend the needed time to make these changes. Indeed, we have to trust the teen because if he or she is not going to make these changes, who will?

When to Begin and When Not to Begin Therapy

We think it best to begin speech therapy with young (as well as older) teens when they begin to show signs of wanting to actively participate in therapy and have reached some degree of emotional, psychological, and social stability. It is probably true that every day these clients continue to stutter makes their stuttering behavior that much more habituated and difficult to change. However, initiating therapy when a teen is clearly not ready is courting clinical failure and frustration. We would prefer that a client actually says to his or her parents, "Dad, I'd like to get some help with my speech," rather than the SLP and parents deciding *for* (rather than with) the client that now is the time, regardless of whether the teen is willing to begin remediation.

With teens (and most clients for that matter) we need to be patient and exhibit trust in the clients' ability to recognize when they are ready for speech therapy. However, this is not to say that some friendly, gentle but firm coaxing and persuading might not benefit a teenager who is a bit uncertain or hesitant to begin therapy. Friendly, gentle persuasion, however, is not the same as threats and browbeating ("If you don't get help, you can't drive the car") into resuming or initiating therapy. Speech therapy that begins when a teenage client is not ready (or is diametrically opposed to it) may leave a nearly indelible mark that subsequent clinicians may be unable to remove regardless of the strength of their therapeutic cleanser. While such therapy may not "make them worse," it may turn them off so badly from the therapeutic process that they want little to do with it, even though they may still need it.

Objectively Changing Speech Behavior

When teenagers are ready to receive speech therapy, it is important to indicate from the beginning that you know that with time and effort on their part change is possible. It is helpful to demonstrate to clients in the first therapy session or two that they are capable of changing their speech, if only temporarily. It also helps if you can make some of your therapy procedure objective and make some of the abstract concepts regarding speech production and change a bit more tangible.

Making speech "visible": The basic concept   An audio tape recorder or even a video tape recorder with a needle deflector or bar indicator VU meter can be used for a variety of clinical purposes. First, you can record the teenager's stuttering while speaking or reading and then play back the recorded tape. The VU meter—whether the needle or bar kind—can be used to show the client the objective difference in vocal level or intensity between her or his stuttered and fluent utterances. You should probably practice this a few times by yourself with a previously recorded sample of stuttered speech so that you can readily and quickly discern instances of stuttering and how changes in the VU meter correlate to instances of stuttering and comparable instances of fluency. An even better way of doing this is with desktop computers and such inexpensive (under U.S. $200) software/hardware devices as the Speech Thing/Voice Master (CoVox, Inc., 675 Conger St., Eugene, Oregon, 97402; Telephone: 503–342–1271). This particular device allows the SLP to quickly and easily digitally record and play back to the client his/her speech utterance; more importantly, it can be used as a digital oscilloscope displaying in real time (that is, as it is happening) changes in the client's vocal level or intensity or loudness over time. This provides immediate feedback to the client that his or her speech is different during a stuttered versus fluent utterance.

As a general rule, *during* a sound that is stuttered (whether prolonged or repeated), the VU meter indicates a *lower* than usual or minimal vocal intensity level. This may tell us one of a number of things, but our research suggests two types of laryngeal behavior associated with this low level meter reading: (1) very closely approximated or adducted vocal folds or (2) widely separated or abducted vocal folds (Conture, McCall and Brewer, 1977; Conture, Schwartz and Brewer, 1985). At the *end* of the stuttered sound or as the stutterer makes the transition into the following *fluent* sound, you may notice either a temporary surge of relatively high level speech reading and/or erratic, normal to relatively high level speech. That is, *during* the stuttering itself the VU meter will often give a *low* reading but at the *end* of the stuttering, as the stutterer makes the laryngeal/articulatory adjustments to move into the following fluent sound, the VU meter will suddenly and sometimes erratically "redline" as the stutterer apparently uses more vocal level "to get it out."

The specific nature of these speaking behaviors need not be discussed with your young client, but you can discuss the fact that he or she may actually become softer when stuttering. Teenagers can be shown the difference between the relatively soft levels associated with stuttering and the more normal (around "0" on the VU meter) as well as louder (above "0" or in the redline area of the VU meter) levels associated with normally fluent speech. Clients can come to realize that it is *their* behavior that is causing the needle deflector to move up and down, go into the redline area, or stay near the bottom or hover around "0." In other words, they can be helped to understand that it is *they* who are stopping their forward movement of speech production, in one way or another, when they stutter.

Making speech "visible": Learning how to change The needle deflector or bar graph VU meter can be used to help the client understand the idea of moving on to the next sound. (The newer, relatively inexpensive digital devices such as the Speech Thing/Voice Master have tremendous potential in this regard.) For example, clients can be instructed to maintain a tight constriction of their lips during the isolated production of /b/ in the word "bee" while watching the VU meter. The VU meter in this case would probably indicate a very low level of vocal intensity. The client would then be gently told to "open up" (to "change") and "move on" to the next sound, say /i/, while still watching the VU meter. As he or she opens his or her lips and articulatorily moves on, the needle will quickly move from the bottom to the top (the green or similar color lights on the bar graph indicator quickly move up into the orange or red area), indicating a sudden rise in vocal intensity that he or she produced by making the appropriate adjustments in speech production behavior.

Through the use of the VU meter, we are trying to help these clients understand that they influence the way they speak and that they can change the way they speak with the appropriate amount and kind of attention and effort on their part. Remember during these types of activities to ensure that the client keeps a relatively constant mouth-to-microphone distance. Otherwise, unpredictable changes in mouth-to-microphone distance will be the cause of changes in the VU meter and not the clients' behavior. A relatively inexpensive tie-tack (for example, Realistic Model 33–1063) or lavalier microphone clipped onto the client's shirt collar or thereabouts will minimize this problem.

Tape recorders as a means, not an end   One major caution in all of this: instruct teenagers (and adults) that the tape recorder is only a means to an end and that it is *not the end.* That is, you are using the VU meter only as a means to help them visualize what is going on when they speak, when they change their speech behavior, or when they work on using more appropriate means of initiating and maintaining speech production. The VU meter is a means to help them *focus on the physical feelings* associated with their speech behavior. It is the *physical feelings* of fluent and disfluent speech (and changes between the two) that they need to attend to. We like to tell them that by watching a visual representation of their acoustic speech output, they can more quickly and accurately attend to and focus on these physical feelings within their vocal tract. If clients are not given these sorts of cautions and instructions, they may become dependent upon the tape recorder or any device used to objectify or feed back what they are doing when they speak. Periodically, turn the tape recorder off or block their view of the VU meter, and observe whether they can do as well without it.

Weaning clients right from the start of their need to rely on such instrumental assistance is very important in establishing the all-important transition between in- *and* outside-of-clinic changes in behavior. This "weaning" is necessary to the development of sufficient carryover of clinical changes to everyday conversation. The young and older client must clearly realize that he or she won't have the VU meter handy when he gives a book report to his English class, asks a girl out for a date, or talks to friends on the phone. Instead, the client must be told by you and come to realize that the VU meter is a means to help him concentrate on his speech and the physical feelings associated with fluent and disfluent aspects of it. (For actual examples of "biofeedback" approaches with stutterers, see Guitar, 1975; for discussion of pros and cons of biofeedback with young stutterers, see Adams, Guitar and Conture, 1979.)

Making speech "visible": Learning easier onsets   The VU meter can be used with teenagers to show them how to make appropriate vocal initiations and transitions. We begin with clients watching the VU meter while we demonstrate a very gradual or "easier" (slower with less physical tension) onset of voicing on a vowel like /i/ or /a/. We point out to the client the relative slowness of onset and the gradualness of initiation. We are trying to help them unlearn what appears to be a problem for stutterers: getting going! While some claim that stutterers begin speaking too fast and with too much physical tension, there are few data to support or refute this contention. We think that this may be a problem but until more data are published in refereed journals, we'll have to reserve judgment.

Helping the teen distinguish between categorical and continuous forms of speech production We think that some stutterers exhibit difficulty going from one vocal state to another easily and smoothly. They seem to want to move abruptly from one vocal posture to another—like going from black to white, night to day, without any shades of gray or twilight or dawn. They appear to want to hop from sound to sound rather than smoothly make the necessary articulatory transition (the in-between "sound") from one sound to the next. Stutterers' apparent tendency toward abrupt, almost categorical (discrete state to discrete state), rather than continuous (discrete state-transition-discrete state) forms of speech production are particularly noted during their initiation of speech. It appears that any place in the utterance where change must be made, whether voiceless to voiced, voiced to voiceless, voiced to voiced, and so forth, is a site where a stutterer may try to move from one state to another *without* the necessary transition (this is a bit like the frog in Chapter 3 attempting to hop from lily pad to lily pad *without* going through the air). It is unclear whether these transitions between sounds are inherently difficult for the stutterer to produce or whether the stutterer has learned, for whatever reasons, to exhibit such difficulties.

Whatever the case, the inappropriateness or lack of these transitions must be emphasized to the client. The client needs to learn how to employ different speech production strategies. One such strategy involves helping the stutterer understand that a word-initial sound can be initiated *without* abrupt, physically tense onsets of respiratory, laryngeal, and supraglottal activity. No matter what the real or perceived time pressures in the communicative situation, stutterers can initiate speaking with an appropriate gesture that moves them from the silence of being a listener to the vocalization of a speaker.

Transitions between sounds can be shown on the tape recorder in such a fashion that teenagers can understand that they must open and move on to become more fluent. The use of cursive writing helps them get the idea that whether they are continuing (prolonging) or reiterating (repeating) a speech posture, they must make movement transitions between letters (or sounds) for their writing (or speech) to look (or sound) smooth. On the tape recorder, the VU meter will probably be at a low level and look stationary during a sound prolongation and then make a rapid change up or down as the client moves into the next sound. The needle will stay relatively still for the prolonged sound but make a quick movement up or down during the transition between the prolonged sound and the subsequent sound. With the rapid technological development of a variety of physiological sensing devices, for example, the electroglottograph, it is already becoming possible for the SLP to more quickly and accurately show the client his or her speech behavior than with an audio tape recorder (see Childers and Krishnamurthy, 1984, for review; see Adams, Freeman and Conture, 1984; Colton and Conture, in press; Conture, Rothenberg and Molitor, 1986; Rothenberg, 1981; Rothenberg and Mahshie, 1988, for examples of application to stutterers as well as procedural/analytical considerations). For the present, the audio tape recorder can be used for a variety of purposes besides recording and playing back of speech, but the SLP should be continually evaluating the rapidly developing technology in this area that promises to influence many of our current clinical practices.

Motivating Client to Make Speech Changes

Emphasize activity rather than the actor   Besides helping clients make the preceding changes in their speech, we must remember to encourage and support them in making these changes. This is done, at least in part, by praising, positively reinforcing, rewarding, and congratulating them for their attempts at changing their behavior. According to Ginott (1969), it is important with teenagers to emphasize events rather than personalities. If the teen makes a nice change in his speech, let him know—"That was a nice change, Tom," rather than, "You've become a good talker." Emphasize activity and not the actor. Make your praise emphatic, be demonstrative in your praise (but not ridiculously so), and use positive emotional tones in your speech, "That was a *good* change, Tom." Tom may not do much but look at you when you say this, but emphatically stated praise for his acts will help him develop the confidence and willingness to work at as well as make change in his speech. The teenage client should, hopefully, come to value your descriptions of his behavior and appreciate your praise. Keep your descriptions and praise focused, as much as you can, on his behavior and try, as best you can, to avoid evaluating and criticizing him as a person.

Sometimes even your best may not be good enough   If, after several sessions, a teenage client does not make change or does not seem to be moving in a positive direction, reevaluate your therapy procedure and the client's parents' role. Parents can make or break an SLP's best laid plans, so you should assess whether your client's parents have a contributing role in the client's lack of therapy progress. Sometimes these teenage-parent problems are so pervasive and complex that family counseling or individual psychotherapy is the only alternative. However, it is quite important to avoid a rush to judgment here because the teenage years can be normally difficult for many. Just because there are friction, fighting, and disagreements at home does not necessarily mean that the teen and his family need psychotherapy.

It behooves the SLP to recognize psychosocial problems in the teenage stutterers he or she remediates and to make appropriate referrals. For example, *frequent* reports by the client or her parents that she stays up all night, cannot sleep, is giving away a number of her valued or cherished possessions, or that she does not seem to be at all interested in food should be thoroughly investigated. Referring the client for psychological services may be warranted if these problems seem frequent and consistent. Such referrals, we hasten to add, will many times be rejected by the client and parents. It is therefore important that you only make such referrals after careful study of the case and the facts. Try not to be confused between *your* (or that of the parents) discomfort with dealing with a typically taciturn teenager (Parent: "Where have you been?" Teen: "Outside." Parent: "What did you do?" Teen: "Nothing.") and the teenager whose concerns are other than those that are typical of an adolescent.

Practice and/or Carryover of Change

Once clients exhibit an ability to make change on isolated sounds, syllables, or words, you should begin to test their ability to make these changes in more *realistic* speaking situations. As any clinician can tell you, however, finding such realistic situations is very difficult. Typically, clinicians take their clients around to other individuals in the building where therapy takes place or into nearby stores or shops. These activities, if not closely monitored, can degenerate into a series of coffee breaks where the client and clinician come to relate to one another in a most cordial, but therapeutically nonproductive, manner (once in awhile this is fine but as a routine event it is a waste of precious therapy time). Phone calls may also be used to help the client practice changes, but this, too, becomes difficult if the clinician shares a phone with others or does not even have a phone and must borrow someone else's.

Advance planning for "road trips" One secret to the realistic speaking situation is advance planning. Before taking clients into a store or shop, we should plan which ones, what is going to be purchased, requested, or inquired about, and to whom the client may be talking. It is a wise policy to discuss in advance with the store employees what you want to do and when and what you will be doing. These businesses/employees are generally willing to help as long as it does not take too much of their time and does not interfere with the routine running of their establishment. Prepare them for the client and his or her problem and ensure that the client asks a simple question such as, "When do you close?" or "How much does this cost?" Be sure to thank them for their cooperation (make it clear to them how much help they have been) and you will likely be welcomed back again with other clients. People generally want to do the right thing if they know what is expected of them and get a little praise for their efforts.

Conducting and evaluating outside assignments Besides advance planning, it is wise to make these activities reasonably short and to the point. Instead of ten phone calls, three may do, especially if they are well-prepared for and each one is immediately assessed in terms of accuracy and correctness of production. Explain to the client why you think he or she hesitated on the phrase-initial sound of the phrase, "What time do you close?" For example, specifically tell him or her that, "You went back to your old way of talking when you began. You first took a deep breath and then held it with your tongue pressed hard against the roof of your mouth" or "You held your vocal cords tightly together," or "You pressed your lips tightly together," or some combination of two or three of these events. Explain and then *show* the client ("show don't tell") what is necessary to initiate that sound smoothly and easily and to smoothly make the transition between sounds. Praise the teen for his or her effort and encourage the client to try again.

Obviously, this much a priori planning and post hoc assessment take time, but it is time well spent. Try not to let the client just go through the motions of talking to strangers over the phone or in stores, but explain to the client when and why he or she was not successful (or was successful) during a particular outside activity. Sometimes it is very instructive to the teen (and adult client) to role-play the situation several times before it actually occurs outside the clinic.

When interacting with a teenager, try to concentrate on the event, the behavior, the activity, and not the personality of the client. For the stranger's (for example, a store employee) sake, try to keep her or his verbal interactions with the client to a minimum. Simple statements that can be answered with either a yes or no response or a short one- to three-word phrase are best. Furthermore, these rather simple, brief statements give the client more control over the speaking situation and minimize elaborate discussions on the part of the client and listener. The emphasis here is on the *quality* rather than the *quantity* of the client's talking. Physically easy, somewhat slower initiations of the word-initial sound are generally, but not exclusively, the item of main import. Try not to allow the client to be continually unsuccessful with the exercise; back up and reevaluate: Is this task too advanced? Have we prepared the client sufficiently? Don't be reluctant to demonstrate repeatedly for the client what you want done and then encourage him or her to do it once more.

The use of the phone in outside assignments   Personally, we prefer the use of the phone as an "outside assignment" since it can be done in the school, home, or clinic and allows the client to experience brief but realistic communicative situations. (Teens understand the phone as an "outside" activity since it is one of the means they have at home of "escaping" parental supervision. That is, parents of most teenagers are familiar with the frequent as well as long phone conversations their teenagers conduct, conversations that allow the teen to be "outside" the home and away from parental supervision while at the same time placating parents by not physically leaving the house.)

Unfortunately, not every SLP has access to a phone, and using the phone costs money. We need to lobby for the use or availability of a phone as part of our professional apparatus; indeed, I would like to see phone companies develop special, low-budget phone services for the SLP that would allow unlimited local phone calls and would provide outlets for the recording of these calls for future study by the client and the SLP. The latter might be impossible since it could be construed as an invasion of privacy, but the former could be easily developed and designed for the exclusive use of SLP's working with teenage and adult stutterers. Making our therapy procedures as similar as possible to those of the outside world makes our chances for successful carryover that much greater. In the the next chapter we further discuss the use of phones with adult stutterers and how procedures like the Relaxation Response (Benson, 1976) in conjunction with our change-of-speech procedure can be used effectively to help the adult stutterer use the phone more successfully when he or she wants to do so.

Difficulties Gauging Changes in Speech

Carryover of inside-clinic change to the everyday world is particularly difficult to assess. That is, we cannot be sure that the significant increase in fluency we observe in the clinic is similarly produced outside the clinic because the speaking situations are so different. This difficulty is in part the reason for the previously mentioned store and restaurant visits; however, even these visits are a bit artificial because the SLP tags along with the clients when they go into the store or sits next to them when they use the phone. These are nice approximations to reality but they aren't reality. Simply put, they are less than adequate for the purposes of assessing the teenage client's ability to use changes during everyday communicative stress.

The need for a fluency stress test   This problem is a bit like the one experienced by doctors when they listen to and measure (electrocardiographically) the activity of the heart while the person quietly sits or rests. These tests may indicate a normally functioning heart whereas the same procedures used while the patient is undergoing physical stress may indicate cardiac difficulties. We need the stuttering equivalent of a physician's cardiovascular stress test: How does the stutterer's speech hold up under conditions similar to those the person finds himself or herself speaking in? The Stocker Probe test (Stocker, 1976) is a step in the right direction of assessing the stutterer's speech under speaking conditions that approximate everyday speaking situations. The well-known Job Task/Home Town procedure (Johnson and others, 1963) is another attempt to obtain speech similar to that used outside the clinic and Thompson's (1983) "survey" of parents' and teachers' observations of the child outside the clinic was developed for similar reasons. This problem—having a meaningful way to assess the client's everyday communication—is one that deserves serious attention and one that makes our therapy carryover procedures difficult to assess.

Related Concerns: Academics, Social Life, and Employment

What may be true for the group is not true for the individual There are numerous references indicating that stutterers are essentially the same as normally fluent speakers in terms of a variety of emotional, social, psychological, and physiological parameters (see Van Riper, 1971; Bloodstein, 1987; Perkins, 1970; Sheehan, 1970b). The SLP should remember, however, that these findings pertain to stutterers as a group. For any one individual stutterer (perhaps the very one the SLP is currently servicing), they may be invalid. Thus, we can expect to observe older children and teenagers who may have significant problems in schoolwork, socializing, and so forth. We should not assume that the other problems exist, but we should be aware of the possibility and if they manifest themselves, plan accordingly. Hierarchical arrangements may need to be made whereby concentrated attention to school problems takes priority over speech therapy for stuttering. Parents and their children should not be expected to attend six different professional settings on a weekly basis. Unfortunately, all too often we are not knowledgeable about these other areas of concern, professional services, or extracurricular activities.

Sometimes, of course, people familiar with the child, including yourself, will decide that the child's stuttering is central to other problems and that with remediation of his or her stuttering the other problems will improve. This is fine and we have seen it happen; however, it is up to you, the SLP, to see to it that business does not go on as usual with all other professional activities as well as extracurricular ones—especially if these other professional services all require that the client take an *active* role in changing behavior or learning new skills.

How many balls do we think the teenager can successfully juggle? The client and parents can only do (and be expected to do) so much. We need to allow the client some free time to think, day dream, and rest. None of us would try to simultaneously learn golf, tennis, squash, sailing, and plumbing; and yet we seem to expect similar types of abilities from teens who simultaneously receive speech therapy, reading remediation, special physical education classes, tutoring in math in addition to regular schoolwork, baseball practices/games, Boy Scouts, and tuba lessons.

Teenage stutterers' concerns regarding future employment shouldn't mean that their SLP must become an employment counselor Employment concerns of teenage stutterers and their parents are many times very serious and need consideration. The two best sources for such services are school guidance counselors or a local rehabilitative counselor. Why, we may ask, is a fourteen-year-old concerned with employment? Generally speaking, the employment concern centers on future, rather than present, employment. The

SLP can provide such professionals, for example, the guidance counselor, with the status and prognosis of the teen's speech problem, and he or she in turn can provide you with information regarding the client's (and parents') employment aspirations. Ideally, you may receive information regarding the client's abilities to do those things he or she professes to want to do for a future job. You must realize that your input into these matters may influence other professionals in their decisions, and thus you need to carefully consider the firmness and accuracy of the data/observations from which you will draw your conclusions.

Whatever the case, avoid getting into employment counseling with the parents and teen in anything other than general terms. Refer, as much as possible, to appropriate counsel in these matters, and keep in touch with that counsel and offer information, copies of reports, and the like. Your job is to diagnose and remediate speech and language and to be cognizant of those events that pertain to these activities. Conversely, it is not your job to help the client determine and find employment best suited for him or her.

In extreme cases, however, there may be a need for SLP counseling to handle the teen's and parents' reasonable employment aspirations; this counseling may have to take place prior to speech therapy. Of course, when employment aspirations are in line with the client's skills and these aspirations seem to be the client's prime motivator for coming in for speech therapy, it may be appropriate to mention these aspirations occasionally. This should help maintain therapy interest through discussion of how speech change will make these employment goals more or less possible. Under no circumstances, however, should the SLP say in effect (no matter how tempting it will be to do so), "You can't expect to become a lawyer [clinical psychologist, politician, and so forth] if you aren't going to work any harder than that at changing your speech." This is an obvious negative evaluation of the teen's personality. More importantly, this is also probably harassing the client in the same way that his or her parents do.

Teenage stutterers with apparent psychosocial concerns Sometimes the teen who stutters appears to, or is reported to, have psychosocial concerns (once again, listeners should not confuse teenage stutterers' supposed concerns with their own level of emotional discomfort or uneasiness felt while listening to the teen stutterer). For example, one thirteen-year old we managed began to act out in class as well as against his parents. He stuttered quite severely, and it seemed that the only way he could get people to listen to him, to pay him some attention (using the axiom that any attention is better than no attention at all), was to misbehave. His stuttering made little change in therapy, and psychological services were recommended to the parents. They declined such services, insisting his only problem was stuttering. (They were partially right; stuttering was a problem, but it clearly was neither his only nor most important one.) They changed their minds, however, when he set fire to his sister's bedroom.

Obviously, not all cases are this dramatic or clear cut, but we need to be aware of their possible occurrence and be prepared to deal with them. Once again, and at the risk of being redundant, the emotional discomfort exhibited by the teenage stutterer when stuttering and that of his listeners should not be misconstrued; the SLP should avoid making a rush to judgment regarding the teen's level of psychosocial adjustment. Most of these reactions on the part of the teen are normal reactions to an abnormal situation, that is, being unable to move forward during speech production.

Sometimes, as Robinson (1964) discussed, all these children may need is the companionship and attention of a significant adult; for some this is an older male, and for others an older female, while for others the gender of the adult is not as important as the adult's personality and warmth. Other times we may need to spend considerable time discussing the mocking and ridiculing these children receive from their peers. It is not uncommon for parents to report, during an initial diagnostic, their concern regarding "other children's reactions to his speech behavior. . .these other children's reactions to his stuttering may have a negative influence on him."

Dealing with the negative comments of peers and other people   These concerns should be dealt with and discussed by the SLP because they are one major reason these children come to avoid talking to others, avoid situations where they may have to talk with others, and in general withdraw from social interactions. While these avoidances and withdrawals may be a normal reaction to an abnormal situation, they nevertheless interfere with these youngsters' development. Telling the teen and his parents to ignore these taunts, jeers, and wisecracks is about as effective as telling you to disregard the negative comments you get from friends and relatives when you have just gotten a new hair style.

Instead of ignoring the comments of other children and adults, the child and parents need to (1) understand why certain people make such comments (the other people actually have a problem, not the stutterer) and (2) how to say something, perhaps slightly humorous, that will defuse the situation and stop the ridicule; for example, "Sometimes my talking will be interrupted due to technical difficulties!" Such concerns, which are the everyday stock and trade of the SLP who remediates stutterers, need to be differentiated from the psychosocial concerns stemming from psychoneurotic problems. To paraphrase an old saying, we need to understand those things we can help with (and change), those things we cannot, and hopefully be able to recognize the difference between the two.

Other concerns exhibited by teenagers who stutter   Reading concerns, language delays, and learning disabilities also occur in this group (stutterers have just as much right to have these other problems as you and I). Learning disabilities is an area where, admittedly, controversy still exists but more is becoming known. In Chapter 2 we mentioned ADD in children—a problem frequently associated with learning disabilities—but it is possible that this problem could also occur with older children and teens who stutter.

The learning disability (LD) specialist and yourself, if you both treat the same child, must come to terms with the significant problems of the child (and his or her family) and try to decide which needs the most immediate attention. Furthermore, you may have to do much in-service training in this area, discussing the knowns and unknowns about stuttering with the LD specialist. Obviously, a child with a learning disability who is finding school a difficult place to succeed and who also stutters is a child with a complex problem, but that may be the reality of the situation. Whatever the case, as an SLP you should try to say nothing to the child and parents that either raises false hopes regarding cures for stuttering or gives an overly pessimistic, hopeless, or inaccurate picture regarding the problem and its origins. Communication between professions is particularly crucial for both client and the involved professionals, especially if the child has several concurrent problems. Such communication can result in a better understanding of each other's profession as well as mutual respect between professions. Other concerns, like language, phonology, or reading, may also need more immediate attention than stuttering, and it is important for the SLP to understand this and set priorities for remediation accordingly. The severity and nature of these problems will dictate, to a large degree, whether they can be treated simultaneously with stuttering or whether one will need to be dealt with before the other.

Maintaining contact with the family physician   The older child's or teen's family doctor or pediatrician should, if the parents so decide, at least receive a copy of your initial evaluation, findings, and recommendations. If reevaluations and therapy are planned, it is also wise to inform the physician. As previously mentioned, although there is always a risk that other professionals may misread (or not read), misinterpret, or poorly understand our communications, they can generally tell when another professional knows what they are about and is proceeding in a reasonable, prudent, and cautious manner. Nothing ventured is nothing gained in these matters, and it is good clinical policy to let the family's main health professional, the doctor, know of your findings and plans for remediation. This is particularly important when you have decided that speech therapy is contraindicated and/or some other professional services seem more appropriate. Furthermore, if the referral comes from the doctor, you are ethically bound to send him or her information regarding your findings (unless, of course, the parents refuse permission).

Maintaining contact with school personnel   While perhaps obvious, school personnel are another group of professionals who need to be considered. Far too often SLPs in clinics fail to communicate with school personnel regarding individual clients and vice versa. The excuse that both groups are "too busy" to communicate is no excuse. While it may take longer than usual because of the differing time schedules of clinics and schools and large caseloads of both, the SLP must take the time to confer with school personnel about individual clients. Our experience with these interactions is that the client typically benefits and our therapy is more effective when all interested parties know what is going on and what they can do to help.

Many times school personnel see the child almost as much as the parents do and certainly more than an SLP in private practice or in a clinic. An experienced school teacher, administrator, guidance counselor, or nurse can often provide you with information and insights that the child and his or her parents cannot. Conversely, some of these personnel may have what we call *long ears* and hear problems when none exist.

We have had situations where every year a particular nursery school or public school teacher sends us a child who stutters. This would not mean much except when you realize that the teacher may only have one class of 25 students every year. Highly coincidental we might say, but experience indicates that these individuals—be they teachers, principals, or other school personnel—probably knew or were related to a stutterer when they were younger or that they have extraordinarily high standards for fluent, articulate verbal expression (and aren't afraid to let children know of their standards). Phone calls, letters, and memos to them explaining the problem of stuttering and what a classroom teacher can do to help should be of assistance. We do not send literature (for example, Ainsworth and Fraser, 1988) until we feel the individual has some basic understanding of the problem. This is because I believe that observations and readings in new areas of information should be a priori guided to be of maximum benefit and the individual should demonstrate some willingness to read and learn. Teachers can become powerful allies to the SLP in his or her remediation of an older child's or teen's stuttering problem; however, allies, like anything that should grow with time, must be cultivated, and developed through continued interactions. We never said any of this was going to be easy.

SOME PARTING THOUGHTS

Clinician as guide, not curer   This chapter shows that older children and teenagers who stutter present a variety of issues to consider in the planning and implementation of therapy. The issue of objective versus subjective awareness of stuttering must be dealt with and appreciated for successful remediation to take place. We have seen with this age group that it is particularly important for SLPs to realize that they not only help and guide people in the changing of their own behavior but that the SLP also must motivate them to want to change that behavior. We have discussed impressing client and parents with our role as guide rather than curer (or magician or wondrous healer) but that this must be done by the SLP in a positive manner, one that explicitly conveys that the client is capable of changing and that the clinician can help in this process.

Objective awareness before speech objectively changes   We have also seen that change in speech behavior involves an objective awareness of the specific things, behaviors, acts, or events the client does or experiences that interfere with as well as facilitate fluency. This objective awareness is followed by discussion and demonstration (hopefully more of the latter than former) as well as practice at opening up, moving on, and changing the word-initial sound or transition between sounds. We have tried to show ways to objectify these changes, for example, the tape recorder, and some of the problems we have when we test these changes inside and outside the clinic.

Some "kinda help" is the "kinda help" teenage stutterers can do without   Most importantly, we have tried to show that it is very helpful to know when to let go; that is, when it is professionally correct to terminate therapy when it is obviously going nowhere. Likewise, it is professionally correct not to begin therapy for stuttering with a teen when all the cards are stacked against successful remediation. It is also professionally correct to prioritize the client's problems and decide that other speech or related issues need attention *prior* to stuttering either because of their severity, pervasiveness, or seeming causal relation to stuttering.

Finally, we discussed related concerns, for example, reading problems, and knowing when and when not to refer to other professionals. We discussed the fact that receiving referrals means making referrals and a cultivation and development of a circle of professionals the SLP can consult and turn to when the need arises. Hopefully, some of these thoughts will help you help others at a point where the problem of stuttering has lingered too long but has not quite settled in for the duration. Anything we can do for these older children and teens to reverse as Van Riper (1971) put it, the "morbid growth" of stuttering, is a step in the right direction for them and their families.

SUMMARY

Teenagers who stutter are teenagers first and stutterers second. They exhibit many aspects of the problem common to younger stutterers as well as some traits common to older, adult stutterers. The period of adolescent disorganization that we all pass through on our way to becoming, hopefully, more organized adults is no less a factor for stutterers than their normally fluent counterparts.

We can try to address the special needs of the teenager who stutters by using age-appropriate language, models in our own speech and nonspeech behavior, and analogies during therapy. We can help the teenager to see that it is behavior, not personality, that we seek to change ("you may stutter but that doesn't make you a bad person"). It is helpful in therapy to engage the teen's intellectual skills for reasonably objective, nonjudgmental analysis of feelings, attitudes, and behavior. The clinician needs to concentrate on helping the teen change behavior and related attitudes while minimizing evaluations and lectures regarding emotions, feelings, and the like. With the teenager, in particular, it is important to provide a nonjudgmental, supporting therapy environment where the emphasis is on what the teen is doing and how he/she can change the same rather than on critiquing the teen's evaluations of his/her feelings.

The clinician needs to understand any events in the teen's everyday life that may have untoward influence on the teen's progress through speech-language therapy (for example, *chronic* failure to make appointments on time; chronic absenteeism or tardiness at school; difficulties with schoolwork; lack of opportunities to verbally communicate at home, school, or with friends; chronic obsessions with acting, looking, thinking, and talking exactly like peers). We may not be able, at least at first, to influence these everyday events, but we should be aware of their presence since they provide the broad context within which the teen fits our therapy program, and as such have potential to facilitate and/or inhibit therapy progress.

The parents' role in the remediating of a teenager who stutters may be minimal, moderate, or considerable, depending on the client's individualistic circumstances. It is probably fair to say, however, that parents' impact on the teenager is at least different, if not less, than it is with younger stutterers. While remediating stuttering in teenagers may be somewhat more of a challenge than with younger children, it is every bit as satisfying to client and clinician, and can be a difference that makes a difference in the young adult's life.

FIVE
REMEDIATION:
ADULTS WHO STUTTER

THE GENERAL LAY OF THE LAND

The Past Many Times Influences the Present

Individuals who still stutter in the later years of high school and beyond qualify as *adult stutterers*. Most often these individuals will have previously received partially to completely unsuccessful speech and language therapy as well as a wide variety of other forms of remediation, for example, hypnotherapy, transcendental meditation, primal scream therapy, traditional forms of psychotherapy or psychoanalysis, or specialized academic or vocational counseling. On rare occasions, however, you may be the *first* professional who evaluates and remediates an adult who stutters, but these adults are the exception rather than the rule.

Naturally, a history of past therapy for continued stuttering means that the adult who stutters may have legitimate reasons for doubting your ability to help him or her at this point in life. These doubts, whether explicitly or implicitly expressed, may threaten the SLP, especially when many such professionals have their own self-doubts regarding their ability to help adults who stutter. Clearly, the SLP who attempts to remediate adults who stutter has her or his work cut out; however, it is just as clear that adults who stutter can be helped: They can be assisted in learning how to speak more fluently and to lead lives that are more enjoyable, comfortable, and productive on both personal and professional levels.

Habitual Inappropriate Behavior May Feel More "Normal" than Novel Appropriate Behavior (or Better to Deal with a Known Devil than an Unknown Angel)

In addition to the doubts are the client's relatively *habituated* attitudes, speech behaviors, and beliefs relating to stuttering in specific and speech in general. Indeed, the adult stutterer may know that his or her stuttering is inappropriate, a major personal and professional hindrance, and the like, but the atypical (stuttering) has become, over the years, typical. Thus, dealing with the devil that is known is often more attractive than risking dealing with an unknown angel. Better to stick with what one knows and is, albeit grudgingly, familiar than to risk the uncertainty of trusting in unknown pie in the sky. These beliefs are not unique to adults who stutter but are part of the human condition, and since these adults are human, one can expect them to feel the same.

The habituation that adult stutterers often exhibit implies that their stuttering and related concerns will be fairly resistant to change because adults who stutter, like all adults, spend many years developing their own personal behavior (neither Rome nor an adult's personal behavior was built in a day). They are, like you and me, most comfortable with their present behavior—the maladaptive as well as adaptive elements—because it is what they know best and routinely perform. Whether an adult stutterer's speech behavior is appropriate or not, it is the behavior that the adult stutterer routinely produces and it is this behavior that feels, looks, and sounds most like him or her. This is the behavior that seems most natural since it is most typically produced even though it is atypical of what others produce. Perhaps the naturalness of the behavior and its familiarity is why the adult who stutters presents the SLP with something of a Catch-22 situation: Clients may ask the clinician to stop their stuttering but they do not as readily request that the SLP help change their means of speaking, reacting, feeling, or thinking. And, of course, to do one (that is, "stop my stuttering") without the other (that is, "change my speaking, reacting, feeling, or thinking behavior") is a bit like trying to stop smoking without giving up cigarettes.

Levels of Emotionality

The possible doubts in therapeutic effectiveness and resistance to change may also be coupled with rather high levels of emotionality concerning the problem. Indeed, for many listeners, it is the adult stutterer's apparent emotionality—this apparent nervousness, uneasiness, lack of self-confidence, unsure-of-oneself or self-deprecating quality—that is the hallmark of adults who stutter. While we all should, from time to time, engage in periods of self-assessment in attempts to change inappropriate facets of our behavior, this should not be confused with continual bouts of self-deprecation where we become not our own best friend but our own worst enemy.We cannot count the number of times we have been told by well-intended (non)professionals outside (as well as inside) the field of communication disorders that such and such an adult stutterer "just needs to get more self-confidence (or be less nervous or more relaxed) and then he won't stutter." While there may be some truth in this advice for some adults who stutter, it is obviously an overly simplistic solution to an extremely complex problem. Besides if such suggestions worked there would be far fewer adults who stutter than there are.

We believe that the emotionality of the adult who stutters is something that should be dealt with by the SLP; however, too many times this dealing is either nonexistent, misdirected, superficial, or too far beyond the bounds of the SLP's training and experience or simply not relevant to the adult stutterer's problem.

The SLP May Have to Encourage
Those Who Are Discouraged

Finally, after the doubts, relative resistance to change, and related emotional concerns, the SLP may also find that the adult stutterer is someone who, on one level or another, is discouraged. Adult stutterers may be discouraged that they do not talk like others, and that speech is not as automatic for them as for others, and that they may never talk as they hear other people do. They may also be discouraged that they have thoughts they'll never be able to contribute to conversations because of their stuttering or that their stuttering makes them unacceptably different from their friends and associates. Like their doubts regarding your ability to help, their discouragement with themselves and their behavior must be addressed by the SLP and somehow mitigated if therapy is to stand a chance of being successful.

Cautious Optimism Is Not the Same as Pessimism

Thus, we approach the adult who stutters with caution but with optimism as well. We believe that the SLP can help adults who stutter but we also know that this is no easy task where success will come quickly. The therapy will require continued review on our part and an ever-watchful eye on those aspects of therapy we should modify, terminate, or introduce. If we can begin therapy with adults who stutter knowing what we know as well as those things we still do not know, we have a better likelihood of helping the adult who stutters change in the long term. We realize, of course, that the adult problem with stuttering differs in both degree and kind from that presented by younger stutterers. And we also know that these differences in the problem create differences in our procedure because the clinical problem generally dictates the clinical procedure.

PROBLEM DICTATES PROCEDURE

Late Onset

In Chapter 2 we discussed the diagnosis and evaluation of stutterers and stutterings, and we do not intend to reiterate these. However, there are a few nuances in the evaluation of adult stutterers that should be mentioned prior to the description of remediation. It will be recalled that stuttering has been described as a disorder of childhood; that is, it has its origins in the developing child; (for example, Beech and Fransella, 1968; Bloodstein, 1987). Thus, adults who tell the SLP that their stuttering just began last year when they were a senior in high school or just after they were married and so forth are adults who do not have what we would consider a run-of-the-mill stuttering problem. Adult "stutterers" who report such late onset of stuttering need careful assessment, a second opinion from another qualified SLP, and perhaps a routine medical or psychological evaluation. We have sometimes been the fool who has rushed into places where angels or at least wiser heads feared to tread, but fortunately we have learned some things from these "rushes to judgment." One of the things we have learned is to be cautious, careful, and reasonably deliberate with regard to remediating stutterers whose stutterings begin in late adolescence or adulthood.

Similarities to Other Problems

A similar but different issue relates to the overlap in the adult population between stuttering, organic-neurological, and psychosocial problems. That is, some stutterings or stuttering-like behavior have organic-neurological or psychosocial origins and do not fall into the category of problem stuttering that this book is attempting to deal with. For instance, some adults with certain types of apraxic disorders (see Darley, Aronson and Brown, 1975) or organic brain damage (Rosenbek, and others, 1978) have stuttering-like behavior, but this does not mean that they are stutterers. Conversely, a person who is actually a stutterer may be referred to a physician, particularly a neurologist, because his or her excessive eye blinking and facial grimaces are thought to be indicative of Gilles de la Tourette's syndrome (Love and Webb, 1986, p. 157; DeJong, 1979, p. 415). Some of these stutterers may even exhibit nonverbal behavior when *not* speaking but careful observation suggests that when this happens (nonverbal gestures without overt speech) that the stutterers may be either silently rehearsing what they are about to say or "talking to themselves" about things that have previously happened.

Likewise, some individuals have deep-seated psychoemotional problems that appear to relate to their speech hesitations. Dealing with these two classes of individuals—stutterers with either psychoemotional or organic-neurological etiology—as if they are typical stutterers does not appear to be a good policy. Indeed, the ability to know when and how to refer these individuals to appropriate agencies or professionals is a skill worthy of development.

Referral from Employers

Some adults who stutter may be referred to us by their employers. For example, an up-and-coming young salesperson who stutters may be told, indirectly or directly, by the employer that advancement (or raises) will be determined by improvement in the salesperson's speech fluency. After discussing this situation with the adult client and directly asking the client if we can discuss this situation with the employer, we may ask the client to have the employer contact us. When we make contact with the employer, we discuss the employer's perception of the client and the client's problem(s). During this conversation we try to impart to the employer basic information regarding stuttering and see how receptive he or she is to such information. We promise no rose gardens, but we do tell the employer that we are positively supportive of clients in their attempts to assist themselves. We try to determine how realistic, supportive, and understanding the employer is with regard to the client, the client's feelings, and the client's problems.

In some cases, we have referred the client elsewhere or declined services because we thought that the situation was untenable in terms of successful therapeutic outcome (for example, the employer was putting unreasonable demands on the client and wanted them fulfilled in a very brief period of time). Obviously, the door to our clinic swings both ways and our services remain open to this client, but we explain that given present conditions, therapy elsewhere or at a later date would seem more appropriate. We, as SLPs, have to continually see to it that we become part of the solution rather than part of the problem. We may be ready and willing to help, but if the client isn't presently capable of being helped, for whatever reason, then declining or postponing services or referral elsewhere may be the best as well as only approach.

GROUP THERAPY FOR ADULTS WHO STUTTER

Until very recently, because of the emphasis on behavioral modification, structured individual therapy, individual instructional plans, and "bottom-line" mentality (that is, exactly how long will it take for the client to be cured and how much will it cost), there has been a movement away from group therapy with adults who stutter. Many times the emphasis has been on getting results as quickly as possible with long-term change seemingly an afterthought. We believe that this is unfortunate because group therapy for adults who stutter can be a positive experience and one that significantly contributes to long-term change as well as supports adults' continued efforts to maintain change once it has been established.

Adult Stutterer Groups

In these groups, adults who stutter can share past as well as present experiences, feelings, attitudes, and beliefs with other adults who stutter, who share the same concerns. The group provides a sheltering atmosphere whereby adults who stutter can say what they want to about their problems and their feelings toward them and others will at least listen, even if they do not always agree. Through a group, adult stutterers come to learn that they are not alone in the world with this problem, that others share their troubles and feel much the same way they do. Groups provide speaking outlets for people who might otherwise go literally for days or weeks without verbally communicating to other nonprofessionals.

Client Reluctance to Participate in Group Therapy

Conducting group therapy for adults who stutter is, however, no easy task. First and foremost, the disorder itself interferes with the very medium the clinician needs to use in group therapy: talking. If it were easy for stutterers to talk, they would not be coming to you for therapy in the first place. Thus, for you, the leader of the group, there are periods of discouragement when it appears no one wants to contribute to the group or talk. However, with patience, time, and support on your part even the most reluctant can be encouraged to talk and contribute to the group.

Based on our experience in recruiting adult stutterers to group therapy, I think I can safely say that group therapy, to the average adult stutterer, appears to be something of an anathema. They may want therapy but only the individual kind. Coming together with a group of people who also stutter seems far less than what they want. They appear reluctant to even see or hear another stutterer; the reasons for this reluctance seemingly vary with each client. The following is a *partial* list of reasons:

1. Some adults who stutter have strong fears about their stuttering that they may be reluctant to deal with, explore, and expose in a group setting
2. Some seem reticent to see themselves in others; that is, they realize that the stuttering problems of others mirror their own problem, and they resist having to face this reality
3. Some may deny or avoid facing the reality that their feelings, beliefs, and attitudes may be contributing to their problem, a reality clearly illuminated in a

group setting but one that may be deemphasized in an individual setting where modification of speech is primary

4. Some seem to believe that by hearing and seeing others who stutter they will get worse or stutter more or regress
5. Some appear to believe that by seeing and hearing others stutter they may catch or pick up more stuttering.

Actually, (5) is just another way that clients state (4).

Logistics of Group Therapy

We have reached a point in our experience whereby we request that all adults who stutter attend weekly group sessions; the only exceptions are the adult stutterer who speaks English as a second language, has receptive language problems, or a significant enough hearing problem to make the group situation an extremely difficult one for him or her to understand. Attendance in our group permits us to monitor the adult stutterers' progress in individual therapy and the specific nature of their speech and related problems.

We have found through experience that the ideal group size is about 7 people, but we have had as many as 12 or 13 and as few as 2 or 3. We try to keep the day of the week and time of the day fixed throughout the calendar year and generally a late afternoon or early evening time works out best. We have also found that an odd block of time, say one hour and fifteen minutes, allows people to arrive late and leave early but still get in about 30 to 45 minutes of group therapy; however, sometimes one-hour sessions are all that can be arranged. With one hour sessions, however, the SLP must learn to adjust to the fact that many clients will come and go in 30 minutes or less. Whatever the case, the SLP must presevere and be patient because, particularly in the beginning stages of establishment of a group, attendance may be erratic and it is the SLP's weekly presence and support that will be the foundation around which the superstructure of the group will be built.

Composition of Group Members

If at all possible to arrange, groups of adults who stutter should be composed of a mix of individuals, for example, college students, laborers, executives, secretaries, and so forth. By forming such "mixed" groups both you and your clients learn how stuttering cuts across all walks of life and how it influences different people in different as well as similar ways. Such variety also ensures that student clinicians, if you work in such a setting, get experience observing and managing individuals from different backgrounds. This is a much more realistic experience and good preparation for their professional careers after graduation. Thus, the SLP working within the confines of a university clinic is going to have to make many different "outreaches" at many different times, to various agencies in his or her area to encourage the type of referrals that will lead to such diversity of clientele.

Group Therapy by Itself

It is possible for an adult who stutters to receive group therapy and nothing else. This is particularly true for the marginally disfluent adult whose level of concern regarding his or her speech does not seem warranted by either the nature, severity, or frequency of presenting speech problem. Through exposure to other members in a group, these individuals quickly realize that the frequency, nature, and severity of their speech concerns are quite different and considerably less than those of others. Sometimes even the most patient, clear presentation of an SLP cannot help them come to this realization as quickly and as surely as an hour spent interacting with three or four moderate-to-severe stutterers. Thus, minimally disfluent clients also benefit from learning that some of their communication concerns are shared by others, but that objectively they have less reason for concern. Also subtle, as well as not so subtle, group pressures ("Why are you in the group, you don't stutter?") influence minimally disfluent speakers to reconsider the level and nature of their concern and think about their problems in light of external reality. And, after all, getting our clients to think and change behavior and related issues is what our therapy is all about.

The SLP as Group Leader

None of the preceding, however, should be taken to mean that group therapy with adults who stutter is a panacea; it will not make a silk purse out of a sow's ear. This becomes obvious immediately as the same problems with tardiness, attendance, and failure to do homework assignments that plague individual therapy bedevil group therapy. The SLP who leads a therapy group must wear many hats and at times be a little bit of all things to most all people. Now a motivator, now an organizer, now a talker, now a listener. At times this SLP group leader must be rather authoritarian in manner and at others very much laissez faire and at still other times turn the leadership of the group, albeit temporarily, to a member of the group. As mentioned above, the group leader is the common thread that runs from one year to the next, the person who provides the anchor for and continuity of the group as individual clients fade in and fade out. The SLP group leader must be sufficiently structured to organize and keep each group going, but be prepared to backtrack and discard all such structured plans if group behavior so dictates. The classic opening line of public speakers—that they have prepared the talk but after meeting the audience or viewing the situation have thrown away their notes—is true when running a group for adult stutterers. Be prepared but also be prepared to do things you haven't prepared for!

Mechanics versus Feelings about Speech

During the group, the group leader must tread a thin line between dealing with, what clients call, *the mechanics of speech* and *feelings about speech*. When there is too much group discussion about attitudes, beliefs, and feelings about speech, some clients seem to lose interest and feel that the group is becoming too esoteric, nonsubstantive, and of minimal relevance to *their* specific problem(s). On the other hand, when there is too much discussion of this or that client's or of all clients' speech mechanics, some clients may feel that we are slighting *their* specific problem(s) or their personal beliefs, feelings, or attitudes.

Indeed, besides the mechanics versus feelings dichotomy, there is also the general versus specific dichotomy that must be addressed by the SLP. The SLP must address specific individual concerns but continually relate them to general group issues; conversely, the SLP must try to help all group members see general or common themes but continually try to relate them to specific individual concerns. The group is a collection of individuals whose understanding of common concerns must be translated through their own individual needs.

As many adult stutterers have told me, in one way or another, "I'm more than just a mouth, larynx...I'm more than just speech, I'm also a person who feels and thinks." Thus, the group leader is constantly shifting within as well as between group sessions from discussions of attitudes to discussions of speech behavior, and back again. The SLP continually shifts from discussions of how a particular individual's concerns relate to general or common concerns among the group members to talking about a particular individual's specific problem and how it can be best addressed by that person.

Group therapy, therefore, is no place for the faint of heart; it is not for the professional who finds it difficult to juggle more than two balls at once! We are convinced, however, based on our experience with adults who stutter, that such groups are beneficial to the client and clinician and should be given serious consideration in the development of a therapy program for adult stutterers.

INDIVIDUAL THERAPY FOR ADULTS
WHO STUTTER: STARTING UP

First Impressions

We previously mentioned the impact that first impressions have on young children and parents we deal with in therapy. As an ad states, "you never get a second chance to make a first impression." First impressions also impact adults who stutter, but the means by which these impressions are made differ with the older client. We hope that it is obvious that our attempts to convey positive first impressions to the adult should not be a show, a forced procedure or performance, or a hype of the wonders of ourself and our approach. Most adults can easily detect a show of insincerity or "sales pitch." Rather, most adults who stutter seek an SLP who demonstrates (1) an understanding of the problem, (2) a willingness to listen, (3) an ability to help, and (4) integrity and confidence.

It is important to the adult stutterer that the SLP make apparent, right from the beginning, his or her *understanding* of stuttering in general, and the adult's problem in specific. Reasonable, clear, and cautious answers to the clients' questions about cause, symptoms, and the like help establish the SLP's credentials in this area. It is also important to the adult client that we *listen* to his or her individual story, concerns, beliefs, and feelings (such listening does not imply agreement with all of the client's beliefs but it does imply acceptance of them). You may have heard similar stories before, but you haven't heard this person's particular version and it behooves you not to give the impression that you have. It is also important to the adult client that we make explicit our willingness and ability to *help* (without exaggerating this ability).

While the client wants the SLP to give signs of support as well as indications that therapy will be of some help, it is important to the client that the SLP be *honest* with him or her. We should make it clear to the client if we are guarded in our belief concerning the client's prognosis for positive change in speaking and related attitudes, beliefs, and feelings. Some clients will need more—some specific concrete, tangible, up-front "proof," no matter how temporary, that things can get better, that they can improve their speech.

Demonstrating to the adult client that his or her speech can be changed, even through an artificial means, for example, a metronome, choral reading, or whispering, can be used to show that (1) the adult client's speech disfluency is malleable and not a fixed, never-changing property etched in stone for all time; (2) that speech fluency, given certain circumstances, is obtainable; and (3) that you, as a professional SLP, can assist him or her in the modification of speech. However, it should be noted that giving early, concrete examples to an adult stutterer that change is possible in his or her speech is not without its problems and these need to be discussed.

We Are Guides, Not Magicians

As mentioned before, when remediating stuttering we use the orientation of *helping with* rather than *curing* the stutterer's speech problem. We want to clearly and emphatically convey to the adult that our role is one of a guide rather than a magician. Furthermore, while we are not Merlin neither is whispering, for example, the silver bullet the average adult stutterer seeks.

Part of being honest with the client is repeatedly and clearly explaining to him or her that quick changes in fluency are generally followed by equally quick relapses and that such procedures as the metronome will not be the principal means by which we will assist him or her change speech and related behavior. We emphasize to the adult stutterer that these procedures were used merely as a means to show that change is possible. Leading the adult client—or any client for that matter—to dream the impossible dream that we can quickly cure him or her of stuttering (while the adult stutterer passively stands around and watches and hopes to absorb "the cure" through osmosis), is, in my mind, the ultimate cruelty because time will show that such a dream cannot be realized.

The short-term gain of wowing the client with clinical legerdemain is counterbalanced by the long-term pain of reality. The quick cure is the domain of the clinical mountebanks and represents procedures that the SLP of integrity and sincerity will want to avoid like the plague. As we point out in the next chapter, quick but total and permanent cures for complex human behavior disorders are not compatible with the present state of the human condition. In short, we want to provide the client from the very first meeting—usually a diagnostic evaluation—with a positive therapy atmosphere where change appears possible and desirable rather than misleading the client that we are able to change lead into gold. Our field needs competent guides willing to stay the course not glib alchemists who fold their tents and move on before the inevitable relapse occurs.

How Many Times per Week?

Assuming the client agrees and we think it appropriate, the client begins therapy. The first question we ask is: How often and how long? This is, of course, not an easy question to answer but hopefully we have told the client in the initial evaluation (see Chapter 2) the approximate time line of the therapy. We must then square the ideal with reality: Therapy every day may be best, at least for quick behavioral change, but our clinical program and the demands on our time may permit only one hour per week.

We recognize that the intensity and/or frequency of speech therapy (see Gregory, 1978) may be of primary significance to our client's improvement; however, while the jury is still out regarding the relative merits of *intensive* (for example, once or twice per day for three weeks) versus *extensive* (for example, once a week for twelve months) therapy, our experience indicates that *lasting, long-term* change of stuttering and related matters may take much longer than we or our clients would like. This is especially true, in our opinion, for adult stutterers. Our observations tell us that *intensive* therapy provides quicker changes in speech behavior but insufficient time for meaningful change in associated attitudes, beliefs, and feelings which, if left unchanged, may impede long-term recovery. Conversely, our observations suggest to us that *extensive* therapy takes longer to achieve changes in speech behavior, but provides the needed time to change associated attitudes, beliefs, and feelings which, if when changed, may facilitate long-term recovery.

These are empirical issues, however, and must await the sort of careful, meticulous evaluation procedures advocated by individuals like Ingham (1984, pp. 433–64). Whatever the case, given the time and space considerations of our own present clinical situation, we remediate adult stutterers on a once- or twice-a-week basis (generally one group and one individual session per week), and the usual time frame (start to end) runs from 3 to 12 months.

Trial Therapy

Before we begin any therapy regimen, particarly one that looks as if it may be protracted, we inform our clients that we plan to initiate what we call *trial therapy*. With adults this trial period usually lasts from three to six weeks. We inform the clients of the beginning and end of this trial and tell them that a judgment regarding the continuation of therapy and its nature will be made somewhere between the middle and end of this period. We emphasize, several times, that the client does not have to produce total change for continuation, but it must be apparent that change seems possible or that the client is moving in the right direction. We stress the positive, but inform clients that before they or we get involved in an extensive therapy program, it must be apparent that the situation warrants the necessary time and effort. It is not unusual in these situations for clients to want to hurry up and get therapy whether or not they are ready and willing to expend the necessary time and effort.

For some adults who stutter there is little connection between their goal (more fluent speech) and the means (time, effort, and work) by which this must be accomplished. It is up to the SLP to explain this connection. For these reasons, and others, the SLP should not be stampeded into untenable therapy situations. Explain to the adult clients that their talk about change is necessary (and appreciated) but not sufficient. The clients need to understand you will be much more impressed by their behavior, by their actions, than all their verbal expressions of good intentions (actions do speak louder than words). Conversely, the SLP should try to recognize a client's sincere and honest desire to commit the necessary personal resources to obtain the type of desired therapy outcome. It's hard to change behavior and you must make it clear to the adult client that you recognize this difficulty and will support him or her in his attempts. Although it is not easy to spot the difference between sincere motivation to change and "talk is cheap" forms of motivation, it is an ability the SLP needs to develop.

If, for the sake of completing this discussion, we find that the client is able to make the necessary effort and commitment and we believe we can assist him or her in modification of stuttering, we begin in earnest. The first step, not unlike what we do with older children and teenagers, is to assist the client in quickly and accurately identifying instances of stuttering and related behavior. The emphasis here, as elsewhere, is on the inappropriate *strategies* and *behavior* the client employs to interfere with fluent speech. For the most part, the problem lies in the strategies the client employs and not in the sounds and syllables the client produces.

INDIVIDUAL THERAPY FOR ADULTS
WHO STUTTER: IDENTIFICATION PHASE

Identifying and Physically Feeling (In)appropriate Behavior

We firmly believe two things about achieving *lasting* change in stuttering: Stutterers need to be able to quickly, correctly, and objectively identify when and what they do when they stutter and this ability to identify must relate to the *physical* feelings of speech movements and muscular tensions. Unless stutterers can do these two interrelated things—quickly correct their behavior and physically feel it—we think it is difficult for adults who stutter to change their stuttering permanently. That is, how can individuals change stuttering when they cannot identify when and how they stutter and what it feels like? As we will see, hearing and seeing these behaviors are important adjuncts to identification, but in the final analysis physically feeling these behaviors is key since, as we've said before, by the time the stutterer sees or hears the inappropriate behavior it has already happened. They need a sensory modality—conscious proprioception or kinesthesia, and so forth—that is associated with the antecedents or at least the concurrent aspects of the behavior rather than its outcome, that is, acoustics.

Many adults who stutter try to improve their fluency without ever becoming aware of what *they do* that interferes with their speaking, but the *long-term* success of these trials is not overwhelming. Indeed, one of the first things we find out in the trial therapy period is whether or not the client is ready, willing, and able to identify instances of stuttering and if so, how quickly and correctly this can be done. While identification—just like modification—requires the adult stutterer to simultaneously monitor the *manner* as well as *content* of speech, the SLP can structure the speaking tasks, at least in the beginning, to make this simultaneous monitoring easier to do.

"Devices" Used with Identification

While physical feelings of stuttering are our ultimate goal, we must still, at this stage of therapy, use devices that give the client auditory or visual information: an audio tape recorder, an audio-videotape recorder (with associated television monitor), magnifying glass, mirrors, language master type tape recorder and/or player, oscilloscopes (signal generated by microphone fed to scope), flashlight with push-button on-off switch, clicker (like those used by children around Hallowe'en), or any other device that quickly and clearly provides a visual or auditory stimulus for the client's observation.

Technology is developing very rapidly in this area as witnessed by interactive computer software and "biofeedback devices." Unfortunately, most computer applications, for example, Visi-Pitch (Kay Elemetrics), Speech Thing (CoVox), or Speech Viewer (IBM), while quite useful, are based on the microphone signal and are not directly related to physical behavior or feelings. Conversely, devices such as the electroglottograph (EGG) and surface electromyography are much closer to the actual movements and tensions of speech musculature and would therefore seem to have a great deal of potential for quickly and accurately informing clients about the physical aspects of their speech behavior.

Perhaps devices that portray acoustic information about speech production could be initially used with the stutterer and then once the client becomes more comfortable and capable of identifying acoustic aspects of speech, he or she could move to such devices as the EGG that more directly measure or monitor speech production activity.

Adults' Reactions to Identification

The previously mentioned devices can be used in a variety of ways. For example, the client and clinician can each employ flashlights or penlights, with on-off push buttons, with the object being to see who—the client or clinician—can push the button first when an instance of stuttering occurs. In the beginning, this procedure works best if the SLP *decides* to identify only more *obvious* instances of stuttering—generally those that are longer and repetitive in nature, for example, sound/syllable repetition, monosyllabic whole-word repetitions.

It is not always easy, however, to get individuals who stutter, particularly adults with a long history of the problem, to listen and view themselves on tape. This is no small concern and must be approached with sensitivity and concern for these clients' feelings. On the other hand, no one ever said any of this process was going to be easy for the client (or clinician), and at times some degree of emotionality and self-recrimination must take place in order for therapy to move forward.

Likewise, some adult clients do not react favorably to clickers, flashlights, or other indicators used to "highlight" or make more apparent or conspicuous their instances of stuttering (see Siegel, 1970, for further discussion of "highlighting"). Adult stutterers may say that this procedure makes them nervous, self-conscious, feel hurried, or other statements to the effect that they are reacting to this aspect of identification with feelings of discomfort.

These feelings, which may be much more central to stutterers than their recognition of instances of stuttering, should be discussed with the clients and the SLP should try to make explicit his or her understanding of these feelings and reactions. That is, the SLP should neither ignore nor downplay these feelings and reactions, but discuss their nature and their possible causes. Explain your appreciation for the unpleasantness of such emotions. ("I know that hearing this clicker every time you stutter is unpleasant and frustrating, but this is one way I have of helping you help yourself become more fluent.")

Amount of Time Spent on Identification per Session

In the beginning do not use these identification procedures for extended periods of time (15 to 20 minutes at a stretch); instead, break them up into smaller blocks of say three to five minutes with a few minutes rest in between to discuss possible reasons for success or failure. You can gradually increase the time of identification exercises as clients become more and more adept at recognizing instances of stuttering, as they begin to get better than you, or beat you at identifying their instances of stuttering. Likewise, more and more time can be spent on identification as the client consistently identifies the stuttering during the middle or toward the beginning of its occurrence.

By no means, however, devote an entire session to identification or a series of sessions to identification. Mix it up with discussion of group therapy events. Or, if group therapy is not part of your adult client's regimen, then talk about success or lack thereof outside the therapy room and situations that are difficult or becoming easier to speak in. Ask the client if friends, relatives, or associates are commenting on or reacting to any changes in the client's speech or the client's therapy progress. Vary the content of the therapy hour to avoid boredom and also because identification of instances of stuttering is hard, intense work requiring focused attention and concentration. Extensive immersion (that is, all session every session) in this procedure is, in the long run, counterproductive to a successful remediation program.

Three Early Signs of Improvement

We firmly believe that long-term recovery, particularly for adults, requires a *gradual* change in speech and related behavior. Sudden improvement is too often followed by sudden relapse. Thus, improvement will not be dramatic, but there are some early signs that are true indicators that improvement is taking place: (1) shortening of the duration of instances of stuttering even though there is little or no change in stuttering frequency (this may or may not be associated with changes in physical tension during speech); (2) individuals in the clients' environment starting to report to the client and/or the SLP or others that they are noticing an improvement in the clients' speech and related behavior; and (3) relatively consistent identification at the beginning and/or middle of stutterings that may or may not be associated with the client's sometimes spontaneously changing his stuttering behavior. This is related to a shortening of the stuttering, but can also lead to changes in the type and frequency of stuttering.

When the SLP notices these early signs of improvement, he or she should tell the client. Make it quite apparent to the client—don't let him guess—that improvement is apparent and that progress is being made.

Continuing with Identification

We begin identification in earnest once the client demonstrates a willingness to see, hear, and feel (especially the latter) his or her instances of stuttering. This demonstration need not be one of absolute but of relative willingness. It should be stressed that it is not only important for your adult client to know why you employ identification, but for him or her also to realize its importance and rationale. Obviously, identifying something is not the same as changing it; however, changing something presupposes that the person who is to do the changing can identify what he or she wants to change (similar to Thorndike's 1913 "specificity doctrine").

The accuracy and speed with which such identification is made is also important. Once again, the *mode* of identification (vision versus audition versus physically feeling physical tensions and movements) needs to be considered. Steps used when employing identification with a client are, therefore, as follows: (1) introducing the concept, (2) helping the client become more objective and less subjective when identifying his or her instances of stuttering, (3) increasing the client's accuracy of identification, (4) increasing the client's accuracy with identifying specific instances or types of stuttering, and (5) helping them concentrate on the mode of identification that is most crucial for long-term change in stuttering, that is, feelings of physical tensions, movements, and positions of speech structures.

Accuracy of identification of instances of stuttering has been covered in other sources (for example, Van Riper, 1973, 1974). Basically, identification with adult stutterers involves giving them an opportunity to observe themselves during speech and then asking them to label through voice or gesture each and every time they perceive a target behavior; for example, all sound syllable repetitions or all sound prolongations that are one second or longer in duration. These opportunities, as mentioned above, can be made available through audio or audio-video recordings of the client's speech productions (*off-line* analysis) or during real time or the actual speech production itself (*on-line* analysis).

Off-line analysis, even though the stutterer's initial reactions may be negative, is the preferred and generally easiest place to begin using identification with adults. Once accuracy of identification during off-line analysis is 80 percent or greater, the SLP can proceed to on-line identification (which we assume has more generalizability to everyday speaking situations). However, remember that most adult clients have difficulty, at least in the beginning, accurately and quickly monitoring their speech productions while simultaneously carrying on a lucid conversation. We might add that clinicians have the same difficulty simultaneously identifying instances of stuttering in the client's speech while at the same time trying to maintain normal conversation with the client. As previously mentioned, this parallel processing (simultaneously monitoring speech production and maintaining thoughts so that a cogent conversation can take place) is a necessary skill the clinician must develop in himself and in his clients.

Off-line Identification

Off-line analysis is best employed when the SLP has a priori knowledge of all instances of stuttering contained within an audio or an audio-video recording. Several rules apply: (1) Start "away" from the client; (2) begin with audio recordings, then video recordings of the client; and (3) progress from more obvious or longer, more physically tense stutterings to shorter, less physically tense, and less apparent stutterings.

Start "away" from the client It is best to start off-line identification "away" from the client, that is, start identifying the stutterings of some other client, preferably an adult. In this way both client and clinician can be objective and say pretty much what they want about the anonymous adult stutterer and his or her stuttering. While the client's objectivity is enhanced by this procedure, he or she also gains experience by being a critical listener and observer.

To facilitate matters even further, the SLP can analyze this recording in advance and even type up a transcript of the recording (this transcript/recording can be used for several adult stutterers at this stage of therapy). The typed manuscript permits client and SLP to easily compare notes and go back into the taped conversation at precise points. Tape counter numbers should be tabulated every ten words or so on the manuscript to enhance the clinician's ability to readily go back and forth through the tape recording, instead of wasting time guessing where a particular section of the recording is on the tape. Most importantly, however, the SLP's a priori listening, analyzing, and tabulating the number and type of stutterings contained on the recording means that he or she can more fully devote their time and attention to the present client's ability to accurately and quickly identify and label instances of stuttering. All too often, the SLP spends precious time in these initial therapy sessions performing off-line identification of instances of stuttering and thus cannot pay as much attention to the client's difficulties with this task.

Progress from audio to audio-video   The next step is to have the client identify his own stutterings on audio rather than audio-video recordings. If audio-video recordings are available, somehow blackout or turn off the video portion and listen to only the audio segment. We recommend beginning with audio for two basic reasons. Audio-video is a rather confrontational medium. That is, it directly and rather starkly portrays the client's behavior and some clients, at least in the beginning, simply aren't ready for this sort of reality. They will be, given time and patience on the part of the SLP, but in the beginning we recommend sticking with audio recordings alone; the client is apt to be far less defensive and more objective when listening than when watching himself, at least in the beginning.

Visually apparent behavior like eyeball movement, blinking, head movements and facial gestures are more apt to be attended to, in the beginning, by the naive client than auditorily apparent behavior like a sound/syllable repetition. In essence, until the client becomes more accustomed to observing him or herself, the visual medium will take precedence over the auditory even though this runs contrary to the SLP's desire for the client to become adept at quickly and accurately attending to disfluent speech behavior.

Progress from obvious to less obvious stutterings   The SLP should next begin identification of longer, more physically tense and aurally apparent stutterings; these are generally, but not necessarily, sound/syllable repetitions. In essence, this makes the client's task easier in the beginning. Success begets success and as the client quickly and accurately identifies longer, tenser, and more obvious stutterings in his speech and the speech of others, then the SLP can change the behavior to identify shorter, less tense, and less obvious stutterings. It is best to start where success is maximized; this not only helps the client learn the task more quickly, but also facilitates motivation as well.

While it is important for the client to recognize the same number or close to the same number of stutterings recognized by the SLP, it is also important that the client recognize the same type of stuttering (for example, sound prolongation versus sound/syllable repetition). Perhaps the difference in number of stutterings recognized by client and SLP relates to the fact that the client easily and quickly identifies all sound-syllable repetitions, but seemingly misses most sound prolongations. Or perhaps the difference in numbers is that the client can readily and quickly identify stutterings of 1.0 seconds and longer, but misses the shorter stutterings, say 0.5 to 1.0 seconds. (It should be noted that stutterings shorter than 0.5 seconds exist, but the beginning client, as well as beginning student-clinician, cannot be expected to readily identify such brief stutterings without some experience and/or guided observations.) Such problems need to be discussed with the client as well as the reason(s) for such successes and failures and exactly what the client calls stuttering in himself or herself and others. In essence, the SLP needs to be clear regarding the client's relative skill as an identifier of stutterings before embarking on more identification.

These conversations between client and SLP—where the client's definition of stuttering and basis for identifying it are discussed—can provide the SLP with fascinating insights. It is not uncommon for the client to identify behaviors the SLP "misses," particularly behaviors that are self-produced, because while the SLP's judgment can be based only on audition and vision, the client can also employ physical feelings that may "indicate" stuttering in the absence of any auditory or visually apparent behavior (for more information on adult stutterers' perceptions of their own stutterings see Kelly and Conture, 1988).

It is very important for the client to be clear on the purpose of these procedures; here, as elsewhere, redundancy of instruction will be necessary. It is not bad policy to continue to discuss with the client, "What are we doing here?" and "Why do you think we are doing it?" You may be surprised at the response. Obviously, your long-range goals are other than merely getting the client to make quick, accurate identification of stutterings, but the client should realize this because you have made this fact explicit. The client needs to be told and periodically reminded that there are short-, medium- and long-range goals. The client also needs to clearly understand—and you need to tell him or her—that learning is a gradual process and the identification step is but one point along the gradual learning curve that leads the client from stuttering to becoming a more normally fluent speaker.

Bridge Between Off-line and On-line Identification

It is time to move beyond off-line identification when the client demonstrates relatively accurate identification of most medium-to-long instances of stuttering from a tape recorded sample of his or her own speech. The client is ready to proceed to the bridge between off-line and on-line analysis. This *bridge* involves using an audio tape recorder or an audio-video cassette recorder that has a pause or instantaneous stop switch.

The object of this bridge is the *speed* of identification which, of course, presupposes accurate identification. Clients are now required to listen to the same audio recordings of their own speech that they accurately identified and quickly stop the forward movement of the tape or cassette as soon as they perceive the stuttering. Another way this may be done, when the tape recorder lacks a pause button, is to use two flashlights or penlights that have instant on-buttons or perhaps a noise clicker. However it is accomplished, the purpose of these procedures is to help clients develop the necessary rapidity of identification that will serve as the foundation upon which clients rest their ability to rapidly change their on-going speech behavior.

Clients are here reinforced for the quickness of the identification to the point where their stopping of the tape recorder or signaling with a light or sound happens *before* or as close to the beginning of the stuttering as possible. Once again, SLPs should practice this themselves until reasonably confident that they have the ability to quickly and accurately recognize their clients' stuttering. Remember to practice the same tasks yourself that you ask the client to do in therapy. After sufficient practice with a variety of stutterers, you will find that you will not have to prepare this aspect of therapy individually; however, some homework, on your part, has to be completed prior to your doing this with the stutterer(s) you manage.

On-line Identification

Once the client is exhibiting 80 percent or greater success at identifying his or her own stutterings on audio and/or audio-video tape recordings, the SLP can begin to help the client identify stutterings during actual conversation. Once again, the SLP wants to start with longer, more physically tense, and more obvious stutterings. The SLP is also advised to encourage the client for any and all approximations to accurate identification. That is, the client will not immediately be 100 percent successful in the accurate identification of instances of stuttering (as well as other speech disfluencies), and the SLP should realize this and reinforce it accordingly.

Demonstrate to the client that you understand the difficulty of the task and that you appreciate the client's attempts. In the beginning, keep the conversation simple and relating to topics the client is familiar with but ones with less apparent emotionality; for example, talk about fixing squeaky doors or sticky cabinet drawers rather than asking the boss for a raise.

Specify stutterings to be identified   Depending on the frequency and types of stuttering exhibited by the client, the clinician may be able to clearly target this phase of the identification procedure. That is, the SLP may be able to target for the client the specific types of stuttering (longer versus short sound prolongations versus sound-syllable repetition) he or she wants the client to attend to and identify. As mentioned above, it is a good general rule to start with longer sound-syllable repetitions, but if sound prolongations predominate, then it is better to start this phase of identification with longer rather than shorter instances. Remember that (1) during normally fluent speech many sounds are produced per second (possibly as many as ten or more sounds per second) and (2) it takes the unsophisticated listener, like your client in the beginning of therapy, a little bit of time to decide and identify instances of stuttering. Thus, give the client a break, and begin with longer, more frequently occurring, and more obvious stutterings. This will ensure that he or she has that little bit of extra time necessary to make accurate decisions and enough chances to succeed in making accurate identifications. With experience the adult who stutters should be able to perceive the shorter and shorter instances of speech disfluency until, with practice, he or she can perceive very short instances of stuttering that occur around a reaction time of 250 ms or less.

The key: Speed of identification The adult client's ability to *quickly* stop the tape recorder upon perceiving instances of his or her *own* stuttering serves as the bridge or introduction into on-line identification. On-line analysis involves the quick and accurate identification of instances of stuttering *during* the actual production of speech. This is not an easy task since adult stutterers must identify their instances of stuttering while simultaneously conducting a conversation with the SLP. The SLP must be very sensitive to the client's feelings about the difficulty of this task and discuss these feelings with the client.

The clinician must also realize that the client may find it very frustrating to have his or her thoughts or conversation continually interrupted by on-line identification. The client may also feel rushed, pressured, or uncomfortable when so much specific attention is being paid to his or her speech production. Again, the SLP must discuss these feelings and let the client know that the SLP respects them. On the other hand, clinicians must not allow such respect to paralyze them or their client from acting in a way that is in the client's best long-range interests no matter how uncomfortable this may be to the client in the short run.

On-line identification as contest between client and clinician One way we have successfully employed on-line identification with adults is by having a simple contest between the client and the SLP. We begin, after conferring with the client, by specifically targeting certain speech disfluencies that the client needs to identify in his or her own speech. Then, while talking with the client, we try to see who first identifies these specific disfluencies. Although we can signal such identity with a simple pointed finger or gesture, a penlight with an instant on-off button is also an effective signaling device. The objective of this contest is the speed with which the client can identify the disfluency. Obviously, clinicians can manipulate their latency of signaling to maximize, at least at first, the clients' chances for identifying their own instances *before* clinicians do.

Facilitating on-line identification To facilitate on-line identification, it is helpful if the clinician selects a topic of conversation that is familiar and of interest to the client. This on-line procedure, at least at first, should be broken up into several short periods, rather than a few long sections within one therapy session. These conversation breaks and discussions of the client's successes and failures with on-line identification enable the SLP to minimize the tension (both physiological and psychological) that may build up when using this therapy method. Better to provide the client with a few successful periods within a therapy session than to spend an entire therapy session working the client so hard that she or he is nearly driven away from therapy. And make no mistake about it, clinicians, no matter how unintentionally, can drive clients away from therapy.

Once again, the clinician's sensitivity regarding the client's ever-changing needs and feelings will dictate the success of this as well as other approaches. With on-line analysis in particular, where the attention to speech production is quick, specific, and quite apparent, the client can easily get the feeling that all the clinician is doing is "picking on" the client. It seems in this situation that the essence of the client's reaction is that the clinician cares only about the "mechanics" of speech and not enough about him or her as a person. It is important to recognize this reaction as it is developing, discuss it, and then possibly mitigate it. The SLP should try to convey to the client the impression not only of seeing the behavior but the person behind the behavior as well.

Further Reactions to Identification

As the adult client becomes more and more adept at quick and accurate identification, clinician latency can be shortened to make the task more and more challenging for the client. At this point, one of several things may be noticed: (1) Clients claim they are stuttering more; (2) clinicians notice clients stuttering more (possibly, because they are avoiding less and/or repeating more often than producing inaudible sound prolongations or within-word pauses); or (3) the duration of each instance of clients' stutterings seems to be shortening. The third observation is, as mentioned above, a positive sign that clients are improving in their objective awareness of stuttering and even without direct modification procedures they are already beginning to change their speech production. The former two observations, however, are a bit more worrisome to both client and clinician and need some discussion at this point.

Client: I'm beginning to stutter more We have previously discussed the client's claim that he or she is stuttering more, and we will not belabor the point. Suffice it to say that clients' heightened awareness of their stuttering heightens their awareness. Stutterers believe they stutter more, we believe, because they have become more objectively and accurately aware of their instances of stuttering through identification. The same thing can also happen to their clinicians; that is, through identification the SLP can actually see and hear more stutterings on the part of the client than he or she originally observed during the diagnostic and first few therapy sessions. The SLP becomes more aware, with exposure to the client, of the depth and breadth of the client's stuttering whereas in the beginning the SLP may miss some the client's speech disfluencies because the clinician must attend to a myriad of

factors that occur in the development of a thorough evaluation and prognosis. In essence, the clinician as well as client changes with therapy and
becomes more adept at perceiving instances of stuttering.

Clinician: client does appear to be stuttering more However, it may be the
case that the client *is* stuttering more now if for no other reason than the fact
that he or she talks more as the client-clinician relation develops (that is, the
more talking the greater the chance for stuttering to occur) as well as the fact
that the client has become more willing to enter into (or become less apt to
avoid) discussions.

What we find of interest in all this is that clinicians often report increases in their client's stuttering and express worry that they—somehow
through their therapeutic procedures—have caused these increases. We
doubt if they would have the same worry if they noticed after several therapy
sessions with a child exhibiting speech misarticulations that the child increased his or her number of speech misarticulations. We would also bet that
clinicians do not have the same worry when they notice after several sessions
with a child with language concerns that there is a decrease in the child's
mean length of utterance or that there are now apparently more missing
grammatical morphemes.

Actually, more stutterings noticed by the clinician after a period of
therapy do not necessarily mean that the client has gotten worse, regressed,
relapsed, or experienced any other such calamities. This observation may
simply mean that (1) the original estimates of stuttering were inaccurate; (2)
the type of stuttering has changed from one that is minimally audible and
visible, for example, silent sound prolongations, to much more audible and
visible ones—such as sound/syllable repetitions; (3) the client is avoiding
less, talking more and in longer units; (4) the situations in which speech is
now elicited differ from those used during the original evaluation; and (5)
any of these reasons and others in combination. Clinicians must stop flailing
themselves when they notice such changes. (They must also stop waiting for
the other shoe of increased stuttering to drop.)

Instead, we should attempt to make the same reactions to increased
stutterings that we make to increased articulation errors, or missing grammatical morphemes, or decreased MLU, or more prevalent hoarseness, and
so forth (for further discussion pertinent to this issue, see Wingate, 1971).
Guilty parents are difficult enough to deal with (for example, "If we had only
given our sixth-grader the Mercedes-Benz convertible he wanted, we know
he wouldn't have started to stutter more"), but guilty clinicians, especially
when there is little or no reason for such guilty feelings, are even more
problematic. The white, hot spotlight of on-line identification seems to exacerbate these concerns, but it is quite unclear to me how we can assist our
adult clients change their stuttering if we and the clients never carefully
examine, touch, and hear those behaviors that are interfering with normally

fluent speech production and need changing. Perhaps it is much like asking a garage mechanic to fix the engine of our car *without* examining it closely and touching and listening to it. While it is understandable that stutterers, unlike some of our political leaders, have met many microphones that they don't love, it is hard to figure how any light other than a limelight can be focused on their instances of stuttering in attempts to help them change their behavior.

BRIDGING BETWEEN IDENTIFICATION AND MODIFICATION

The client's ability to temporally beat the SLP at identifying instances of his or her own stuttering *as they occur* is the bridge between identification and modification. With careful explanation, clients should come to understand and physically *feel* the various things they do wrong during speech as they are doing them. I want to stress that the key here is *as he is doing them,* not several seconds or five words ago, but during the right here and now. We want the stutterer to do this at the exact moment of stuttering. Sooner rather than later. The physical feelings of interfering with speech and the rapidity of these behaviors must be carefully examined and accurately recognized. Once again, we try to stress to the client (and ourselves) that the problem is *not* within the sound or syllable, but involves the strategies used by the stutterer to produce those units of speech (as Shakespeare said, "the problem is not in our stars but in ourselves").

Spontaneous Modification

For some adult stutterers, simply identifying stutterings as they are being produced is sufficient to enable them to start modifying these very same instances of stuttering. For some stutterers it seems that on-line identification of stuttering—recognizing stutterings as they are occurring—facilitates their attempts to change stuttering. One of the first signs of such facilitation, as previously mentioned, is a decrease in the duration of the instances of stuttering. We have taken this decrease in duration to mean that the stutterers are beginning to realize that they can change their stuttering midstream, that they can use less physical tension in the production of a particular sound or sound-to-sound transition.

Another sign is when the stutterer stops in the middle of producing a stuttering, perhaps a brief pause, and then initiates the same sound or syllable in a more appropriate fashion. These signs essentially mean that the client is taking an active, direct approach toward coping with or changing his or her inappropriate speech behavior. By shortening the duration and/or stopping and reinitiating in a more fluent manner, these clients are giving the impression that they are beginning to come to grips with their stuttering and are beginning to do something to change their behavior. These are signs that adult stutterers are beginning to do battle with their stuttering—that they are taking an active role rather than running and hiding from the situation.

To be effective in this battle, we try to arm the adult stutterer with an objective understanding of stuttering as well as an ability to quickly and accurately confront instances of stuttering. Sometimes when I see an adult who stutters begin this self-confrontation process, I am reminded of a Pogo quote: "We have met the enemy and he is us." Rather than ducking and weaving, the adult stutterer has started to "face the music" and circumscribe the boundaries of his or her speech problem. The adult who stutters can now begin to operate from a position of understanding rather than ignorance, one of relatively clear vision rather than hazy insight.

If Identification Fails to Develop

Some adults who stutter never seem to develop the ability to identify and subsequently modify instances of stuttering. We are not sure why this is, but several reasons may exist. First, for some there is so much emotionality associated with the actual sight, sound, and feel of their stuttering that these individuals find it quite difficult to actually confront occurrences of their own stuttering. Many times these clients try to keep therapy on a subjective, fairly abstract discussion basis (cf. Johnson, 1946, for discussion of individuals who employ high levels of verbal abstraction), rather than a get-down-to-specifics approach. Some of these clients use an "intellectualization" (cf. Vaillant, 1977, pp. 132–35, 385) method of coping with the problem and this too gets in the way of their actually coming to terms with their problem. Sometimes, a break from therapy helps so the clients have time to think about whether they are willing and able to specifically confront their instances of stuttering.

Second, other adults who stutter do not appear to have the ability to concentrate to the degree and for the length of time necessary to identify and modify instances of stuttering. They may be "tuned-in" to emotional feelings surrounding their stutterings, but the stations they receive broadcast mainly subjective, emotional messages rather than programs that directly and specifically deal with their own behavior.

Third, some adults who stutter may be fairly able to see and hear their instances of stuttering but appear relatively unable to physically *feel* these same instances. It is as if this third group of clients is physically as well as emotionally insensitive, or out of touch with their own bodily feelings.

Of course, the possibility also exists that the clinician is not very effective in assisting the client to identify instances of stuttering or that the clinician has not sufficiently and clearly explained the rationale for identifying instances of stuttering. We sometimes need to face reality: Some clients cannot or will not easily, readily, or accurately perceive their own instances of stuttering. These clients will either need different approaches or must wait until such time that they are more receptive to our therapeutic approaches.

INDIVIDUAL THERAPY FOR ADULTS
WHO STUTTER: MODIFICATION PHASE

Modification of stuttering is actually not that hard; it is just that neither we nor our clients appear to realize this fact. What is hard, on the other hand, is providing the necessary intellectual and/or emotional environment in and around the client that *continually* facilitates, fosters, and encourages the client to modify his or her own speech. Once again, as Williams (1978) suggests, our goal is change of speech *outside* therapy, not merely *within* the therapy room. As we've seen, quick, accurate identification of stuttering is one important aspect of this environment. So is the notion that specific speaking strategies, rather than specific sounds, are the main ingredients of stuttering.

Movement between Rather than Movement
within Sounds

The client must be helped to understand that stuttering involves an interference with or disruption of the appropriately timed, smooth, physically easy movements from one articulatory gesture to another. Emphasis is on movement from one posture to the next. Stress is placed on movements between sounds rather than the specific nature of the movements needed to produce each sound. We want to facilitate the stutterer's making connections between sounds rather than concentrate on making the specific sounds.

The Problem Relates to the Nature of Speaker's Speech
Behavior, Not the Nature of Speech Sound Spoken

The client needs to realize that speech is something produced by him or her as the speaker and as such it is something he or she, as the speaker, can modify and change. For example, a simple waltz enjoyed by most couples on a dance floor was not so simple when these various couples were first learning to dance. In the beginning they practiced, with and without a partner, the basic box, or rectangular, step until they felt reasonably comfortable with it. They practiced the specific movements of body, legs, and feet as well as placement of arms, hands, and feet. They did not practice "waltzing" because this would have been too vague or too macrocosmic to learn. Instead, they practiced the specific movements, placements, and postures of their bodies and body parts that constitute the act of waltzing. During practice, the end product—waltzing—was not as important as ensuring that each subpart of the act of waltzing (for example, this foot moves here, the arms are placed so, and leg or the foot follows like that) would be adequate and that, with further time and practice, he or she could become a better and better dancer.

This dancing analogy is not exactly identical to replacing maladaptive speaking behavior with appropriate speaking behavior; however, neither is this analogy that far removed. Like the beginning dancer, the adult who stutters needs to focus on the specific postures, movements, and placements of speech production and be able to initiate them or change them when he or she so desires. If such movements and postures are produced, the end product (speech) will almost take care of itself. The person's speech will be appropriate, perhaps not excellent at first but adequate and, with time and practice, it should get better and better.

Helping our adult clients focus on their speech behavior and breaking this behavior down into its constituent parts is one of our primary responsibilities in therapy. Toward these ends, Webster's (1975, 1978) management program employing fluency targets is a move in the right direction; however, only through more empirical research will we be able to more clearly circumscribe those aspects of stuttered speech production most in need of changing as well as those aspects of fluent speech production most in need of adopting.

Modification: Where and What to Begin Modifying

As with identification, we first emphasize during the modification phase those aspects of speaking that are the most apparent, longest, and clearly disruptive to the forward flow of fluent speech. While we could start with less apparent, shorter, and less physically tense speech behavior, most of these lesser stutterings will escape the attention of most adults who stutter, at least at the onset of therapy. Thus, we have found it better to start modifying the more easily recognizable stutterings because once change is effected with these stutterings, it is much more noticeable to the stutterers and their listeners.

Which stutterings are easily recognizable?   This is not something that is readily explained on paper, but it is most likely a longer stuttering that is associated with apparent physical tension in and around the face, neck, and upper chest. Along these lines, however, we would like to point out that it is not usually necessary to *directly* remediate such behaviors as lack of eye contact, turning of the head, or constriction of the external throat muscles. These inappropriate behaviors are most likely a reaction to, rather than cause of, instances of stuttering. Therefore, when modifying stuttering itself (the actual disruptive speech behavior), the basis for these inappropriate reactions will diminish, which means that the reactions themselves will cease.

We must remember that there are just so many hours during the therapy day and that we must wisely choose our battles and battle sites. That is, we must wisely pick and choose those issues we want to deal with in order to maximize the effectiveness and efficiency of such therapy. Thus, starting a therapy program by trying to change a stutterer's lack of eye contact (its obvious nature is apparently one reason it is frequently selected by beginning SLPs as a behavior to modify) is not an effective use of therapy time when so many other speech-related events need remedial attention, for example, inappropriate tongue movement, lip closure, laryngeal abductory gestures, and so forth.

One example of an easily recognizable stuttering Cessation or fixed-articulatory posture disfluencies, for example, audible sound prolongations, are excellent places to start modification with adult stutterers. This gamma behavior (see Chapter 1) is most likely the stutterer's reaction to sound-syllable repetition and is thus a complex behavior. Careful study will show you that a restricted number of inappropriate speaking strategies constitute the basic physiologic aspects of these types of speech disfluencies. You will probably note the relative fixed or stationary or stabilized speech production gesture (that is, there are minimal amounts of the rather wild oscillations of speech musculature commonly associated with sound-syllable repetitions) during audible or inaudible sound prolongation and, particularly with longer instances of prolongation, a relatively high degree of physical tension in the client's speech musculature.

The "anatomy" of one easily recognizable stuttering Listening to these cessation or fixed-articulatory posture types of speech disfluencies, you may hear: (1) little or no sound (high probability but not certainty that vocal folds are closed); (2) breathy, whispered, or noisy vocal quality (high probability of open vocal folds); or (3) a glottal fry-like, popping, or pulsing sound (closely approximated, but to some degree vibrating vocal folds with false vocal folds perhaps being medially compressed and/or "loading down" the true vocal folds). While these various laryngeal behaviors are going on, you will also probably notice that the stutterer's jaw, lips, and/or tongue are set or fixed or stabilized in the posture for the sound being audibly or inaudibly prolonged; however, the stutterer is not using these supraglottal structures to make the necessary transitional or connecting gesture ("they aren't moving on") to the next sound. The stutterer has "locked" his speaking gestures in place on the sound and is not making the between-sound or syllable transition. During all this, we can make the reasonable assumption that the stutterer's rib cage and abdomen are also relatively locked or fixed or stabilized or if anything, slowly deflating.

All these details about these behaviors cannot, of course, be easily explained to the client and in some cases would not help even if we were to do so. However, you, as the client's SLP, should clearly know the nature and frequency of these behaviors because this will help you recognize changes in their quality and quantity as the client progresses through the modification stage of therapy. Furthermore, because the rate of speech is so fast—relative to our ability to identify and modify it—in the beginning of therapy, we need to help the client change inappropriate behavior during or slightly after the instance of stuttering. Making these changes during and after the stuttering is not a place of choice but when starting to modify stuttering it is a place of necessity.

Modification: After and Then During the Instance of Stuttering

What to work on, what not to work on   To begin this discussion, let us assume that an adult stutterer is holding for too long a period of time the speech posture for the word-initial /s/ in the word *see*. This would probably result in an audible sound prolongation on the /s/. We might see the physical tension in the face, particularly the lip area, and neck muscles and possibly the movement of the eyeballs to the left or right together with blinking or closed eyes. As mentioned before, it is less than helpful to try to modify these "nonverbal" facets of the problem regardless of their maladaptive nature. Likewise, we hear the air rushing from the lungs, through the larynx and over and through the restricted space formed by the tongue approximating the cutting edge of the central and lateral incisors. However, it should be stressed that we should not instruct the stutterer to "take a deep breath and start over" because we think he or she has or is about to run out of air.

Instead of watching these grosser behaviors—facial gestures and air escaping—what we should be observing is the lack of speech posture movement from this prolonged sound to the next one (a lack of transitional or connecting gestures). We should be observing the client's failure to make the necessary transition from the word-initial /s/ consonant to the /i/ of the subsequent vowel. The client is probably pressing his or her tongue tip tightly against the alveolar ridge behind the incisors but is not moving it into position for the subsequent sound, in this case a vowel. Again it needs to be pointed out that we are not witnessing a problem with producing sounds, but a problem with connecting sounds—stuttering involves the inability to go from sound to sound, rather than the inability to produce particular sounds.

We speculate that these problems of connection are based on inappropriate strategies. In the case of our sound prolongation example, I think that one inappropriate strategy has been developed in attempts to override or mask or change another previously developed inappropriate strategy involved with the production of sound/syllable repetitions. That is, rather than continue the reiterative or repetitive attempts to begin or end a speech posture without making necessary connecting gestures to the next sound (a sound/syllable repetition), the stutterer now changes the reiterative gestures to a "frozen" or fixed or stabilized speech gesture (sound prolongation). However, the outcome is the same: The stutterer fails to move on to the next sound. As SLPs we need to work on helping the stutterer *move on* to the next sound, not move their eyelids, eyeballs, or facial muscles in a different fashion.

Modification during and/or after the stuttering   Using again our example of the adult stutterer prolonging the word-initial /s/, we would first try to help the stutterer change or move on to the next sound while he or she is in the middle of prolonging this sound. This would be our first attempt. However, since many stutterers do not like to be *stopped* once they *begin* talking, it is not unusual for the stutterer to continue saying more than a few words rather than make the necessary change. If this happens, and change during the middle of the stuttered word is not possible, then we would allow the stutterer to finish the word (or subsequent words) but immediately repeat the stuttering on this word and encourage change this time.

Obviously, this procedure is not particularly new (see Van Riper, 1973; Starkweather, 1974); however, what we do believe is slightly but importantly different is that we emphasize in lay person's terms the type of speech production that is being inappropriately used by the adult who stutters. Rather than use such terms as *blocks*, or *pullouts*, or *bouncing*, which have a place in therapy but can become too vague too quickly, we try to help clients *feel*, see, and hear the exact thing or things they are doing with their speech apparatus that interfere with speaking (for example, "John, you aren't moving your tongue from the /s/ to the /i/ position and that's why you aren't finishing the word"). We also try to emphasize the common thread that runs through all these behaviors and focus attention on the client's strategies, rather than the sounds being prolonged or repeated.

Clinician signals to client: "Change," "Move on," "Now," or "Easy"   It is not easy to help the client change his or her speech behavior in midstream, but after a successful identification problem, this can be implemented rather successfully. We can shorthand the procedure somewhat, once the adult client appears to understand what you want them to do—"When you *feel* yourself holding that speech position, move on, slowly and easily, to the next speech posture. With practice, you'll be able to do this quicker and smoother." At the point in time during the stuttering when we have been saying, "change" or "move on" to the client, we can, as the client gets the point and demonstrates that fact, simply say, "Now" at the same point in time. Of course, we have previously spent some time explaining and showing the client what we mean when we say "move on" or "change" (that is, go on to the next sound).

In a sense, we become, at this stage, the clients' external monitoring device by helping them tune in to the type of speech behavior they are producing in error and then reminding them when and how to change this behavior by moving on to the next sound(s) (we also, of course, want to make it clear to clients what type of behavior they should change *to*). Here again, the client and clinician enter into a kind of contest to see who can first recognize the stuttering. Once it is recognized, the client is reminded to change and is verbally rewarded by the SLP for any and all attempts to do so. This procedure requires the SLP to be very supportive and sensitive to the client and his or her feelings. Clients must be verbally rewarded by the SLP for successive approximations to change and the clinician's "now" must be clear, kind, and rapid, but not repulsive. We do not want to harass clients verbally about their speech the same way everybody else does. Instead, we want to objectively and systematically recognize their instances of stuttering and then help them modify (on-line) their inappropriate or stuttered speech production behavior while they are actually producing it. We are not expecting instant success and we tell the client this. We do not expect perfection but we do tell the client that we expect him or her to give this a try. These "trys" will be greatly facilitated by our support, reinforcement, and understanding for the difficulty that any human being has in changing something about her- or himself. I can easily say that the modification of speech behavior, particularly that which has been habituated over a period of several years, is just plain hard work.

Modification: When the Client Fails to Change

If the adult who stutters fails in his or her attempts to change inappropriate speech behavior when you clearly, but in polite and supportive tones say, "Now," do not persist with this procedure. Backtrack and *demonstrate*, once again, for the client the actual or specific change you are referring to; *show* the client how; don't just *tell* the client to change. *Show* the type of change you want. *Demonstrate* the behavior you want him or her to change to. Far too often we seem reluctant to actually show or demonstrate to the client—through actual positioning as well as moving our own lips, tongue, jaw, and larynx— the inappropriate speech behavior we are talking about and the specific means by which we are asking the client to change this behavior. Perhaps we fear that doing so may be construed by stutterers to mean we are mocking or teasing them. However, if our feelings toward that client are right, if we have demonstrated good faith to the client in terms of our sincerity to help the client change, then we have little to fear on this score (in Chapter 6 we further discuss clinician attitudes).

Instead, we think that some of our reluctance stems more from our lack of clarity regarding *what* behavior is in need of changing and *what* behavior should be substituted. This is due, in part, to our history of concentrating on "stutterings" or "repetitions" or "prolongations" or "blocks" without bothering to examine the actual speech production behaviors that make up or underlie our perceptual labels for these behaviors. This concentration, on our part, reflects the past zeitgeist (spirit of the times) in the field of stuttering that essentially implied that examination of the speech production of stuttering indicated that the examiner is seeking an organic or physiological or "nature" cause of stuttering. This zeitgeist, which we can more objectively evaluate with hindsight, has led us away from studying a rich source of information regarding stuttering: the actual disruptions in speech production that are associated with stuttering as well as the more subtle, perhaps imperceptible, disruptions in speech production that may accompany stutterers' perceptually fluent speech.

We are only fooling ourselves if we believe that we can capture the essentials of the stuttered speech production more precisely by minimizing our usage of the term *stuttering* in favor of using terms like *sound prolongation, sound-syllable repetition,* or even *block.* This is similar to believing we have captured the essentials of oranges, lemons, grapefruit, kumquats, and so forth by calling them *citrus fruit,* rather than merely *fruit.* Surely, a term like "sound prolongation" is a more specific descriptor than "stuttering," but it may still be too broad, too nonbehavioral, and too vague to help our adult clients help themselves become more fluent. We must strive to become more and more *specific* in our understanding of what our stuttering clients actually *do* when they interfere with their speech production (for an example of a research study that tries to do this, see Caruso, Conture and Colton, 1988). Such specificity should help us become clearer and clearer when we talk to ourselves about our clients' behaviors. It should also help in our talks with our clients (particularly those adult clients who want and need such specificity) regarding what they are and are not doing when they exhibit behavior that listeners label as "stuttering."

Modification: When the Client Produces Real Change

We have some clue that our clients are beginning to make significant change when we notice them effecting change in their maladaptive speech production strategies *during* the actual instance of stuttering. This is a rather ethereal event that is quickly over and done with as the client moves on to the next sound, syllable, or word. The SLP must, therefore, quickly recognize such change and clearly and *immediately* reinforce it. Perhaps no other aspect of therapy with stutterers places a higher premium on quick and accurate SLP observational abilities than this phase. While the demands on SLP observational skills are high, the rewards are great as most clients respond with increased frequency of change.

Reinforcement of these client changes by the SLP is quite important. Reinforcement, here as elsewhere, serves to both *confirm* ("Your behavior is as it should be") and *inform* ("That is the type of behavior you and I want to see") the client about his or her exhibited changes. Such reinforcement, particularly during conversation, can be somewhat disruptive to the forward flow of communication, but it is better to interrupt than to allow this very positive sign that the client is changing to go unnoticed. The actual change during the stuttering may take even longer than if the client had simply "bulled" his or her way through the particular speech posture. However, this is a clear sign that the adult has taken it upon him or herself to make this change, and the SLP should clearly and emphatically reinforce this self-initiative. Besides, the client's willingness to take slightly more time to make the change, if this is the case, demonstrates an ability to deal with time pressure, to become more independent of real and perceived reasons for "full steam ahead and damning the torpedoes."

In essence, these first changes by the adult stutterer are the true beginning of the end of the problem, but this implies neither a cure in the traditional sense of the word (more on the issue of cure later in this chapter) nor a time to relax on the part of the client and clinician (to paraphrase Robert Frost, both still have to travel many miles before either of them sleep).

Changes in disruptive, inappropriate, or maladaptive speech posture that occur during the stuttering can then be continually reinforced in restricted utterances ("Tell me everything you know about this ballpoint pen"). During this phase of therapy, try to provide the client with a restricted or closed set of thoughts, ideas, or topics to deal with so that he or she can concentrate on these changes in stuttering to the exclusion of conjuring up elaborate conversation. Specifically target and demonstrate the change or the types of inappropriate speech behavior you expect or desire the client to modify. The client will be far more successful, at this point, if you don't ask him or her to attempt to change *all* forms of disruptive behavior or every instance of stuttering. Failure, like success, has a way of spreading and influencing its surroundings.

We stress to the clients (many of whom already believe that they are either all right or all wrong) that consistent change on one specific type of inappropriate speech production, for example, longer sound prolongations, is a very good first step and *is* what we would call success at this phase. They may still be holding for too long and with too much physical tension the posture for production of the word-intial sound, but the client is making real progress if he or she can consistently demonstrate a rapid, easier movement into the posture for the subsequent sound.

As we have previously stated, our belief is that much of what we would describe as an instance of stuttering results from inappropriate strategies, rather than specific difficulties with particular sounds or syllables. This belief is supported, we think, by the observation that many clients' ability to change certain instances of stuttering, such as reduction in the length and physical tension of their longer sound prolongations, generalize, and they begin to demonstrate similar change in other disfluencies. The inappropriate strategy is being replaced by an appropriate one in every place the original or inappropriate one was applied. This can generalize to the point where almost overnight, it seems, the client becomes markedly more fluent. This initial burst of speech fluency may be what is sometimes called *lucky* or *false fluency* and is not to be confused with increases in speech fluency that result from a more lasting appreciation and ability to apply the "how and the why" of speech modification.

It would, however, seem a bit silly to look a "gifthorse in the mouth," so to speak, and reject out of hand the initial success the client has demonstrated. At this point in therapy, what is in order are words of praise mingled with words of caution as well as discussion of what is going on and why. Try to use this success to motivate clients toward the further work that must follow, particularly the work involved in "maintenance" or "carry-over" aspects of therapy.

What the SLP needs to avoid, however, is premature dismissal from therapy and/or premature expressions of euphoria. Honesty at this juncture is the best short-, medium- and long-term policy. The client should be supported and encouraged for his or her progress to date, but should not have expectations raised to unreasonable heights. When people suddenly fall from heights, no matter how pretty the view, their injuries generally hurt more and last longer than when they stumble over the curbs and potholes of life. The SLP clearly doesn't want to become, as one of our politicians once said, "a nattering nabob of negativism." Rather, he or she should praise the client for the present as well as facilitate the likelihood of future progress, but at the same time try to help the client understand that occasional setbacks and slippages may occur along the road to improved fluency.

Modification: Within-Therapy Carry-Over

Clients who change with you but not by themselves   Some adults who stutter seem to make change quite easily and effectively when you are monitoring their speaking behavior, but seem to do little on their own, even in your presence (this is somewhat similar to current discussions of *co-dependency*, Beattie, 1987, whereby person A gets person B to do the thinking, worrying, and the like for her or him). We are not talking about a carry-over problem in the traditional sense of difficulty in transferring, maintaining, or carrying-over changes in speech behavior from one therapy session to the next; instead we are discussing carry-over problems *within* the therapy session itself.

An adult who stutters who can quickly and accurately identify and then change during an inappropriate or disruptive speech posture or movement *only* when the SLP is assisting in the monitoring and changing is a client who obviously is not ready for dismissal ("I just can't get the feeling of fluency by myself"). This client has a problem since he or she is not ready to transfer his or her changed speech to the external, everyday environment where the SLP is nonexistent. To understand this situation we should first examine the client's understanding of the meaningfulness and rationale for your procedure. Ask the client if he or she knows what is going on and why. If need be, explain again, perhaps using different terms, why you are doing what you are doing and why you think this particular procedure is important. Do not be afraid to retrace your steps and travel over old ground. It is not uncommon that reexplaining "old" issues may give the client new insights since he or she has now had the time and sufficient experience with which to evaluate these issues afresh.

Examining the nature and number of your rewards   Second, examine the frequency and manner with which you are reinforcing the client for successful approximations and achievements in his or her own speech and related behavior. Does your reinforcement or reward seem to come too infrequently? Does your reward seem to mean anything to the client? Does he or she seem to understand not only when you reward, but what you are rewarding? Perhaps, your rewards are neutral because your relation with the client is rather neutral. Perhaps you are too businesslike and professional in manner, and the client has trouble relating to this sort of approach. However, this is not to say that you should go completely to the opposite extreme and become the client's buddy. Instead, we are merely suggesting that you study these aspects of your clinical dealings with the client.

Client's specific understanding of specific desired changes   Third, do you make it clear what elements of the client's inappropriate strategy must be changed? Do you actually *show* the client what must be changed or do you simply *tell* him or her to change? As we have said before, all too often too many clinicians fail to specifically *show*, or *demonstrate*, or *do* for the client the actual behavior they want to achieve. Rather, these clinicians do a lot of talking about change, and a lot of telling the client to change, or lecturing the client on change. It makes intuitive sense to me that a client who is quite hazy about the specifics of changing his or her speech behavior is a client who is very unlikely to make these types of changes and/or put out the necessary effort to make these changes. The client is neither asking for nor should be given a course in the anatomy and physiology of the speech and hearing mechanism; however, the client does want and needs specific instructions on how to change. For example,

> During your sound prolongations, you hold your tongue tip tightly against the roof of your mouth in the front. You then fail to move your tongue into the position for the first position for the next sound. During this time, you're also holding open your vocal cords in your voice box. I want you to try to begin closing your vocal cords and moving your tongue tip into position for the next sound when you physically *feel* yourself holding them in that "stuttered" posture. It looks like this. (You demonstrate several times or until the client seems to have the general idea; for the client to get the specific idea, he or she will have to try it several times him- or herself.)

Clients who simply fail to make change on their own Obviously, even the best laid clinical plans can go awry, and some clients, for unknown reasons, simply cannot or will not make the shift from clinician-monitored change to change on their own. These clients are problematic, but some of them respond better to approaches where they are *given* a procedure to use to change their speech. Such procedures are amply covered elsewhere (for example, Van Riper, 1973; Wingate, 1976), but they all have a common thread running through them: The client is provided with some internally or externally generated means for minimizing stuttering. The relation of these various procedures to our present understanding of the speech production characteristics of stuttered/fluent speech is, at best, unclear. Most such procedures are advocated because of their expediency and their ability to improve the client's fluency, if only for a while. The client achieves fluency after a fashion, but this is not to be confused with an approach where the client is viewed as the *perpetrator* (however unintentional) of the stuttering and as such has the means to make the necessary change in speaking behavior (what is done by the stutterer, in this case, *can* be undone).

In other words, if we take the approach, as we have done throughout this book, that clients have the means within themselves to effect change in their own speech—without the use of external devices like metronomes, miniaturized or otherwise—then it makes the most sense to help them understand and observe what they are doing that interferes with their speech. This should help them try to produce more and more of those strategies which are appropriate for the production of fluent speech ("to do more and more of the things that normally fluent speakers do when they talk"). This does not mean that we are saying that all clients will react positively to this approach—it is doubtful that some clients will react positively to *any* approach—but that this is the conceptual or philosophical base from which we start remediating.

Modification: Changing Speech during Conversation

Once the adult client begins to consistently change stuttering (shortening the duration and moving on to the next sound more easily) in restricted conversations and situations with the clinician, the clinician can begin to help the client effect change in his or her speech in more naturalistic settings, for example, talking over the phone. Some role playing of these situations, in advance of their occurrence, may help the client deal with and become appropriately desensitized to the actual speaking situation. This is where a group therapy situation, which may be conducted in parallel with individual therapy, is quite useful. Both you and the client get a chance to see the extent to which the client can make the change in front of the group. Selected phone calls can also help clients test their developing ability to change in the presence of time pressure. Having the client go into stores (with the cautions mentioned in Chapter 4) is another good experience and means of testing the client. Talking to the clinical secretary, building janitor, local shopkeepers, or fellow clinicians—if these people have the time, and seem willing, and have been previously briefed by you—is another good experience and test.

Activities should be brief but planned   Remember to keep these situations brief, to the point, and allow time for the client and yourself to discuss the results. Do not simply do this for the sake of doing it. Nothing is less appreciated by clients, particularly adults, than activities that merely take up time in the session, that seem to have no real focus or purpose, that appear to be so much "busy work." Instead, plan these "real world" conversations in advance and try to reinforce as well as critique, if necessary, the client's performance after each and every experience. If the client's performance in more than a few phone calls or conversations is less than successful, you may want to return to the therapy room and spend more time on basics. Obviously, this activity, like any other therapy activity, will not work if the client is "sleeping" between therapy sessions.

Trying to gauge improvement   You can get some idea if the client is changing the frequency, duration, type, or severity of her or his stuttering by asking, "What does your wife (husband, father, mother, boss, fellow workers, teacher, and so forth) think about your speech now?" "Has anyone mentioned anything to you lately about your speech?" "Has anyone noticed or said anything to you about your speech since you have been in therapy?" If the client reports that associates, friends, or relatives are actually starting to notice or mention positive change in his or her speaking behavior, you have some idea, in our experience, that positive change in speaking behavior is actually starting to occur where it should be occurring, that is, outside the confines of the therapy room.

If you can, you might give the client's associates outside therapy a call and ask their opinion regarding your client's progress. Of course, this presupposes that you have previously established some minimal working relations with them. These calls should not be construed, by the client, as your snooping into his or her personal life, but rather as your sincere and honest attempt to determine if other individuals in his or her environment are beginning to notice positive changes in speaking and related behavior. Often these associates will note positive change when you believe therapy is at a standstill and this, we think, should provide you with some encouragement to continue the client's therapy (clients aren't the only people who need reinforcement). Obviously, you would not want to make these phone calls frequently, but they can be made at appropriate times with very positive results on present as well as future therapy plans. Conversely, if such calls indicate little change by the client, but you seem to be noticing considerable change by the client in the therapy room, you have gained valuable information and direction for present and future therapy.

Modification: Homework or Further Work Outside Therapy

The purpose of homework   The basic reason for doing homework—in the context of therapy for stuttering—is to provide the client practice with and habituation of behavior being discussed and dealt with in therapy. A secondary reason is that such homework assignments foster an acute awareness of speech behavior and the need as well as the means to change speech. Third, homework assignments, especially those that are successfully completed, show clients that they can actually change the way they speak, that they can really do something on their own to help themselves. There is a great deal of truth in two old sayings: "If you want to roll the dice, you gotta pay the price," and "Before you sing the blues, you've gotta pay your dues." Part of the price as well as the dues the adult who stutters must pay to achieve more fluent speech is completion of homework outside the clinic.

Some realities of homework assignments   No one likes to bring home work from the office and adults who stutter are no exception. Therefore, avoid setting yourself up for frustration, anger, and feelings of resentment: Don't assign your adult client *large* amounts of between-therapy work. Make these daily assignments short and easily accomplished in a nontherapy setting, for example, in front of a dressing mirror. Make sure that the client clearly understands how, why, and when he or she is to do these assignments. Be sure to monitor these assignments; write down at the end of the therapy session the exact nature of the assignment so the client realizes that you are evaluating his or her completion and relative success with these assignments. If homework assignments involve speaking outside the home, for example, talking to strangers, make sure that the client has an opportunity to encounter strangers during the week. If this is not possible, switch assignments because neglected and impossible assignments will surely influence in-clinic therapy and most clients in a less than positive way.

Homework assignments where the client uses the phone are excellent opportunities for the client to practice identifying, monitoring, and changing speech behavior. The client's number of calls can easily be counted, the client can control the length and nature of each call fairly easily, and the exercise can readily be completed at home (in some cases, at work). Calls don't have to be complex; they can be to restaurants, pharmacies, department stores to see when they open or close; or they can be in response to newspaper ads about items the client knows something about (for example, asking one or two specific questions about cars: How many miles has the car been driven? does it have front- or rear-wheel drive?); or they can be to restaurants asking the price range of their meals. With experience and increasing success, the number, length, and nature of phone conversations can be modified to provide the client with larger numbers and varieties of speaking opportunities.

Modification: Some Client Reactions to Change

Speech should be automatic or why do I have to think about it all the time? About the time clients are beginning to change their inappropriate speech strategies more and more on their own, some of them may start to show signs of backsliding. One way or another the client may express the notion that, "Your procedure works, but only if I think about it all the time. If I don't think about it, it doesn't work. Am I going to have to think about my speech for the rest of my life?" This is obviously a frustrating state of affairs for both client and clinician.

When do conscious changes in speech become less conscious or more "automatic?" While we do not have good objective information on how long after initial change in speech an adult stutterer needs to continue consciously monitoring and changing, it does seem that this period of time is longer rather than shorter. That is, there will probably be at least a six- to twelve-month period or longer of behavioral habituation. Some period of time is also needed for the client to generalize his or her increasingly fluent strategy to more and more speaking situations with more and more success. This period of habituation will, therefore, be a period where change in speech strategy is not automatic, and clients will have to be somewhat conscious of their speaking behavior and their relative success or failure at changing and monitoring it. We believe that it is wishful thinking—on the part of both the client and clinician—to expect anything different, to believe and expect quick establishment of new strategies for speaking when it has taken years to establish the other, inappropriate strategies which create the instances of stuttering.

As we've said before, misleading our clients that change in their speech behavior will be a quick, easy, and painless process is doing them a great disservice and is more a sin than providing ineffectual therapy. While we don't subscribe to the modern "no pain no gain" school of thought, we do believe that the other half of inspiration is perspiration. It is simply going to take some time and effort on the part of the client to change maladaptive, habituated speech strategies that have been used to initiate speech over many years. For example, when beginning speech, the client might habitually fix, lock, or stop the respiratory system during mid-exhalation simultaneously with opening the vocal folds in association with stabilizing the lower jaw and pressing the lips together. This sort of inappropriate response pattern is going to take some time to change. One does not learn to drive a car in two weeks, but must spend considerable time behind the wheel in various traffic and weather conditions. For example, the process of learning to drive must first involve conscious monitoring of motor behavior until the motor behaviors necessary for steering, accelerating, shifting, and so forth are established and become more automatic. Even when established, these behaviors will become continually refined with further experience. Learning never stops; it just becomes less noticeable as refinements and subtleties rather than basic behavioral changes are made.

Creeping before walking Even though some clients initially exhibit a lack of automaticity when changing their speech, these same individuals may want to rush out and use their newly found fluent strategies in *all* situations at *all* times. One can hardly blame them, but the SLP should restrict this tendency somewhat, at least at first, until the client has demonstrated the ability to do this in more controlled situations where the probability for successful implementation of appropriate strategies is maximized. Using the car analogy again, we explain to the client that after you first learn to drive, you do not want to practice during the time trials for the Indianapolis 500. Instead you practice your driving skills in low-traffic, side-road situations until you get more and more of the feeling for the strategies of driving. We stress patience and try to focus on success in more restricted situations. However, we also tell clients that with time and additional experience, they will be talking in more and more difficult situations. At first, however difficult it is to restrain oneself, go slow. We must creep before we walk.

Modification: Knowing When to Dismiss

In an ideal world, dismissing adults who stutter from therapy should be like the old response parents gave their children when the youngsters asked, "Mom, how will I know when I'm in love?" The sage parent supposedly replies, "Don't worry; when it's real love you'll know it." In other words, when an adult stutterer is ready for dismissal from therapy, we should know it. Unfortunately this is not an ideal world, and we do not always know when to dismiss our clients. Thus, we have to take an educated guesstimation which is just that: a considered hunch based on our education, training, and clinical experience.

What sort of nonspeech, behavioral "signs" does the client exhibit? Is the client giving you signs that he or she is ready for a break (either temporary or permanent)? Is he or she calling in more often than in the past with excuses for not coming to therapy? Is he or she arriving late and leaving early more regularly? Do other adults who stutter begin to question why this client continues to come in for therapy because he or she is very fluent now and/or exhibiting little change? Does therapy seem to be playing more and more of a second fiddle to other activities? Is therapy becoming less and less of a priority for the client? (This may suggest resistance to as well as lack of motivation for further change.) Or is the client seemingly interested in helping others with similar speech problems? As mentioned in Conture, 1983, we think that this is always a good sign (for further discussion of "altruism" as a coping or adjustive mechanism, see Vaillant, 1977).

What sort of speech "signs" does the client exhibit Is the client consistently demonstrating in therapy a quick, accurate, and relatively easy ability to identify and change instances of disfluency? Does the frequency of stuttering hover at or below 3 percent to 5 percent? (As previously alluded to, these sort of percentages would be problematic when we are making decisions with very mild or nearly fluent stutterers.) Does the clinician have to give minimal or no verbal, auditory, or visual cues before the client begins to change? When the client lapses back into old speech strategies, is he or she able to quickly, easily, and without much emotionality reverse directions and become more fluent again? Do you find yourself, if you have group therapy, using this adult client as a good example or role model for the other adults who stutter?

How does the client manage "breaks" from therapy? Does this client, during breaks from therapy, continue to make improvements, albeit small, on his or her own? Do you find that this client, after a longer-than-usual break from therapy (say, three to five weeks or longer), is able to maintain progress to date or has he or she slipped back a couple of rungs? Does the client appear anxious or uncertain about maintaining his or her gains just before a scheduled break from therapy? Sometimes, if you have real doubts about dismissal, a scheduled break from therapy might be a viable alternative; you could terminate therapy for a fixed but relatively brief period of time, say a month, after which the client returns to therapy. This way you can observe how the client can effect changes on his or her own away from your watchful eye and the "healing" ambience of your clinical situation. As always, of course, make it clear to the client that the door to your clinic will remain open and that you will be willing and able to receive phone calls and visits.

Dismissal may result from lack of, as well as demonstration of, success Dismissal from therapy, for some clients, may not mean that they have been successful in therapy or that their therapy is completed. Some clients may have to be dismissed before they actually achieve normally fluent speech. These clients may not be able to receive maximal benefit from therapy at this point in their lives for a variety of reasons: too many other professional and personal obligations vying for their attention, concomitant problems that may be ongoing but show signs of future resolution, unavoidable and unresolvable schedule conflicts, and so forth. This situation must be handled carefully by the SLP because he or she does not want to engender hopes of future success (or, conversely, dash all hopes for improvement) when the SLP is just plain unsure. It is better, in most of these cases, to keep your uncertainties to yourself, but make it apparent to the client that the door is always open for further discussion and consultation. In the end, you have to have some faith, which I think you can have, in your client's future ability to know when it is right for him or her to re-enter speech and language therapy.

Modification: Maintenance/Follow-up Therapy

As the various contributors to Boberg's (1983) edited text on the maintenance of fluency indicate, there's much we don't know but would like to find out about maintenance/follow-up therapy. One thing that most clinical investigators do know, however, is that some form of maintenance/follow-up therapy is quite important to long-term improvement in stuttering. In essence, once our clients have left therapy, their work has really just begun. As Williams (1978) points out, "the goal of therapy is not change within the clinic but change outside the clinic." The client, in his or her everyday world, must now try to apply the information, insights, and new behavior that he or she has gained in therapy. For some, this outside-of-clinic effecting of change will go fairly smoothly, but for others it will be problematic. Hopefully, the client has developed a sufficiently sound problem-solving orientation and will be able, although not always 100 percent successfully, to change and adjust independently.

You can't hit a home run every time up to bat   You should let clients know that neither you nor they should expect success each and every time they have to speak. We realize that this instruction may sound a bit heretical because it appears rather pessimistic. It may sound to some that we are saying that the client will stutter forever and ever. Well, perhaps, but in our opinion this advice is more realistic than pessimistic. It is based on what we believe is the reality of the situation. As previously mentioned, adults who stutter have taken many years to develop their speech problem and their social, emotional, psychological, and intellectual reactions and attitudes to it. This behavioral-attitudinal complex will not be changed overnight, and at this stage we think that the client should be prepared for some future moments, hours, or days of difficulty. We said prepared (forewarned is forearmed), and not excused.

Follow-up therapy: Some logistical considerations   The SLP can help the client through the adjustment from daily/weekly therapy to no therapy by scheduling follow-up or maintenance therapy sessions. Much of what we know about the number and nature of these sessions has come from experience with clinical practice and there are very few hard and fast rules in this area. While there is clearly a need for empirical, objective investigations into the quantity and quality of maintenance therapy, there are still a few helpful observations that we can pass along at this point, although they are rather imprecise guidelines.

First, and perhaps most obviously, maintenance therapy sessions should be spaced far enough apart so that the SLP is not merely duplicating or recapitulating the original therapy schedule, only under a different guise. Second, it is probably better to phase out therapy gradually than to make the client go "cold turkey" and then return. We have used two different plans: (1) once a month for 6 months following dismissal; then once every 2 months for 6 months, followed by once every 6 months for 1 year and then periodic phone calls for another 12 to 18 months; or (2) a 3- to 6-month break from therapy after dismissal, then once every 3 months for a year, once every 6 months for one year, and then periodic phone calls for one more year. We prefer the former maintenance schedule because it is more gradual during what we believe is the crucial post-therapy period: the first six months following dismissal.

Generally speaking, however, if the client's outside-of-clinic fluency is maintained 12 months post-therapy, then the probability is high that significantly increased fluency will be maintained for the long term and maintenance sessions can be spaced even farther apart, if the SLP and client so wish.

Third, the basic point behind maintenance therapy is that the client not be set adrift, so that he or she feels there is a place where contact can be made with a caring professional who can and will answer questions and help the client work through problems that arise as the client becomes a more fluent speaker. And, it should be noted, there can be problems.

Problems during follow-up therapy   We've already mentioned the tendency on the part of some clients to feel discouraged, during the latter parts of therapy or maintenance therapy, when they are not 100 percent successful in changing their speech and/or speaking more fluently. This problem should be addressed so that the client can learn how to cope with this situation.

Another problem, that some clients encounter, is when the client's new found fluency begins to influence his or her relations with relatives, friends, and associates. A bit like a child with a new toy, some adults who stutter may begin to use their new, more fluent speech any and everywhere and at all times, much to the consternation of those around them. Whereas previously these associates may have felt that the adult client wasn't talking enough, they may now complain—and we've had this occur—that the client is talking too much.

Naturally, such problems need to be discussed between client and clinician and if possible, and where necessary, between client and concerned relatives and or associates of the client. While these associates must be helped to realize that they can't have it both ways—having the client talk *and* be quiet only when *they* so decree—the adult client must also realize that normally disfluent speakers listen just as well as speak. Their increased fluency is not a license for monologuing, monopolizing the speaking floor, interrupting other speakers, and the like. Follow-up sessions provide a natural vehicle for discussing these issues and can be used by clients to tell themselves and others, "I'll ask my speech person what she thinks about that when I see her in a couple of weeks."

Of course, when real pressing concerns arise, the telephone can be used with the client being clearly and explicitly told that you will welcome such calls. We have found that it is better to head off little problems when they begin, before they develop and evolve into bigger ones that require more work on the part of both the client and clinician.

SOME PARTING THOUGHTS

"This Is What We Think Needs to Be Considered"

In the two preceding chapters, we discussed our thoughts and those of others regarding the evaluation and remediation of younger individuals who stutter, with particular emphasis in this chapter on the adult who stutters. We have tried not to provide a recipe orientation, but rather a "this is what needs to be considered" approach. Obviously our approach was derived from our clinical and research experience, training, education, and biases regarding stuttering. However, we make no apologies for the selection of our considerations because all that one can do is present what appears most appropriate and important, given his or her considered opinion.

Needless to say, other approaches do exist, and others will be developed and should not be slighted (for example, note Gregory's, 1978, description of the "stutter more easily" versus "speak more fluently" forms of therapy). However, given the orientation of this book, we thought it most appropriate to give the reader a *common thread approach* rather than one fractionated among a variety of approaches.

Its the therapist, not merely the technique   Regardless of the specific approach, it is the clinician's intensity of purpose, his or her concentration on the task at hand, his or her ability to attend to relevant detail, ability to listen to the message behind the client's words, and his or her demonstrable caring for the client that will significantly determine the outcome of therapy. While we have come a long, long way from the days when therapy for individuals who stutter (children, teenagers, or adults) was much more of an art form than a science or trained skill, the clinician still remains central to this science and skill. Even though clinicians' personal, experiential, and professional qualities are central to the long-term success of their clients, clinicians must resist the temptation to divorce themselves from the seemingly esoteric world of empirical research. Simply put, the quantity and quality of objective data pertaining to stutterers and stuttering has and will continue to develop to the point where clinicians must, regardless of their clinical persuasion, at least give it some consideration.

While the art and skill of the clinician in handling people, expressing concern and care for the clients, listening to their needs, and so forth, should never be denied by any thinking individual, neither should clinicians disregard basic, objective empirical evidence regarding stuttering and stutterers. Granted, not every clinician can and should become an experimentalist testing out this or that hypothesis or collecting this or that normative piece of information. However, as highly trained, educated, and up-to-date practioners, we should all try to understand the objective information that tells us more and more about the nature of stuttering and the people who stutter. Such attempts at understanding are preferable to simply proceeding with clinical game plans derived from data bases that have little or no factual support or that current information refutes or casts significant doubts upon. Thus, I believe that the future will be a time when the art and the science of stuttering therapy can become more closely aligned. As such alignment becomes more and more of a reality, we can begin to hand down, from one generation of clinicians to another, clinical procedures that are based as much on fact as they are on tradition.

Avoid being too certain about the uncertain   We have discussed in the preceding chapters some of the complexities, subtleties, and vagaries involved with the clinical management of stuttering. One of the intentions behind these writings is to help people become clear on their points of unclarity and confusion. If we have done this, if only in part, then we have contributed to the reader's abilities to identify areas of uncertainty that should, in turn, help us to formulate relevant questions whose answers may truly advance our knowledge. Clarity, however, is not the same as certainty.

If we, on the other hand, are certain about the uncertain—if we think that we have all the answers—we will never bother to ask needed questions because we are so certain we understand that we never question. We are neither advocating questions nor disagreements for their own sake. Rather, we need to ask ourselves questions. Surrounded by this imperfect world, can we realistically expect that our therapy with stutterers will be perfect, that it will contain within it no points of uncertainty, that *all* of our clients will *always* improve for *all* time? I think not. While we should and cannot harbor such expectations, we can work toward improving and providing the best possible clinical services. I welcome your joining me in these efforts, for this is the material from which we formulate purposeful and interesting lives as professionals as well as people and help improve those of our clients. If we can do this, I am convinced that the best is yet to come for our clients.

SUMMARY

We have discussed what we have think "needs to be considered" when remediating stuttering in adults. We have tried to place as much emphasis on the clinician's abilities and experiences as we have on the specific therapy techniques used by the clinician. However, it was also emphasized that the art and the skill of the clinician should not lead the clinician to disregard basic, objective empirical evidence regarding stuttering, particularly when that evidence runs contrary to accepted beliefs and practices. At present, there are *too many uncertainties* about remediating adults, particularly regarding relapse, maintenance, or long-term recovery, for any clinicians *to be certain* that *all* of their adults who stutter will *always* improve for *all* time.

Typically, adults who stutter exhibit the most habituated form of stuttering and related behavior. Many of them have had prior experience with therapy, with varying degrees of success. However, adults who stutter can often be very rewarding clients to work with because of their motivation to change, seriousness of purpose, their desire to finally "do something" about and for themselves, and their more refined intellectual and social skills coupled with their increased maturity.

Adults who stutter, like all other adults, *behave* in ways which influence the way they think and, conversely, they *think* in ways which influence the way they behave. Because their behavior influences their thinking, it seems reasonable to assume that therapy for adults should *ideally* involve three interrelated procedures: (1) some form of *discussion* ("talk therapy") to deal with attitudes, beliefs, emotions, and ideas which engender and maintain inappropriate speech production strategies; (2) objective, nonjudgmental *identification* of those strategies used to interfere with speech production; and (3) systematically *changing* those behaviors which interfere with speech production by using those strategies which normally fluent speakers use to produce normally fluent speech. In essence, we want to couple identification and modification of the client's inappropriate strategies for initiating and continuing speech production with exploration and modification of the client's attitudes, beliefs, emotions, and ideas which foster and perpetuate such strategies.

It is our belief that clients can't effectively change, on a long-term basis, behaviors which they do not know how or when they produce. Thus, we believe that relatively quick, accurate identification of inappropriate speech production strategies must precede and continue together with effective modification of the same. Initially, identification is based on auditory and visual feedback. With continued effort and experience the stutterer should come to *physically feel* what is being done to interfere with speaking, and how that differs from and can be changed into strategies that can be done to facilitate speaking.

While changes in the adult stutterer's speech patterns may be quite sudden and occur very shortly after the onset of therapy, experience indicates that the *lasting* change is not generally as rapid. Thus, patience for the rather slow manner in which changes occur in adult human behavior is a virtue that both client and clinician should develop. Much can be and is being done to help adults who stutter, but the length of time in which this help occurs may need to be realistically assessed and discussed with the client *prior* to the initiation of therapy.

SIX
CONCLUSIONS

DROWNING IN A SEA OF INFORMATION

Even a cursory reading of textbooks in the area of stuttering suggests that information is pouring into the pool of knowledge about stuttering at an alarmingly fast rate. Rather than suffering from a lack of information, it sometimes seems that we are in danger of drowning in a sea of facts, figures, and speculation about the problem. Increasingly, the consumer as well as disseminators of knowledge, (that is, students and their teachers) need to wear a personal flotation device to avoid going under. Hopefully, the following guidelines will help.

Data Is Not Always Reflected in Discussions

One thing that should be kept in mind when swimming through this sea is the difference between data *and* discussions about that data. The data are as factual and as objective as the experimenter could obtain. The discussion can be as subjective and as fanciful as the experimenter feels comfortable with and his or her peer reviewers (and journal editors) will tolerate. While discussion can be closely grounded in observable fact, it can also range fairly far afield from actual facts. Readers should try not to blur the distinction between data and discussion of the data. The common thread that runs through studies should be the findings. Once these findings have accumulated to a point where a picture starts to emerge, researchers generally find that the speculations contained within their discussions have a more solid base of support.

Science Advances by Small Increments in Knowledge as Much as It Does by Quantum Leaps

Because clinicians are people as well as professionals, it is understandable that they sometimes hope against hope that someday, somehow, someone will find the silver bullet that cures stuttering. Likewise, because researchers are people as well as professionals, it is understandable that they may hope against hope that someday someone will publish the breakthrough study that shows what causes stuttering. While silver bullets and breakthrough studies may indeed emerge, we shouldn't hold our collective breaths waiting. Indeed, the trouble with the advancement of knowledge is the trouble with life—both are so daily.

Our clinical and theoretical knowledge advances in gradual steps as much as it does by quantum leaps. Gradually the story unfolds as independent investigators replicate findings and refine methodology. Sometimes, of course, in the gradual accretion of knowledge, earlier findings are buried in the blitz of intervening journal articles, but this is where careful scholarship should play a part. For an example of how knowledge advances in small, incremental steps, we will examine one variable, VOT, that has been studied for nearly ten years.

Early research suggested that stutterers' VOTs differed from those of normally fluent speakers (for example, Agnello, 1975; Hillman and Gilbert, 1977), but further study in this area found no significant difference between the VOTs of stutterers and their normally fluent peers (for example, Metz, Conture and Caruso, 1979; Watson and Alphonso, 1982; Zebrowski, Conture and Cudahy, 1985; Pindzola, 1986; McNight and Cullinan, 1988). Gradually the story unfolds. To determine whether stutterers' VOTs significantly differ from those of normals, a great deal of care must be taken when matching subjects as well as when designing speaking material (Healey and Ramig, 1986; Adams 1987).

But the real story, in my opinion, is that looking for differences in VOTs is similar to the person who, when asked why he was looking under the corner streetlamp for his lost keys, replied "I'm looking here 'cause the light is better." VOT may be a good street light, but we'll probably have to look elsewhere to find out more about stutterers' speech production abilities. VOT may be relatively easy to measure and seems to have an important relation to something stutterers supposedly have trouble with—temporal interactions between glottal and supraglottal behaviors. However, if stutterers' VOTs were *appreciably* different from those of normals, we would perceive when we listen to stutterers, which we don't. A lot more of their voiced sounds would sound unvoiced and vice versa. Rather, our gradual buildup of knowledge in this area suggests that other measures and/or aspects of laryngeal-supralaryngeal behavior need to be investigated. This insight has taken over ten years to develop but is becoming a solid building block in the foundation of our knowledge about stuttering.

Number of Subjects Versus Replication by Independent Researchers

Much is made about the fact that this or that study had one, two, three, or thirty subjects. Should we, as readers of research, disregard findings from studies employing small sample size? While sample size can influence the generalizability of findings, the size of the sample is many times related to the question(s) under investigation. Piaget, for example, developed a vast number of observations and a rich theory based on a sample size of one to three subjects (that is, his own children). Likewise, our knowledge of "normal" VOT values were, for many years, based on a total sample size of well under ten subjects, but this did not stop many investigators from positing elaborate speculations based on these findings. This is neither a call for small sample sizes nor a dismissal of the importance or relevance of sample size to the generalizability of findings. Rather it is an attempt to get us to see that sample size is less of an issue than whether independent researchers obtain similar findings.

Indeed, replication by independent researchers was one of the decision rules applied by Andrews and his colleagues (1983) in their review of stuttering research. Is it not more impressive that three *independently* conducted and reported studies, each containing only three subjects apiece, obtain identical findings than one study of ten subjects that is never replicated? If our understanding of stuttering advances by an accretion of knowledge, it also advances when more than one investigator observes the same phenomenon. If this sort of agreement requires 3 or 33 or 103 subjects, so be it. Big is not necessarily better.

ORIENTATION

In the preceding chapters, we have attempted to discuss the diagnosis and remediation of stuttering and how these activities change with the individual, the duration of the problem, its severity, and concomitant variables. My orientation towards diagnosis and remediation of stuttering as presented during this discussion may be summarized as follows:

1. The need to consider that people who stutter are people first and stutterers second.

2. The need to understand that while behaviors or events may have a central tendency, there is always a "normal" dispersion of values that surround that central tendency.
3. The need to know what issues are typical for most stutterers, but to be able to recognize important individual differences in etiology and symptomatology among stutterers.
4. The need to recognize that for clients, clinician and parental models for and demonstrations of behavior speak far louder than all their verbal explanations, instructions, or admonitions.
5. The need to develop the ability to make quick, accurate behavioral observations of people and their communicative and related activities.
6. The need to understand how the psyche and soma interact with stuttering and how to deal with the speech production and language characteristics of stuttering within the context of the stutterer's psychosocial activities and concerns.

This orientation may seem a bit abstract. This abstraction, however, is as much due to the nature of stuttering as it is to the nature of my orientation. While abstraction is not necessarily a virtue neither, in some cases, is specificity. Clearly, it would be preferable to enumerate, quantify, and objectify all that we could about stuttering. Such quantitative specificity, however, may currently be neither possible nor feasible, at least for certain aspects of stuttering. Thus, as aspects of the preceding five chapters indicate, I decided not to ignore the reality of such abstract, hard-to-quantify psychosocial factors as anxiety, parental guilt and concern, coping strategies, motivation, personality variables, and so forth. Ignoring the reality of such nonquantifiable factors would seem to be akin to ignoring the reality of love simply because we have not as yet been able to quantify, measure, or empirically investigate it. Factors like love and motivation may represent some of the untidy, elusive details of life but they are part of life and therefore need some, albeit less than objective, consideration.

EVALUATION PRECEDES REMEDIATION

Far too often SLPs begin to remediate individuals who stutter *before* they have a good handle on the number and nature of the individual's concerns. While we can never know everything there is to know about our clients, this should not excuse us from beginning our therapy program *before* we carefully evaluate the client. We have tried to show that generating an effective therapy plan for stuttering necessitates an adequate evaluation of the stutterer, his or her stuttering speech problem, and related (non)communicative concerns.

We have also tried to show that besides the speech disfluency problem, SLPs need to recognize that various other speech and nonspeech events should be evaluated, such as parental standards for child behavior, parental rates of utterance and length and type of turn-switching pauses, the child's articulation, language, voice, hearing, reading, and academic abilities. Below we illustrate how difficult it is to develop such recognition by showing a classic example of the saying, "Do as I say, not as I do." This example will make apparent the fact that I myself have not always recognized that there can be more to stuttering than stuttering and have occasionally forgotten that stuttering is not the only or even principal concern of each and every stutterer I clinically serve.

Do as I Say, Not as I Do: An Example

My example, from my early days of clinical practice, involves a four- and one-half-year-old boy I was remediating for stuttering who frequently exhibited a hoarse voice quality. My ears heard—it was even noted in the original diagnostic report—but I really did not listen or pay attention to the possibility that the child's hoarseness might be a problem. Instead, I continued to focus on the child's stuttering. One day another SLP watched one of the child's therapy sessions and mentioned the boy's seemingly inappropriate voice quality. This woke me, to some degree, to the reality of the situation and I referred the boy to an otolaryngologist for determination of whether there were any physical or physiological reason(s) for such vocal symptoms. Fortunately, the physician observed no significant laryngeal pathology, but he did observe some slight superior vocal fold surface edema and reddening of tissue coloration. This physician's observation, based on his careful indirect laryngoscopic examination of the boy's laryngeal structures, is the type of information that one naturally expects the medical specialist to provide, rather than the SLP. However, there is more to this story.

This physician also provided information that I, as an SLP would and should have known, had I not been so focused upon the child's stuttering. The physician did this by carefully questioning the boy's mother who indicated that the *voices* I sometimes heard the child produce while waiting in the lobby (once again, I heard, but I wasn't listening) were a routine home occurrence. The child appeared to be physically tensing and straining with his vocal folds to achieve these voices (a high-pitched squeaky voice of a mouse, a low-pitched voice of a frog, and a loud voice of a monster). To compound the child's problem, he sometimes yelled when he produced these voices. The mother was cautioned—first by the ENT and then with follow-up talks by me—to help the child cut back on his use of these voices and his yelling. He eventually curtailed his use of these voices as well as inappropriate yelling and his vocal quality gradually returned to within normal limits.

Our point with this example is that my concern for the child's stuttering clouded my judgment and kept me from asking some simple but pertinent questions of the child's mother. It also obfuscated my thinking since I had heard the child's "voices," but didn't pay any attention or see them as related to the child's voice problem. Fortunately, in this case, the child's concomitant voice problem was neither serious nor apparently contributory to stuttering, but I wonder how many serious and contributory concomitant problems clinicians may overlook in their sincere, but perhaps overly focused, concerns regarding a client's stuttering. Truly, an objective, thorough evaluation of our clients who stutter is something toward which we continually strive but as yet have not achieved.

IDENTIFICATION

The Importance of Physically Feeling Behavior That Interferes with Speech Production

We have stressed in the preceding chapters the importance we place on helping stutterers develop the ability to identify and *physically feel* what they *do* when they interfere with their own speech production. If we make the reasonable assumption that the goal of stuttering therapy is to help stutterers transfer their in-clinic fluency to the "real world," we should try to provide them with a means to insure this transfer. Identification of their own behavior is one means to this end.

We have previously said it is difficult to change, on a permanent or at least a more consistent basis, what you do not know that you do when you do it. This specificity, akin to Thorndike's (1913) "specificity doctrine," relates to the stutterer indentifying or physically feeling his or her interfering speech behavior and influenced by such factors as (1) the severity and nature of the stuttering behavior; (2) the client's ability to assess objectively and analytically his or her own behavior; and (3) the client's willingness to objectively come to grips with what he or she does to interfere with speech.

The Clinician's Ability to Identify Will Influence What the Client Gains from Identification

As we have mentioned, stutterers can be helped to identify and physically feel their interfering or disrupting speech behavior by using audio and audio-visual tape recordings, mirrors, magnifying glasses, and clickers, buzzers, flashlights as well as hand gestures or simple statements like "there," "now," or "that's one." All these "devices" serve to signal to clients their interfering speech behavior. While perhaps obvious, we need to stress how important it is for the SLP to have the ability to quickly, accurately, and nonemotionally recognize and point out to the stutterer the stutterer's inappropriate or interfering speech behavior. This ability by the SLP really determines, no matter what technology or equipment is used, the success of the identification procedure.

The clinician should also realize that he or she is *only* using auditory and visual information to identify the stutterer's stutterings while the stutterer, besides audition and vision, also has available the internalized physical feelings (kinesthesia, deep touch, and so forth) associated with his or her speech behavior. Therefore, the clinician must make a concerted effort to obtain some degree of appreciation for what instances of stuttering feel like as well as sound and look like; this is best done by the SLP imitating, as closely as possible, the stutterer's stutterings and asking the stutterer if it *feels* like thus and so (for example, "John when I prolong the "s" as you just did like this [clinician models /s/ prolongation], I have this tense feeling in the front of my tongue. Is that what it physically feels like to you when you do that?"). An older client, particularly one who is sensitive to his or her own behavior and is reasonably articulate, can help the clinician learn much about what it feels like to stutter.

As well as having the ability to identify stutterers' stutterings, the SLP also needs to be able to provide the stutterer with some reasonable rationale for identification. The SLP will probably, particularly with the silver bullet-seeking client, have to repeat this rationale, supplying more detail as the stutterer progresses through therapy.

Helping the Client Identify Stutterings Should Not Take the Place of Helping the Client Learn to Modify Stutterings

Simply put, identification of stutterings does not and should not take the place of modification of stuttering. They are related processes. Identification is the beginning and is part of the platform upon which we help the client build a lasting change in speech fluency. Change that passively happens to the client because of what you make the stutterer do is change that will fade with time. In stutterers' everyday life, when they need to change their speech, they will need to recognize quickly and nonemotionally how they are interfering with the forward flow of their speaking behavior. While it is important to learn a different, more fluent way of speaking, it is just as important, if not more difficult, to know when to appropriately effect such learning. Identification provides some of this knowledge as well as a means by which the mystery and vagueness of the problem can be removed.

Doing It for Clients versus Having Them Do It for Themselves

The objective insights gained by stutterers from a detailed examination of their stutterings and related behavior and then rapid identification after, as well as during, its occurrence cannot be overlooked. We want to help the clients learn these abilities in an independent, problem-solving fashion. We are not interested in their becoming *dependent* upon us for identification and modification of their speech. If the SLP changes the clients' speech fluency *for* them, without their objective awareness of what they *do* to interfere with their own behavior and what *they must do* to change, the SLP is using, we believe, a short-sighted procedure.

To draw an analogy, let us suppose that you were learning a foreign language. Could we realistically expect that you would be ready and able, by passively repeating the words, phrases, and sentences of the foreign language, to use these phrases effectively when the situation calls for you to use the foreign language? The number, nature, and complexities of the situations are never predictable, and neither is the learner's emotional-intellectual state at the time when the situation occurs. Thus, learners, to be maximally effective across a wide variety of situations, need to be able to actively generate a strategy to effect or change behavior when they realize the situation demands such action or when they are producing inappropriate behavior.

MODIFICATION

Behavior Modification: Thirty Years Old and Still Limping Along on the Rim

The 1960s brought to the field of stuttering a panoply of new terms and concepts from the area of learning theory and behavioral therapy (for example, Shames and Sherrick, 1963; Brutten and Shoemaker, 1967). Although the 1970s witnessed some critical assessment of this approach (for example, Siegel, 1970), during the 1970s and into the early 1980s clinical investigators employing behavioral modification methodology with stutterers seemingly concentrated on refining this methodology (for example, Ryan 1978, 1980) rather than empirically investigating underlying theory.

More recently, there has been some thoughtful attempt (Guitar and Peters, 1980) to integrate and/or combine traditional and behavioral modification approaches when remediating stuttering. Although the theory and methodology of *behavior modification* continue to generate interest, particularly with regard to clinical practice, there are, as Prins and Hubbard (1988) indicate, a variety of unresolved theoretical issues in this area. Whatever the case, *behavioral modification,* in some form or other, will probably continue to generate interest and controversy for some time to come.

Behavior modification, broadly defined, is a clinical procedure stemming from conditioning and learning principles used to change a client's behavior. Some have expressed the belief that behavior modification for stuttering is akin to old wine in new bottles (for example, Sheehan 1970b), whereas others appear to believe that behavior modification is a sound, more systematic means of remediating stuttering (for example, Ryan 1978, 1980). There is, as usual, some truth in both opinions; however, we believe that there are other issues that are just as, if not more, germane to the topic of behavior modification of stuttering.

Being Able to Modify Stuttering Behavior Does Not Mean We Know What Stuttering Behaviors Need Modifying

Simply put, how can we modify something we don't understand? Do we really know what an individual does with his or her speaking mechanism just before and during an instance of stuttering? Are all behavioral aspects of stuttering equal and the results of similar underlying processes? The idea that not all aspects of stuttering are similar is, of course, somewhat akin to Brutten and Shoemaker's (1967) speculation that some aspects of stuttering, such as within-word disfluencies, result from classically conditioned "negative emotion" whereas other aspects, such as facial gestures, represent maladaptive adjustive or coping behaviors that are learned and/or reinforced through instrumental conditioning processes.

What We Know about Stuttered Speech Production

In our scurry to modify stuttering, we may have lost sight of one important fact: specifically, what aspects of stuttering need to be modified to achieve long-term recovery. Recent research provides the beginnings of an objective data base describing what *actually* happens to speech production *during* stuttering—rather than what informal observation suggests happens (for example, Conture, McCall and Brewer, 1977; Freeman and Ushijima, 1978; Conture, Schwartz and Brewer, 1985; Caruso, Conture and Colton, 1988). These studies have helped us understand, among other things, that (1) different types of stuttering may be associated with different types of disrupted speech production; (2) there is a complex relation between the type of stuttering, the phonetic elements being stuttered, and the resultant observed speech production behavior; (3) the larynx is clearly a part of stuttering although there is little evidence to indicate that it "causes" stuttering; and (4) the "discoordination" hypothesis (cf. Van Riper, 1982, pp. 396–453), while still an interesting and potentially sound explanation of stuttering, is not supported by existing empirical findings (for example, Conture, Colton and Gleason, 1988).

The Need for Pre- versus Post-therapy Research

However, regarding the long-term recovery from stuttering, it is still unclear what aspects of stuttering are the most crucial to modify. Very much related to this issue is the pre- versus post-therapy research of Metz and others (Metz, Onufrak, and Ogburn, 1979; Metz, Samar, and Sacco, 1983; Robb, Lybolt and Price, 1985) who have attempted to assess what aspects of acoustic correlates of speech production appear related to therapy-induced changes in stuttering.

While it appears that changes in the temporal domain of speech production are most related to improvement in fluency, it is still unclear how these acoustic variables relate to *long-term* improvement in stuttering, that is, improvement that lasts five years or longer. However, acoustic measures as some have suggested (for example, Caruso and Burton, 1987) may neither accurately nor precisely reflect underlying supralaryngeal or laryngeal movement. Furthermore, as Atal, Chang, Mathews and Tukey (1978) show, it is difficult to relate changes in acoustic measures to changes in speech production since the articulatory-acoustic relation is less than simple; for example, identical format frequencies and amplitudes in the acoustic signal can be produced by different vocal tract shapes.

What would appear to be needed, therefore, are instrumental procedures that directly measure speech production behavior (e.g. Conture et al., 1988), *used in conjunction* with the pre-, during, and post-therapy designs employed by, for example, Metz, Samar and Sacco (1983) or Robb, Lybolt and Price (1985). However, what is needed is a post-therapy period that covers the five years after therapy. This sort of "longitudinal" followup work would, of course, be difficult as well as expensive but it is, nevertheless, work that needs to be done.

If we knew which aspects of speech production are most clearly related to long-term recovery from stuttering as a result of therapy, it would obviate much of our debate regarding what forms of remediation are most appropriate. Indeed, the nature of these behaviors would dictate the nature of our modification procedures. For example, if faster, less hesitant coordinations between laryngeal and supralaryngeal behaviors seemed to be most highly related to long-term improvement in stuttering, then therapies could be designed to maximize changes in these laryngeal-supralayrngeal interactions.

Of course, a number of people have already stated what "behaviors" they believe are most importantly related to improvement in stuttering. For example, some have suggested that stuttering results from or is related to a conflict in presentation of the role of the self (Sheehan, 1978); therefore, we should logically employ procedures appropriate to resolving or modifying such a conflict. Unfortunately, we have no evidence that role conflicts or a variety of other behaviors, advocated as "key" for changing stuttering, are any more or less associated with long-term recovery from the problem.

If we, as SLPs, hope to assist stutterers permanently change what they do when they stutter, it seems apparent to me that we need a vastly superior understanding than we currently have of what stutterers *do* when they stutter. We also need to know a good deal more about what they *do* when they change stuttering as well as what they *do* that is related to long-term recovery from their problem. Telling our clients, "You prolong the /s/ when you stutter," is a bit like telling them "You get nervous when you are anxious." A prolongation of a speech sound in time is almost by definition a stuttering and vice versa; at best, using this approach, we could describe for the client that the sound is *prolonged* and then evaluate it as a *stuttering*.

However, we need to ask ourselves questions. What are we saying to ourselves with regard to *how* the stutterer actually produced the sound prolongation? Do we talk to ourselves as we do to our clients, using this same rather vague almost circular form of reasoning and manner of description? The answer, we are afraid, is all too often *yes*.

Starting with "Simple" and Working toward "Complex" Behavior

Behavior modification might be appropriate for all stutterers if we knew more precisely what aspects of the stutterers' speech production need modification for long-term recovery. (Of course, in the strictest sense, to use behavior modification methodology we would also have to assume that the stuttering speech behavior results from or behaves in accordance with the laws or principles of conditioning and learning.) A reasonably observant individual can see and hear the stutterer reiterate, cease, or prolong various speech postures, but how, when, and where within the vocal tract are such reiterations, cessations, and prolongations initiated, maintained, and terminated?

At present, what too often passes for behavior modification appears to be the result of clinical expediency and or experimentation, rather than a clear understanding of what needs modification. This problem is compounded by some behavioral modification approaches that appear based on very rudimentary, and probably inaccurate, conceptions of the *simple to complex* continuum of speech behavior. Many times this rudimentary understanding appears to be based more on an understanding of written, orthographic communication behavior than it does on an understanding of the articulatory, laryngeal, and respiratory behavior of disfluent and fluent speech (see Faircloth and Faircloth, 1973, pp. 77–78 for description of orthographic versus articulatory sounds and syllables).

Spoken versus Orthographic Behavior

One good example of such rudimentary understanding is typified by clinical approaches that modify speech at the isolated vowel level first and then proceed to the sentence level without apparently once considering if this progression makes sense in terms of *speech production*. One can't quibble with the fact that such a progression, at least some of the time, significantly assists stutterers to become more fluent. However, one cannot help but wonder if this progression is inappropriate and whether it may somehow contribute to the oft-reported relapse that many stutterers experience post-therapy. It is, after all, *speech*, not *orthographic*, behavior that needs modification and while related, like walking and running, speech and writing are two different acts and need to be dealt with accordingly.

How to Behave before All the Data Are In

Clearly, stutterers' speech needs to be modified, changed, or to coin a term, metamorphosed. Given this need, employing behavior modification procedures may make the most sense: These procedures are systematic, relatively quantifiable, and permit reasonably clear communication between clinicians and clients regarding therapy goals and procedures.

However, to advocate behavior modification—or any other procedure—to the relative *exclusion* of other approaches is unwarranted, particularly when we still are so unclear regarding the precise behaviors that need modification for long-term recovery and the relative effectiveness of different therapy approaches to bring about long-term recovery from stuttering. Too often with stuttering therapy, we have had to put the cart before the horse and provide therapy without strong justification for its particular use. This, of course, is understandable because we have a practical need to develop ("before all the data are in") therapy procedures despite our recognized incomplete understanding of the nature of stuttering. In this regard, stuttering is similar to cancer, where many possible causes exist, but where therapies for the sake of practicality are more often based on what works or arrests the development of the problem for at least a while, rather than being based on a clear understanding of the cause and true nature of the problem.

Obviously, we must and should continue to provide such clinical services, but we should, in our writings and lectures, make it apparent to our professional audiences (as well as ourselves) that the present state of the art is less than an exact science. Before all the data are in we have to help our clients the best way we know how based on our current understanding and accepted practice. However, we must not confuse what is expedient with that which is most appropriate, given the best of all possible worlds; clinical reality requires us to tolerate the former but it need not make us abandon our continual search for the latter.

SLPs Modify Stuttering, but Can Stutterers Maintain the Modification?

Regardless of the specific approach, therapy that follows the evaluation of stuttering has two general concerns: (1) producing meaningful in-clinic change in the nature and number of stutterings and related behavioral events that then are (2) transferred and maintained outside the clinic in a variety of speaking situations. As we've mentioned before, and as Williams (1978) agrees, the goal of our therapy with stutterers is much more importantly related to transfer of change to the outside environment than change within the therapy setting. Effective therapy procedures (that is, effective = long-term change) involve a continuous monitoring of the client's outside-of-clinic change; for example, surprise or unannounced post-therapy phone calls and actively trying within the clinic to bring about such "real world" change. Ideally, our therapies should be structured to optimize the bridge between in-clinic change and outside-of-clinic performance. Developing such bridges is, of course, no easy task, but one that should be a main goal of stuttering therapy. Our therapies should continually strive to assist stutterers, should they so choose, to speak as fluently as possible in their *everyday* environment and to effect the necessary behavioral change that will facilitate more fluent speech.

Realistically, even if we are effective in planning for the client's transfer of speech behavior, we should not maintain the hope that each and every one of our clients, particularly those with a more habituated stuttering problem, will *immediately* and *dramatically* become fluent outside the clinic. Our experience, which is consistent with Perkins' (1978) comments, is that real transfer will take longer than any of us would actually like or sometimes even admit to. Speech-language pathologists dealing with stutterers, particularly those with a more established or habituated problem, would be well advised to develop patience for the length of time it takes a human being to effectively change a central or even peripheral part of themselves, especially when that part is stuttering. Change is quite possible, but seldom easy or quick.

There Are Carry-over Problems with Other Problems

We must keep in mind, however, that stuttering is not all that unique in terms of its relative resistance to change as a result of therapeutic intervention. In fact, human resistance to change appears to be the rule, rather than the exception, no matter if the behavior is cigarette smoking, obsessivecompulsive traits, study habits, or sexual dysfunction. For example, Zilbergeld and Evens (1980), in a critical appraisal of Masters and Johnson's (1970) sex-therapy research, state that "the main problem for brief therapy is not inducing change, but maintaining it."*

Thus, clinicians, dealing with other types of human behavior, in this case sexual dysfunction, are extremely concerned with the amount of relapse or lack of transfer they observe in their clients shortly after termination of therapy. (Studies of sex-therapy relapse report, not unlike reports of stuttering-therapy relapse, rates of 37 to 54 percent relapse after termination of therapy.) SLPs remediating stuttering are not alone; relapse cuts a wide swath across the human condition.

The point of this comparison of stuttering to other human problems is to caution against our suggesting to ourselves and our clients that quick cures from stuttering are readily possible. We've already said that we believe it unethical to encourage our clients, particularly those with a habituated problem, to expect easy, quick cures. Based on current information, this is not a pessimistic, but a realistic approach to stuttering and the individual who stutters. We later mention that thoughts and feelings create behavior, and that behavior creates thoughts and feelings. Behavior and thinking are inextricably related. Speech-language pathologists who want to assist stutterers to produce

*B. Zilbergeld and M. Evans, "The Inadequacy of Masters and Johnson," *Psychology Today* 14 (1980), p. 37. Reprinted by permission of B. Zilbergeld.

lasting change must take into consideration the circularity of influence between an individual's thinking and feeling and his or her behavior.

Regardless at which end of the behaviorist-nonbehaviorist continuum a particular therapeutic approach rests, each encounters relapse in stuttering and the amount commonly observed across *all* such approaches—regardless of press releases to the contrary—indicates that a change in approach is needed. We would like to suggest that this change reflects a movement away from the classic "t'is-t'aint" war waged between behaviorists and traditionalists towards a meld of the "mentalistic" insights and procedures of traditional approaches and the systematic, objective methods and principles of the behavioral approach. Both approaches have some validity, but neither, by itself, appears sufficient.

Psyche versus Soma

The idea that stuttering should be treated either *this* way or *that* way is very much related, we think, to our "t'is-t'aint" views of what causes stuttering. Typically, the battle lines have been drawn between the *psyche* (essentially a nurture idea) and the *soma* (essentially a nature idea).

One of the central tenets of the *psyche* philosophy is that stuttering is caused by a nervous overflow into the peripheral speech structures and musculatures (perhaps even influencing central processes as well) that is caused by an individual's psychosocial problems. Thus, for whatever reason, there is a disruption or disturbance in the stutterer's psyche, attitudes, emotions, and beliefs on some level, and what listeners hear and see as stuttering is nothing more than the fixations, cessations, and repetitive shakings or oscillations of peripheral structures and muscles manifested during other psychosocial problems.

The *soma* philosophy views stuttering as the result of some inherent physiological, biochemical, or organic defect within the stutterer that creates, in as yet unknown ways, cessations, fixations, prolongations, and reiterations of speech postures, but that generally differs in degree and kind from the more profound nervous system damage of a problem like cerebral palsy, which also fosters certain types of speech dysfunction. Either approach—psyche or soma—seemingly views the problem as having a singular cause.

A third, perhaps, *equatorial* or *interactionist* approach (an example of which we discussed in Chapter 1) is to view the stutterer as an individual with a minimal, marginal, subtle, or very difficult to detect organic concern. During most situations this concern is of little bother, but may become exacerbated, thus disrupting initiation and/or continuation of speech production when the individual speaks under certain forms of emotional communicative or environmental stress. What is so attractive about this third approach is that it bypasses the "t'is-t'aint" arguments of the psyche versus soma theory proponents and even the traditionalist versus behaviorist therapy approach, and assumes that both the stutterer *and* his or her environment will require attention. While the proportion of attention may vary when dealing with children versus teenagers versus adults who stutter, this middle-ground approach *assumes* interaction between stutterer and environment and takes each client as they come. Sometimes this approach would focus on one's environment where the environment seems key, other times concentrating on one's speech production strategies when those seem paramount to long-term recovery, and still other times dealing with both stutterer and environment when the interaction between the two seems key.

While we will discuss below the elements that we believe are central to changes in stuttering, we want to make it clear that focusing on speech does not mean we disregard stutterers' attitudes, beliefs, feelings and environmental reactions. Unfortunately, even though these non-speech issues are important, we are less clear about their commonalties across stutterers than we are about events that seem highly related to changes in stuttering.

CHANGES IN TIME AND TENSION: THE COMMON THREAD THAT RUNS THROUGHOUT CONDITIONS THAT DECREASE STUTTERING

We have established the idea that the speech behavior that listeners typically perceive as stuttering (within-word disfluencies) is readily changeable, if only temporarily. We are not alone in this belief. It is expressed by such other experienced clinicians as Shames and Florance (1980). We believe it instructive, however, to consider briefly the common threads that run through the means by which stutterers, albeit temporarily, positively change their speech fluency. Bloodstein (1949, 1950) previously attempted to do this and hypothesized that most conditions that bring about a reduction in stuttering are also associated with a reduction in anxiety about stuttering. Although this is an interesting and possibly valid hypothesis, there has been little empirical research conducted by independent investigators that would support or refute Bloodstein's speculation.

More recently, Cooper (1978) discussed some of the common means by which fluency is increased and described these means as *fluency initiating gestures* (FIGs). Cooper's FIGs, while also interesting and possibly valid, have also received very little empirical attention by independent researchers. We want to avoid the "t'is-t'aint" polemic and state that it should be possible to meld Bloodstein's "mentalistic" interpretation with those of a more behavioral nature. However, currently most data in this area (for example, Brayton and Conture, 1978; Adams and Ramig, 1980; Klich and May, 1982) support some of our own hunches—which happen to be more behavioral—as well as those of fellow SLPs like Cooper (1978). Thus, what follows is not an eschewing of the thoughts-feelings-and-attitudes hypotheses, as represented by speculations like those of Bloodstein's (1950) that still await experimental assessment.

Rather we will discuss those behavioral changes that occur when stuttering changes and for which some empirical evidence exists. We believe these changes involve changes in *time* and *tension,* two terms we use frequently but misunderstand just as often.

We Need to Spend Some Time Discussing Time

Conture, Colton and Gleason (1988, p. 640) mention that "time is not a single concept, but a multifaceted one encompassing a variety of experiences and events, for example, relatively short versus long interval events (for example, Dossey, 1982; Hall, 1984; Ornstein, 1969), and it is by no means readily apparent which of these various temporal experiences or events is most relevant to the study of stutterers' speech production." Indeed, it is hard to envision speech sound production (disturbed or otherwise) as unrelated to time since, as Furster (1985) mentions, "Human action, much as human experience is indissolubly anchored in time" (p. 57). Thus, while we may agree with those (for example, Van Riper, 1971; Kent, 1983) who have mentioned the centrality of "time," "timing," or "temporal events" to the problem stutterer, we still are relatively clueless as to what facet of "time" we should study: stutterers' perception of passing time or their perception of temporal aspects of speech production or both? Stutterers' actual rate of speech production or the duration of the steady-state or transitional aspects of their speech sounds? It's almost like trying to put together a jigsaw puzzle when all the pieces have been painted white.

Understanding time is no simple matter since it is quite clear that time by the clock does not equal time by the head (Hall, 1984). Our precise micro- and millisecond measures of this or that aspect of speech production may not be the aspects of "time" that are central to understanding the role of time in stuttering. We, as SLPs managing and researching stuttering, would profit from reading the literature in the field of chronobiology, a science dedicated to the study of time and how humans interact with and are influenced by it (for example, Campbell, 1985; Dossey, 1982; Hall, 1984). But I get ahead of myself.

"Time is of the essence." "Don't get tense." How mutually contradictory are these two statements. It is a bit like saying, "Swimming is good exercise" in one breath and then, "Don't get wet" on the next. Chronic concerns, worries, and fears about the passing of time ("time is speeding by"), either small, medium or large units of time, can lead the "time worrier" into habitual states of psychological and physiological tension and distress (Dossey, 1982). It is quite possible that with regard to stuttering that time and tension are interrelated and that they may contribute to the onset, development, and perpetuation of stuttering. However, before we launch into the relation of time/tension to stuttering, perhaps we should explore a bit further the meaning of "time" and "tension."

What Is "Time"?

This is an easy question to ask, but a very difficult one to answer. Our first reaction is that time is what the clock measures. Well, to some extent this is true, but is this the only way time can be viewed or measured? What of other cultures either within our own country, for example, the Native Americans of North America, or those who live outside our own country such as individuals living south of the equator. Do these people view time as we do? And if they don't, whose "temporal orientation" is correct? We hope to show that differences in temporal perceptions—within and between cultures—are the main issue rather than this or that perception's being more or less correct. We believe that understanding such differences should give us important insights into the problem of stuttering and its treatment.

Let us start with our concept of time. If you are like most of us in the United States and other industrialized countries, you carry a calendar or appointment book with you or have one on your desk. If you can, take a look at that book right now. You'll see that it divides each weekday into 15-, 30-, or 60-minute blocks. Your 10:00 A.M. appointment is directly followed by your 10:30 A.M. meeting which leads to the 11:00 A.M. class you must attend and so on throughout the day. You may ask, what is wrong with that? You have to keep a schedule book to keep your days straight and organized because without one your life would be a mess. Your daily routine, as you look at your schedule or appointment book, is organized like a straight line that extends into the future away from you as far as you want to envision. This linear flow or sequencing of temporal events is part of our culture; its cultural acceptance, however, should not construed as a law. While we may, at some level of our consciousness, understand that people in other parts of the world do not operate according to such a strict, linear time flow, it is a bit harder to appreciate that some, within our own culture, operate according to a different "temporal perception." In fact, we have to look no further than the average physician to see how time is dealt with in a different manner.

Let us assume that you have a bad cold and call your doctor's office and get the only available appointment for 1:30 P.M. that day. Although 1:30 is in the middle of your workday, you are feeling sick enough to make the effort to show up at the office on time. You announce your arrival to the doctor's secretary and take your seat. One-thirty comes and goes and then 2:00 and then 2:30 and finally your name is called and you go back to one of several examining rooms. There you sit and wait while out in the hall you hear nurses and the doctor (you presume) busily scurrying around. Around 3:15, your doctor pokes his head in, says hi, sticks a thermometer in your mouth, and quickly leaves again. After two more quick visits with you over a 15- to 30-minute span of time, he gives you his diagnosis and prescription around 3:45 P.M.. By now, 2 hours and 15 minutes after your 1:30 appointment, you are so furious because of the wait and waste of your time that you wouldn't be surprised if your upper respiratory infection spontaneously recovered! You walk out muttering to yourself that you are going to seriously consider changing doctors. What has happened here?

Disregarding the possibility of overbooking, let us say that it is flu season and that many acutely ill people wanted to see your doctor today. And, when someone is ill, they have to be evaluated and treated to the best of the physician's ability. The clock on the wall can't dictate his length of stay with the patient; the patient's problem(s) dictate the length of stay. However, each patient is scheduled in accordance with a strictly linear time-flow appointment book, that is, one at 8:30, one at 9:00, one at 9:30, and so on. Each patient expects to be seen at his or her appointed time in the appointment queue (without anything's diverting the doctor's attention); however, the doctor is running his patients in parallel or simultaneously in time. He deals with each one a little bit at a time while moving quickly from one to another until each appointment is completed regardless of the time taken up by the clock on the wall to do this.

The point is that different people view and use time differently and when these different views and uses must interact, when they must be coordinated or meshed with one another, it is not uncommon that friction, misunderstandings and other difficulties ensue.

Outside of the United States, particularly in countries closer to the equator, similar differences in time views and uses can be seen (Hall, 1984). One good example is the market bazaar or open-air market where everything and anything is sold. Within the market bazaar may be a farmer who is dealing with many people at once (no tickets are given). The lines of customers, with which we are so familiar, are typically not formed; rather, the farmer/seller deals with the various people a little bit at a time, now telling the price of carrots to this one, now helping that one pick out a nice head of lettuce, haggling with this one over the price of apples, and then back to the first customer who now wants to pick out a dozen carrots. Time is handled differently here in the market bazaar than in a typical busy American bakery where individuals pick a number and wait in line for their turn. Time in the market bazaar is dealt with simultaneously whereas we typically deal with it in a linear, sequential fashion: Now is the time for this, then it is time for this, and after this it will be time for that. Once the time allotment is used up ("Hurry up, there are people in line"), whether or not the task was completed or completed satisfactorily, we must move on to the next block of time and do within it what was scheduled for it.

How Stutterers' Perceptions of Passing Time
May Relate to Their Stuttering

It is important, we think, to understand our own perceptions and dealings with time if we are to help people (that is, stutterers and their families) whose sense of time may be hurried or faster than our own. The stutterer may be an individual who routinely (and unnecessarily so) hurries from one situation to another, who continually does several things at once (for example, reading while driving because he or she feels that time is lost as it linearly flows by). This is a person whose clock seems to be running faster than usual and whose schedule book seems to dictate his existence. For this sort of an individual, getting things done is more important than getting them done correctly. Clearing calendars and agendas, doing something, anything, is better than waiting and thinking about what must be done. There is a price to pay for all this "promptness"; these individuals will often be under stress. These people seem driven by time; they are "time urgent." For them everything should have been done yesterday. They have never met a clock they didn't like, unless, of course, they get behind their arbitrarily determined schedule. These people don't watch the clock as much as they feel that the clock is watching them!

What should we do with these clients if they are stutterers? If we were to tell them to slow down and take their watches, clocks, appointment books, and the like away from them, they might be visibly agitated. For some of these people, time by the clock and schedule book brings order, security, and a sense of well-being. However, despite the regularity and security these time pieces may give to our lives (it is no coincidence that a widely-used, old-fashioned pendulum wall clock was called the "Regulator"), nothing is free. For some, the price paid for chronic and slavish devotion to temporal regulation, is, what others have termed "hurry sickness" (Dossey, 1982). Emotional, psychological, and physical problems can result from inappropriate concerns regarding the passage and use of time.

Am I saying that stutterers now have a new disorder—"hurry sickness"? Hardly. However, we do need to understand that each person, be he or she a doctor, lawyer, or Indian chief, appears to perceive time through his or her own perceptual windows. For example, when judging a minute, some of these windows stay open for only 45 seconds while for others the window stays open as long as 75 or more seconds. And each individual stutterer, just like each individual nonstutterer, has a perception of time that is relative to him or her. For some stutterers, the temporal aspects of life and speech in particular are intricately bound up in the cause, perpetuation, and remediation of their stuttering. While some, such as Sheehan, (1958), have cited such factors as "time pressure" as having a relation to stuttering, the issue of time is more than just, on the one hand, a mistiming of the supralaryngeal and laryngeal systems, or, on the other hand, simply an inappropriate reaction to everyday "time pressures."

We believe that one of the reasons that stutterers' dealing with time generally and with speech specifically has escaped most of our attention is that we take for granted the absoluteness and the appropriateness of linearly flowing time. After all, the day is followed by the night, our workdays are eight hours long, it takes three minutes to boil an egg, and so forth. Such familiarity has not actually built contempt as much as it has lent to our developing a complacency and acceptance of a linearly arranged time schedule that is purely arbitrary. Sixty-second minutes, we seem to say, must exist in nature because we can use our clocks to accurately and reliably record and predict events; for example, how long the average three-year-old horse takes to run the Kentucky Derby. But what did we do with ourselves before the pendulum and now the digital clock? Did farmers crops suffer less heat and damage before the invention of daylight savings time? How did we function before the ubiquitous wristwatch? Differently, that is to be sure.

What Our Perceptions of Stuttering May Suggest about the Problem

Listen to the average stutterer stutter. What disturbs you the most about his or her speech? Is their speech unintelligible? Generally not. Are their language structures and vocabulary words outside normal limits for their chronological age? Sometimes, but generally not. Are their voice and articulation abilities below normal limits? Sometimes, but generally not.

Rather, when a person stutters you may notice something else, something that may be distracting, annoying, or otherwise less than pleasant to listen to. What disturbs you when you listen to someone stutter? Does the stutterer sometimes seem to be talking far too fast for his or her ability to coordinate speech production? And sometimes does he or she seem to be talking too slow? Does he or she seem to be taking so long to "get it out" that you feel like supplying "it" for him or her? Does he or she seem to be using too much physical tension to speak? Do you feel justified in interrupting and talking for the stutterer since "they are taking so much time and are having so much trouble." Perhaps what is going on here—at least in terms of your reaction and feelings of discomfort during a stutterer's stuttering—is that your own time urgency or sense that speech (and the thoughts it reflects) should be moving along faster or more steadily are being violated by the stutterer's stuttering. Your desires to now "speed him up" and now "slow him down" suggest that somehow some facet of time is being disturbed, at least from your perspective. It is as if listeners think that things would be better for the stutterer if the temporal domain of their speech production could be rectified.

When any aspect of our behavior breaks down, when we find it difficult to perform any complex act, or when we become concerned about our performances, we frequently go slower, minimize extent or range of movement, and stretch out each movement a bit longer than usual. For example, a young child who is really trying to learn to use a spoon to pick up small pieces of food will go very slowly, be very deliberate, and exhibit a reduced range of movement. This minimizing-of-extraneous-movements-temporal-expansion strategy seems to be a very human response when faced with stressful situations or situations where we find it difficult (for various reasons) to adequately perform a developing or newly acquired skill. We seem to simplify the necessary movements and perform them at a somewhat slower rate, making each aspect of the behavior as deliberate and discrete as possible.

Thus, it does not seem particularly unusual that stutterers may do likewise and that when they do—as either a result of therapy, their own initiative, or exposure to conditions like rhythmic stimulation—they become somewhat, or in some cases, completely fluent. The big question, of course, is why doesn't the fluency last? Well, many times it does but some times it doesn't and the answer to this question probably lies in the nature of the causal as well as perpetuating factors of stuttering, factors that are still not certain.

Manipulations of Time and Spatial Movements: The Essence of Changing Fluency

Research clearly demonstrates that stutterers become more fluent, at least temporarily, if there is a temporal expansion of sound segment transitions and durations. For example, during metronomic or rhythmic stimulation—a powerful if temporary influence on stutterers' stuttering—the time between adjacent syllables or vowels is expanded and made less variable (Conture and Metz, 1974) and each syllable's vowel duration is increased (Brayton and Conture, 1978; Klich and May, 1982). Increases in vowel duration have also been shown to be related to decreases in stuttering associated with therapy (Prosek and Runyan, 1982; Mallard and Westbrook, 1985). This is not to say that rhythmic stimulation or therapy do not influence other aspects of speech production, for example, fundamental frequency, and vocal sound pressure level. But when these other aspects, such as fundamental frequency/fundamental frequency contours (Sacco and Metz, 1987) have been studied, they have been shown to not change significantly and/or have little relation to changes in stuttering.

The earlier explanations for these changes, for example, the "distraction hypothesis" essentially holds that anything "novel" or "different" that distracts the stutterer's attention away from his or her speech, albeit momentarily, is capable of producing an increment in fluency (see Bloodstein, 1987, pp. 275–278 for discussion of this hypothesis; see letter exchange between Bloodstein, 1988, and Siegel, 1988, for some current thoughts regarding this hypothesis). The distraction hypothesis is somewhat similar to Pavlov's (1920) "investigatory" or "What-is-it?" reflex whereby a dog, conditioned to respond to a bell or light by salivating, would either reduce the frequency of or entirely stop responding when some change in external stimuli, (for example, changes in room illumination as the sun comes out from behind the clouds) occurred that made the dog "orient" to the novel or changing stimuli. Interestingly, relatively recent empirical studies of the "distraction" hypothesis or the influence of "distraction" on stutterers' stuttering have failed to find evidence to support this hypothesis (for example, Mallard and Webb, 1980; Thompson, 1985). Thus, as Thompson (1985, p. 35) suggests, "stutterers' perceptions may account for the popularity of the distraction explanation," but empirical data to support this explanation are currently lacking.

It should be pointed out, however, that while many different conditions lead to some change in stuttering, very few bring about the consistent and dramatic reduction in stuttering (75 percent to 90 percent or better), like conditions such as rhythmic stimulation, speaking under delayed-auditory-feedback, singing, and a few others. Clearly, not all conditions that change stuttering do so to the same degree. To consider speaking with a foreign accent along with rhythmic stimulation is to blur important distinctions. Not all "fluency-inducing" conditions are created equal. Some will bring about a sudden, dramatic reduction for almost every stutterer almost every time they are used whereas some, for example, taking on a role as in a play, will work for some only some of the time.

While all such conditions may have only a temporary effect, the means by which the more "powerful" ones change speech are noteworthy. Although some case studies show little that is common in terms of temporal changes in speech production (Andrews, Howie, Dozsa, and Guitar, 1982) other, quantitative assessments of the acoustic records of stutterers during these conditions and/or therapy indicate that *temporal* changes are the main if only change in speech production that occurs. (Conture and Metz, 1974; Brayton and Conture, 1978; Metz, Onufrak, Ogburn, 1979; Adams and Ramig, 1980; Klich and May, 1982; Metz, Samar and Sacco, 1983; Mallard and Westbrook, 1985).

Although the temporal changes in speech production are important to changes in stuttering, they may not be apparent. It is quite likely that the temporal changes in speech of greatest import will be minimally noticeable, if at all perceptible, to the casual observer. Changes in such events as speaking rate are easy to measure and have a great deal of face validity, but stutterers stutter on sounds or syllables. It is the sound and syllable level that needs to be addressed, not more macroscopic events such as the amount of time spent phonating during an utterance or how fast their overall speaking rate is. We are specifically referring to temporal changes in the durations and relations between consonant and vowel durations, consonant to vowel (and vice versa) transition rates and durations, and a variety of sub-segmental events such as stop gap frication and aspiration duration. When these measures of brief temporal events have been made, they have indicated that the *relations* among these events, for stutterers, is dissimilar to those of non-stutterers (for example, Zebrowski, Conture and Cudahy, 1985; Borden, Kim and Spiegler, 1987). Interestingly, when quantitative assessment of therapeutic induced fluency has made similar measures, some of these same temporal events, frication durations, are the ones seemingly most influenced by therapy (for example, Metz, Samar and Sacco, 1983).

Naturalness versus Amount of Fluency

It should come as no surprise, therefore, that many therapy procedures that have been shown to bring about significant increments in stutterers' fluency employ reduction in the rate of movement between and within sounds and encourage the use of more gradual onsets and offsets of speech with less physical tension (for example, Shames and Florance, 1980; Webster, 1975, 1978). Although, at least initially, other aspects of speech behavior such as fundamental frequency are changed, these changes often drop out. If not, they may contribute to the perceived "unnaturalness" of speech some of these therapies seem to create (see Franken 1987; Franken, Boves, Peters and Webster, 1988).

In fact, we predict that research into changes in stuttering are going to involve two parallel but different lines of investigation: (1) investigations of variables most highly related to decreases in stuttering, and (2) investigations of the naturalness of the stutterers' improved speech as a result of therapy. Both aspects—*improvements* in as well as *naturalness* of speech fluency—are inextricably related to one another with some therapies perhaps better at achieving one versus the other. Indeed, clinicians may concentrate on improving the stutterer's fluency while the stutterer may be more interested in the naturalness rather than amount of fluency he achieves.

We Should Eschew Differences for the Sake of Difference

Easy-hard speech, easy-gentle onsets, or *smooth speech* are terms used by different clinicians to refer to slightly different but essentially similar behaviors. Figure 6–1 shows how we roughly equate these therapy terms or procedures to one another, break them down into their constituent parts—*time* and *tension*—and then describe, for children and their parents, the extremes of the two aspects—time: fast versus slow; tension: tense versus relaxed. Whether these temporal as well as musculature tension/movement changes in speech production result from psychological, social, or some as yet unknown mechanism, there is no escaping the fact that they occur. As we learn more and more about stutterers' fluency (for example, Conture, Colton and Gleason, 1988; Prosek, Montgomery and Walden, 1988) as well as stuttered speech production (for example, Caruso, Conture and Colton, 1988), we will begin to focus on those behaviors most likely associated with changes in stuttering. What this eventually should show us is that there are many ways to skin a cat, but in the end, no matter how it's done, the fur has to be removed.

Creativity Involves Novel Use of the Commonplace and Not Necessarily Novel Ideas

We must, therefore, not be too eager to claim novelty for any one clinical procedure since they all may be manipulating the same variables only using different means. Conversely, we should not be too eager to totally cast

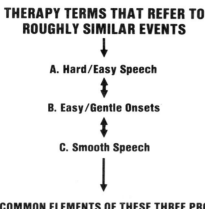

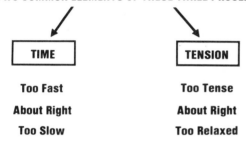

FIGURE 6-1. Relation of common therapy terms or approaches to one another and to the two key elements (time and tension) that need all three employed to achieve increased speech fluency. With these approaches a slowing down of time is used to allow physical tension to return to within normal limits which allows the person to move on to the next sound or syllable. Some of these approaches may, however, sacrifice perceived "naturalness" of speech to achieve increased speech fluency; the relation of changes in speech fluency to changes in speech naturalness is an issue that will receive much clinical and research attention in the years ahead.

aside procedures like rhythmic stimulation—which may shed needed light on the variables of import—simply because these procedures have been around for years. These procedures deserve, at the least, continued, careful empirical study as well as systematic clinical investigation. What we need as a discipline is more explicit, documented evidence that there are commonalities among our clinical approaches rather than the casual but oft-made remark that all therapies are alike, regardless of theories.

If they are so much alike, we should make explicit to each other, our students, and fellow professionals how they are similar, instead of giving the appearance of vast differences in approach when, in fact, the names may be different but the game essentially the same. One very meaningful attempt at exploring commonalities among various stuttering theorists and/or therapies is presented in an edited book by Gregory (1978). Gregory and his contributing authors discuss their various approaches to stuttering, and it is evident to the reader that they do share certain common ideas despite their more well-known differences of opinion. Guitar and Peters (1980), through their attempt to meld behavioral and traditional approaches, also show that they feel some need to explore the commonalities of stuttering therapy.

Explicating a Common Thread Gives the Lay Public Something to Hold Onto

While differences may be healthy, lead to constant exploration, and are the "stuff" that fosters theoretical as well as therapeutic progress, unnecessary differences can also give the lay public the impression that no one really knows what is going on with stuttering. If everybody is right but different then everybody must be wrong. However, despite this public impression, nothing could be further from the truth.

As mentioned in Chapter 1, much has been and continues to be discovered in the area of stuttering, and we need to make this fact apparent. We also need to clarify and explicate the degree of similarities among our various approaches. Charlatans would appear to have far less chance of dealing with stuttering, for the most part, if we who conscientiously deliver clinical services to stutterers would put more of a concerted effort into explaining how much consistency there really is among approaches to stutterings used by SLPs who specialize in this disorder.

The common thread among our therapies must be there because too many seemingly different therapeutic approaches appear to have a similar ameliorative influence on stutterers' speech. If nothing else, keeping this common thread notion in mind when we evaluate and remediate stutterers should help us, as individual SLPs, clarify what variables most of our colleagues are trying to manipulate or modify. Of course, clarification of these parameters is not a solution, but at least it is a start.

THE CLINICIAN

Six Characteristics of Successful Clinicians

Besides discussing the evaluation and remediation of stuttering, we need to be concerned with the SLP's knowledge, motivation, and personal characteristics as they pertain to clinical involvement with stutterers and their associates. Van Riper (1975) described three personal characteristics that successful clinicians appear to possess: accurate empathy, nonpossessive warmth, and genuineness (see Appendix C for more general discussion of clinician concerns and characteristics). We would like to add three of our own: the ability to listen, the ability to adjust to changing circumstances, and the ability to make quick, accurate behavioral observations.

Briefly, *empathy* relates to our ability to understand or imagine how other individuals feel about themselves and events that surround them. It is the ability to "walk a mile in my shoes" and to view events as others do that successful clinicians make so apparent. Being able to take the perspective of the other person is key to understanding how he or she is reacting and coping with his or her circumstances. The second characteristic, *warmth*, is something we all feel, to greater or lesser degrees, in our daily interactions with people, and it is another feature that successful clinicians seem to exude and establish in their clinical relations. Warmth relates to the ability to imply or make explicit our desire to help our clients, to make them know we care and that we think they are OK—perhaps best done when we, ourselves, can say, "I'm OK—you're OK" (Harris, 1967). The third characteristic, *genuineness*, relates to the clinicians' openness, the ability to expose their unique human traits, and be, in essence, themselves. It is difficult to like your clients when you demonstrate in one way or another that you do not like yourself. Clients don't expect a superhero for a clinician but they do expect clinicians to be honest and straightforward with them regarding their assets and liabilities.

The fourth characteristic, *listening*, is very much related to the first (empathy). Listening involves attending and responding to the denotative aspects of communication as well as the connotative, the message behind the message, the message that is written between as well as on the lines. Clients want a clinician who can listen to them and attend and respond to the subtleties of their verbal and nonverbal communication. If a client feels that there is no "use talking when nobody is listening," there is little chance that therapy will be successful. The fifth characteristic, the ability to *adjust* or to be *flexible*, is required in order to deal with the dynamics of the constantly changing circumstances of therapy. A clinician can be well prepared, like a coach with a game plan, but within minutes after therapy begins (or after the game begins), circumstances change and the clinician must adjust (the coach must scrap the game plan). For example, the clinician must adjust and be flexible when the client is not feeling well, has regressed, hasn't done his or her homework, doesn't understand or can't seem to deal with today's lesson plan, the therapy plan is obviously inappropriate, and so forth. These are situations requiring a clinician to work smarter, not harder. Successful clinicians "roll with the punches" and go where the client takes them. Unsuccessful clinicians, to paraphrase an old proverb, are a bit like swimmers who continue to fight their way upstream, seemingly expecting that at any moment the river will change direction for them.

The sixth characteristic, *quick, accurate behavioral observations,* is an attribute/skill that definitely improves with age but only if the person tries to improve the skill. The clinician who is a keen observer of behavior is readily able to "ballpark" the client's stuttering frequency, duration, most common disfluency type, and severity. This skill comes from recognizing the need to be accurate but quick in observing and assessing the client and the client's behavior. While few clinicians can be like the observant Sherlock Holmes, many more could be far better at observing what is in front of them if they would apply themselves more and concentrate their efforts on learning how to recognize behavior. The successful clinician recognizes the "silences" before speech initiation as part of the stutterer's stutterings, the unsuccessful clinician only understands that the client appears "nervous.".

Certainly, other attributes are correlated with successful clinical practice; but these six seem to be among the most common we've observed exhibited by those clinicians we think are successful. While it is not the purpose of this book to help clinicians develop the above six attributes and skills, it does seem appropriate to spend some time discussing how some of these clinician skills interact with the clinician process.

Problem-Specific Empathy

Of the three personal characteristics of a successful stuttering therapist, the one that seems the biggest challenge for normally fluent SLPs to acquire is that of empathy. I am referring to problem-specific empathy: what it physically feels like to actually stutter and to be a stutterer. This is a particularly challenging attribute for the normally fluent SLP to develop, but if the SLP has decent general empathetic and listening skills and is a keen behavioral observer, problem-specific empathy can be readily developed.

The old classroom practice of having undergraduates go out and stutter openly for a day or two in front of ten different strangers was a small step in the direction of developing problem-specific empathy. We can, to greater or lesser degrees, empathize with people who have various problems that we do not have ourselves. However, as SLPs, we are not called upon to professionally help these various people; instead, it is our responsibility to assist people (stutterers, in this case) who feel that they are unable to move forward when speaking. How do you, as a normally fluent speaker, get the feeling of what it is like to be "stuck" when you talk? Clearly, the ideal way is by doing; however, this is not to say that stutterers are the only ones who can do stuttering therapy (any more than it says that heart attack victims make the best cardiovascular surgeons or bank robbers the best criminal lawyers). What we are saying, though, is that normally fluent speakers must realize that problem-specific empathy is not going to "happen" to them; normally fluent speakers with problem-specific empathy for stuttering are made, not born. They will have to work diligently to grasp some of the feelings—physical, cognitive and psychological—that stutterers experience when they stutter.

In attempts to develop and refine my problem-specific empathy, I frequently ask the client who stutters: "Tell me what it feels like to you—in your own words—to stutter? Do you feel terror? embarrassment? anger? fear? pain? fright? hurt? frustration? a numb sensation? Do you feel a tightness in your chest? your throat? your mouth? Is there anything else you do, for example, lift weights, hold your breath, try to open a hard-to-open jar top, that makes you feel the same sort of tightness or constriction in your upper torso and neck? Is it anything like having a close accident in your car? Is it anything like suddenly touching a hot stove burner you thought was off (demonstrating the quick pulling back of the hand/arm and the quick, forced inhalation of breath)? Do you ever want to run out of the room and hide?" and so forth.

In this way, over the years, I have gained a measure of appreciation for the feelings of individuals when they stutter. I say *measure* because truly no one can totally understand what it feels like to be someone else. We can come close to such understanding, we can get a pretty decent idea, but we never fully know and we should know when we don't know. Indeed, one of the hallmarks of clinicians whose listening skills are less than they should be, whose general as well as problem-specific empathy is less than ideal, is that they don't know that they don't know.

An analogy to help with empathy One way we have found that seems to closely describe the feelings that stutterers experience when they stutter is to analogize it to the momentary panic, terror, and fear people encounter when they pull back from a ledge or high place from which they almost fell. During the physical maneuver back from the ledge, people attend to emotional elements and have little awareness of what they did that got them safely back from the edge. We've discussed this before and described it as a *mental whiteout*. Ironically, during this *whiteout* is the worst time for stutterers to objectively concentrate on what they are doing that interferes with their speech production; however, it is precisely at this very point in time—during the whiteout—that they need to concentrate objectively on their behavior. We try such analogies out on our clients—and invite them to develop their own—and listen to what they say. We use these analogies in attempts, albeit a bit artificial, to "walk a mile in their shoes."

Clinical Art Interacts with Clinical Science

We try to be as honest with our clients as possible when they ask us questions about stuttering. We try to make it clear that we don't totally understand everything about stuttering (an example of genuineness) but we also try to make it clear that we really want to know about the clients' feelings so we can understand their problem and help the client help him or herself (an example of warmth). We hear the client out when discussing a routine problem he has when ordering coffee at a diner (an example of listening) and essentially scrap large parts of our lesson plan trying to help the client problem solve a situation—ordering a cup of coffee—which, although it seems relatively trivial, is of major daily concern for the client (an example of flexibility).

It should be clear, however, that the aforementioned personal characteristics and skills are necessary but not sufficient for successful therapy. As Van Riper (1975) mentioned in some detail, the personal characteristics of the SLPs who work with stutterers must be built upon a solid foundation of knowledge about stuttering and then refined through a series of experiences with stutterers. Perhaps, describing the clinician's personal characteristics and skills is just another way of talking about the art of stuttering therapy. Likewise, describing the clinician's knowledge of and experience with stuttering is simply another means of discussing the *science* of stuttering therapy. When the art and science of stuttering therapy are viewed from this perspective, it is a bit easier to see that each is necessary but only together are they sufficient for successful remediation of stuttering. All the warmth, empathy, and listening skills in the world won't help the clinician who doesn't understand what stuttering is about; conversely, all the knowledge in the world about stuttering won't help the clinician who doesn't understand that they are dealing with humans, not automatons.

FUTURE DIRECTIONS

The Future Is a Carte Blanche We Write On with Hope

The team that loses the championship game is many times quoted as saying, "wait until next year." The future is a carte blanche that we often write on with hope. Things are always going to work out or be better in the future.

We, too, as speech-language pathologists who work with stutterers, continually anticipate and hope that new approaches and information, "just around the bend and over the horizon," will improve our clinical acumen and methodology. While, as the saying goes, tomorrow is promised to no one, our field has been paying its dues and the future does hold bright promise for those who stutter and those who professionally manage them. Thus, I would like to predict what some of those new ideas and procedures may be.

Two Trains Running in Parallel

To understand these predictions better, however, you must realize one basic fact about individuals who work in the area of stuttering: The employment setting dictates much of what these professionals do and think about stuttering. While professional conferences, journal articles, books, and the like continually bring these professionals together throughout the year, the fact cannot be denied that individuals who clinically serve stutterers and individuals who empirically research stutterers have different perspectives, interests, and needs. It is as if there were two trains running on parallel tracks whose passengers occasionally look out the window and wave at one another or who even disembark and mingle together at common stops but who get back on the train and ride toward their separate destinations. Clinicians have an interest and need to know about the most effective way to manage stuttering and researchers have an interest and need to know the most they can about stuttering, whether or not such information has immediate application to treatment.

Granted, there are scientific clinicians as well as clinical scientists who routinely bridge the gap between treatment and theory, between applied and basic science, but most workers *daily* find themselves on one side or the other. We mention this distinction since future directions will come not only from the laboratory but will also emanate from clinical practice. Thus, scientists will need to monitor the results of clinical practioners just as clinicians will want to monitor the findings of experimentalists. The complexities of stuttering are such that neither group of workers can afford to ignore the efforts of one another.

The Brain

Although Orton (1928) and Travis (1931) are generally cited as being among the first to explore and suggest possible differences between stutterers and their normally fluent peers in terms of central nervous system (CNS) function, it has only been in recent years that advances in technology for the study of CNS function have permitted the type of investigations necessary to assess Orton and Travis's earlier speculations seriously. (For a clear and not too technical overview of such technology, see Fincher, 1984 and Sochurek, 1987.) Moore (1984) and Moore and Boberg (1987) have nicely summarized the more recent work in this area; indeed, Moore (1986) himself has contributed much of the recent empirical work in this area. Recently, speculation based on stutterers' speech motor control (Caruso, Abbs and Gracuo, 1988) and bimanual handwriting performance (Webster, 1988) has also contributed to our thinking regarding stutterers' cortical activity during speech and non-speech behavior.

Our understanding of this work leads us to also predict that although some future studies may report findings that can be interpreted to suggest differences in *structural* asymmetries in stutterers' brains, far more studies will show that these differences in hemispheric asymmetries are *functional* in nature. That is, differences between stutterers and their matched controls in cortical asymmetries will be found only during active processing or handling of meaningful speech or linguistic stimuli. Thus, stutterers' central nervous system functioning may be found to be different but this difference will be differential; that is, it will differ according to what (non)linguistic activity and associated "cortical strategy" the stutterer is required to employ at the time of testing. While a variety of behavioral (for example, bimanual handwriting [Webster, 1988]) versus electrophysiological (for example, study of hemispheric alpha wave asymmetries via means of electroencephalography) means will be used to indirectly or directly study stutterers' CNS function, it is most likely that future breakthroughs in this area will come through the application of new electrophysiological technologies (for example, the brain electrical activity mapping [BEAM] work of Pool, Freeman and Finitzo, 1987) since they actually record brain activity rather than infer it as with behavioral measures. This is an exciting area of study and one, as technology continues to advance and data accumulate, should help us better understand stutterers' CNS function—whether it differs among stutterers as well as between stutterers and normally fluent speakers and (the $64 thousand question), how CNS function may relate to disruptions in speech fluency.

Temporal versus Spatial Disruptions in Speech Production

CNS functioning is not the only area where technology is rapidly advancing. Technology to study speech acoustics and production (cf. Kiritani, 1977; Folkins and Kuehn, 1982; Childers and Krishnamurthy, 1984; Baken, 1987) is becoming much more sophisticated. Information about various aspects of speech production that heretofore were extremely time-consuming and laborious to collect, analyze, and process have become with computer-assisted or even computer-automated methodology, much more "doable" within a reasonable period of time. While the number of subjects assessed in any one study of speech production can for the foreseeable future never be as large as that studied via perceptual means, the sizable number of data points typically gathered per subject, the relative stability of speech production, and nature of questions asked in this area generally permit smaller sample sizes.

We predict that research in this area will increasingly indicate that stutterers are grossly similar to the normally fluent in terms of temporal as well as spatial aspects of speech production. Differences, we think, will be found as researchers and their methodology permit the study of briefer and more "molecular" aspects of speech production. The temporal discoordination hypothesis (see Van Riper, 1971; Perkins, Rudas, Johnson and Bell, 1976), no matter how seemingly attractive or high on face validity, has received very minimal support from empirical studies of stutterers' speech production (for example, Caruso, Conture and Colton, 1988; Conture, Colton and Gleason, 1988; Prosek, Montgomery and Walden, 1988).

Clearly, the "discoordination" hypothesis needs refinement in light of present data. In the future, we predict that researchers will begin to realize the following:

1. "Discoordinations" can occur within one speech structure, for example, the lips, as well as between different structures, or the laryngeal and supralaryngeal systems

2. "Coordination" and "discoordination" represent terms that are widely used but just as often misused and definitions of these terms must encompass thinking and work from related areas of speech motor control and the like

3. Speech structures move through time as well as space and both aspects—time

and space—will have to be considered when investigating and theorizing about stutterers' speech production abilities

4. Time encompasses much more than the mere durations and transitions of speech production gestures and that the stutterers' perceptions of passing time during speech and nonspeech behavior probably plays a role in this problem

5. Methodology will continue to be developed that permits investigators to non-intrusively, noninvasively study the speech production skills of young stutterers

6. It will become clearer and clearer that one can not readily extrapolate information from the speech production behaviors of adults who stutter to those of children who stutter and vice versa; these are two related but different groups

7. The computer will increasingly find its way into the clinic, first in the way of feedback of stutterers' acoustic output and then laryngeal behavior (by means of EGG methodology) and finally through feedback of muscle tensions/activity through surface electromyography.

The application of the computer, like work on stutterers' CNS function, is an exciting area and one that workers in the area of stuttering will want to continue to monitor through journal articles and conference presentations in the years ahead. While understanding CNS functioning may tell us what initially may go awry, only through study of the peripheral speech production mechanism will we know what is or what is likely to go awry. We need both types of information.

Nature Interacting with Nurture

More and more clinical investigations will attempt to study the very difficult to understand *interactions* between the stutterer and his or her environment, particularly in children. These studies will not be as much addressed as *initial,* or *originating* or *precipitating* causes as they will be trying to circumscribe and understand *maintaining* or *perpetuating* or *exacerbating* or *aggravating* factors. More and more studies of mother-child interaction, before the child reaches seven years of age, will show that mothers of children who stutter are grossly similar to mothers of children who don't stutter, but that subtle aspects of their verbal and nonverbal behavior are associated with changes in the number and nature of their stuttering behavior. Stutterers will increasingly be viewed as subtly different people raised in subtly, but importantly different environments. This is an area desperately in need of study and although there are many difficulties in conducting this work in a careful, meaningful way, the potential rewards in terms of new information and insights are truly great.

Subgroups of Stuttering

More and more workers will try to uncover—on perceptual, acoustic, physiological, and other levels—differences among stutterers that make a difference. These differences will be explored both in terms of etiological subgroups as well as behavioral subgroups with the latter receiving more attention and probably more consistency from study to study.

On the basis of empirical research (Daly, 1981; Preus, 1981, Schwartz and Conture, 1988; Van Riper, 1971), it has become increasingly clear that "childhood stuttering may not only begin from different origins but once begun the problem may develop along parallel but different routes" (Conture, 1989, p. 33). As work in this area progresses and the number and nature of these various "subgroups" of stutterers becomes clearer, this information will be very useful to researchers in terms of subject selection and matching and to clinicians trying to differentially diagnose stuttering and plan therapy accordingly.

Clinical Data Bases Will Emerge

With the proliferation of the computer in every facet of our daily personal and professional lives, clinicians will start to develop their own data bases on the clients they evaluate and remediate. While we have always had these data bases in the form of clinical records and folders, the computer, with its ability to rapidly count, sort, and organize, will greatly expand the accessibility of these records. Subtle and not-so-subtle trends will emerge as clinicians scroll through these data bases looking for past clients similar to those with whom they are currently confronted. Heretofore ignored behavior, for example, phonological processes, may emerge as variables highly associated with either protracted therapy or relapse. Some of these data may challenge wide-spread clinical hunches about stuttering and will be interesting to see whether clinicians and researchers alike will allow factual information to ruin "good" theory.

Concomitant Problems of Stutterers

While the current "zietgeist" in this area is that stutterers have a "language problem," very little research supports this oft-made remark. Instead, research will accumulate to show that one of the more common problems is phonological difficulty, particularly in children (for example, Blood and Seider, 1981). First, the number and nature of stutterers' phonological problems will be carefully documented and any phonological difference these children exhibit from those children who only exhibit phonological impairments will be clarified. Second, theories will arise to explain the overlap between phonological difficulties and stuttering, and data and speculation in this area will contribute to a further understanding of the subgrouping notion discussed above. Third, longitudinal studies of young stutterers in therapy may show that children *with*, versus *without* concomitant problems, particularly phonological concerns, may differ in terms of the length of therapy and whether or not relapse occurs (for an excellent overview of the concept of "co-morbidity" or co-occurring problems see Feinstein, 1970). "Special" therapies, based on information gathered from tests such as the OMAS test developed by Riley and Riley (1986), will emerge to manage stutterers with concomitant problems.

Systematic Study of Transfer

More and more applied researchers and clinicians will systematically investigate the issue of relapse, "slips" in behavior, and transfer (see Ingham, 1989 for excellent and germane view of issues pertaining to therapy efficacy). Parallels will be drawn between stuttering therapy and other therapies used to remediate human disorders, for example, sexual dysfunction, and it will become increasingly apparent that *changing* behavior is much less difficult than *maintaining* it. It will also become increasing apparent that "slips" in behavior or reverting to old, inappropriate behavior do not a relapse make. The common problems with relapse and transfer, which many, many different therapies share, will become a very obvious concern and one to which attention and thought will be applied.

Melding of Behavioral and Traditional Therapies

The traditional therapies and behavioral therapies will begin to edge toward one another and meet in the middle. Increasingly, we will recognize that thoughts, feelings, and attitudes influence behavior *and* that behavior can influence thoughts, feelings, and attitudes. Thus, the insightful, perhaps sometimes a bit abstract and hard to objectify, approach of the traditionalists will be blended with the more empirical, perhaps sometimes needlessly specific, approach of the behaviorists. This melding or meshing of approaches will benefit from two divergent events: (1) the increasing amount of information generated from the empirical study of stutterers' fluent as well as stuttered speech production, and (2) the growing trend in some physical sciences, for example, biology and physics, toward more humanistic approaches to science. While the pendulum of thought in the field of stuttering will probably never completely stop in the middle, it is believed that the extent of its swing from one side to another will never again be as great as it has been observed to be in the past.

Dealing with this midground, however, means that students, in both their academic and clinical training, will need to be exposed to and learn about divergent bodies of information, for example, behavioral versus humanistic studies, principles, and practices. It will also mean that students and clinicians alike will need to become and remain knowledgeable regarding speech production in order to be able to read current literature, meaningfully attend workshops and conferences as well as apply such information to the evaluation and remediation of stuttering.

Slow, but Gradual Improvement In the Public's Sophistication

Although individuals will continue to claim clinical and theoretical monopolies on the truth, the public will slowly come to recognize and discriminate between the reputable professional and the montebank. While everyone would like to believe the purveyors of fast fluency, as the true complexities, nuances, and subtleties of stuttering are made increasingly apparent to the public and professionals alike, it will become more and more difficult for any one individual to try to claim a clinical or theoretical monopoly on the truth about the cause and remediation of stuttering. Such phrases as "overnight success," "100 percent success rate," "complete cure," and the like will become repellants as the public becomes more and more adept at seeing through the smokescreen and mirrors of the latter day "great and powerful Oz."

The facts relating to stuttering will simply weigh so heavily against the "great and powerful Oz," and so many professionals will recognize the untenable nature of such a therapeutic or theoretical monopoly, that only a few will dare to claim such omnipotence and those who do will receive scant attention. This widespread recognition of stuttering's complexities and nuances will counter the inappropriate, self-aggrandizing approaches of a few and should mark the true advancement of stuttering from an interesting object to be kicked around among different disciplines to a recognized discipline with its own standards, approaches, and body of knowledge based on clinical and laboratory endeavor. Our clients deserve no less.

SOME PARTING THOUGHTS

Harbingers for future remediation of stuttering are quite bright. We have gained considerably more basic understanding of stuttering in recent years (for example, Caruso, Abbs, and Gracco, 1988; Conture, Colton and Gleason, 1988; Moore, 1986) and an ability to evaluate claims of therapeutic success systematically and objectively (for example, Adams and Runyan, 1978; Metz, Onufrak and Ogburn, 1979; Metz, Samar and Sacco, 1983; Samar, Metz and Sacco, 1986; Sacco and Metz, 1987, in press; Robb, Lybolt and Price, 1985). These increases in our basic knowledge and understanding of clinical process in the area of stuttering can lead only to more appropriate and effective approaches to the diagnosis and remediation of stuttering and to the development of research projects that should bring us ever closer to understanding the truth about stuttering. It will be recalled that the reader of this book was offered *no* guarantees, recipes, quick fixes, or total solutions for curing stuttering, and, to my knowledge, none were given.

Guarantees, cures, and total solutions for complex human problems like stuttering are ideals to which one might like to aspire; however, one must also recognize that such ideals are not compatible with the present state of the human condition. While an overly realistic view might actually have a depressive influence on a person, an altered state of consciousness resulting in overly optimistic feelings does not provide sufficient motivation to improve our lot.

Instead, by recognizing the imperfections of the human condition, we at least have a reasonable backdrop against which we can develop and work toward improving our understanding as well as diagnosis and remediation. We are confident that speech-language pathologists will develop an even better understanding of the human condition that will enable them, in their daily dealings with stutterers, to realize "what cannot be changed . . . what should be changed, and wisdom to distinguish the one from the other" (Niebuhr, 1934).*

SUMMARY

This book examined the nature of stuttering, its onset and development, and how it may be assessed, evaluated, and remediated according to the nature of its manifestation and the chronological/developmental level of the individual client. The approach throughout has been a behavioral, problem-solving orientation; a "this is what needs to be considered" rather than "cookbook," "recipe," or "prescriptive" approach. Emphasis has been placed on viewing the individual who stutters as an individual first and a stutterer second; the individual has been viewed, as much as possible, within the totality of his or her abilities and environment rather than solely within the component given over to speech fluency. Assessment and evaluation are considered to be key to effective therapy, indeed as merely another form of therapy, and as a continued need throughout the time of therapy.

Changes in *time* and *physical tension* of speech production were viewed as essential to effective modification of stuttering, and are thought to be central to all procedures and therapies that increase stutterers' speech fluency, if only temporarily. Although time by the head ("subjective" time) as well as time by the clock ("objective" time) are considered central to our understanding and remediating of stuttering, it was shown that time is a multifaceted concept and that it is far less than clear what aspects of time are more or less related to stuttering and its modification. The direct or indirect result of many therapies is the lengthening of intra- and intersegmental durations and transitions which probably gives the stutterer additional time with which to bring the physical tension level of speech and related musculature closer to an appropriate level for smooth, forward speech. However, the means by which these "improvements" in speech fluency occur may result in a deterioration of overall naturalness or quality of the stutterer's speech, for

---

*J. Bingham, *Courage to Change: An Introduction to the Life and Thought of Rienhold Niebuhr* (Boston: Little, Brown, 1961), p. iii.

example, there may be a reduction in the natural variability of vocal pitch and intensity levels.

Clinicians who have a suitable personal approach (for example, individuals who exhibit empathy for the feelings of others) and who possess an adequate technical understanding of stuttered and fluent speech can employ a variety of procedures and achieve reasonable results. Obviously, however, for a speech-language pathologist to arrive at a point where "reasonable results" with most stutterers are the rule rather than the exception, takes some degree of clinical experience and perserverance as well as appropriate technical/professional knowledge and interpersonal skills. SLPs who manage stutterers must be keen observers of human attitudes, behaviors, and feelings, and be able to change procedure according to the needs of the clinical situation. Recognizing what *needs* to be changed and in what direction is no more important than recognizing what *can* be changed.

Future directions in stuttering will involve further delving into: (1) *cortical* and *sub-cortical* activities associated with fluent and disfluent speech; (2) studies of the *temporal* and *spatial* parameters of fluent and disfluent speech production; (3) advancements in the nature and number of of *computer-assisted* diagnostic and remediation procedures; (4) refinements in procedures for systematically assessing listener-speaker *interactions,* particularly those between mother and young stutterer; (5) clarification of the number and nature of behavioral as well as etiological *subgroupings* of stutterers; (6) refinements in our understanding of *co-morbidity* as it pertains to stuttering (that is, the number and nature of problems that co-occur with stuttering); and (7) systematic, long-term assessment of therapy *efficacy* and *transfer.* Although difficult to predict their specific nature, other topics will surely emerge in the years ahead, with some topics reaping greater dividends than others, but serendipity is as much a part of research as it is daily life and only hindsight can truly tell us which paths were best initially traversed.

As discussed in the first chapter, our honest recognition of what doesn't work, of what doesn't make sense, and of what doesn't pertain to stuttering helps us to better understand that simple solutions to complex problems like stuttering are ideals toward which we aspire but may not always be compatible with the present state of the human condition. And this human condition, for stutterers and their families, looks increasingly brighter. We are making headway in understanding and treating stuttering, and continuing this progress is, in my opinion, worthy of the best efforts of all involved.

APPENDIX A
INTERVIEW QUESTIONS FOR THE PARENT(S) OF A DISFLUENT CHILD

Remember: These questions are a *guide* for you. It is *your* job to organize the questions in a logical sequential manner. Furthermore, they may be adapted and modified for use with older children and adults.

Introduction

What can we do to help you? or Tell us (me) about why you are here today? or Tell us (me) about the (your child's) problem? or What seems to be the matter or the problem?

How did you find out about our Clinic?

General Development

Tell us a little about his/her general development from birth to present. (Don't strive for detail at this point.)

How does this compare with his/her sister's and brother's development?

Other children his age that you may know?

Are you satisfied with his/her development?

Family History

Are there any speech, hearing, or language problems in other family members (mother's *and* father's side?)

(If so) did they receive speech therapy or other professional assistance (help)?

Speech Language Development and History

When did he/she begin to babble? (You may need to define the term babbling.)
Begin to imitate (non)speech sounds?
Begin to say first words?
Begin to say first phrases, for example, "milk all gone."
Does he/she have any articulation or language problems? (May need to explain these terms.)

Academic Information

How is he/she progressing in school? (Be sure to know if child is in school before asking this question.)
Which subjects does he/she like the best?
How does he/she do in the subjects?
Which subjects does he/she like the least?
How does he/she do in these subjects?

Social Behavioral

What are his/her interests or hobbies?
Who are his/her playmates? Ages? Younger or older?
(At this time you may present selected items of the Vineland Social Maturity Scale or else intersperse them during the interview.)
Is there anything (other than speaking) that particularly concerns you about your child?

History/Description of Problem: Part 1

Describe what you see to be your child's speaking problem(s) at this time.
When did this start?
Who noticed the problem first? Under what circumstances?
Were you worried or concerned about it at the beginning?
What was your reaction at that time?
Did you bring this "problem" to his/her attention?
What did you call it?
When did *you* begin to use the word "stuttering"? If not you, *who* did?
Did you or do you ever notice the same behavior in your other children at any time?
Children or relatives, neighbors, or others?

Speech/Language Abilities

Did you child have any trouble saying words? Sounds? Syllables? Letters? (Or, does he/she have any speech sound articulation problems?)
Can you *describe* your child's speech (stuttering) behavior when you first noticed the problem?
Is it the same now?

Has it changed? That is, duration, type, frequency-cyclical-stablized. (It may be necessary to provide examples, for example, sound repetitions, sound prolongations, word, part-word or phrase repetition. Clinician should know how to produce these various disfluency types.

History/Description of Problem: Part 2

Any body movements? Before? Now? Other concomitant behaviors?
Eye contact? Has this changed since beginning of problem?
Facial grimaces?
What aspect of the problem concerns you the most?
What was/is different that he had/has never done before?
Since the "onset" of this speech problem has your child done this everytime he/she has spoken? Is he/she ever fluent?

Anxiety Situational Hierarchy

a) In certain situations?
b) On any particular words? sounds? letters?
c) With certain listeners? for example, authority figures
d) Strangers, friends, mother, father, and so forth.
Does he avoid any situation to avoid speaking?
Why do you think the problem developed?
Do you think it will change?
How?
If it were to change, do you think there would be any other changes in various aspects of his/her behavior? Would the child be different, for example, in his interactions if he/she didn't stutter?
What have you been told previously about your child's "stuttering"? Other problems? (Advice from relatives, teachers, friends, doctor, speech pathologist, etc.)
Has your child had any speech therapy? Other counseling? Has anyone else in your family had any kind of counseling, for example, psychological? academic?

History/Description of Problem: Part 3

What have you done to help your child stop stuttering?
Does/did it help?
Who recommended this?
Why do you do this?
Do you think that your child reacts to his speech behavior? Does he/she get embarrassed or show concern?
Is he/she aware? How do you know?
How does he/she react to your recommendations, promptings, "help"?
Does he/she try to improve his/her speech?
Results?
How do you react to your child's stuttering? (For instance, looking away, speaking for him, interrupting, punishing?)

What about children, relatives, friends, strangers, and others?

Is someone more critical of his/her speech?

How do you react when your child is speaking in front of others?

Do other children ever tease him about his speaking? How does he/she react to this teasing? How do you react? Does this teasing hurt you?

Family Interaction

What kinds of things do you do as a family? What things does your child enjoy the most? The least?

Do you talk with your child very much? (read, play, etc.?) Your spouse? (This is an important question—dwell on it if there is any hint of inadequate communication.)

How does the child get along with sister(s) and brother(s)? Any hostilities or jealousies or rivalries?

How do you (or spouse) handle these?

Social/Behavioral

Does your child play well by himself?

Does he/she have may friends? Do they visit him/her at home? Does he/she visit them?

Does the child require much attention? More than normal? Needs more from mother or father?

How does he/she adjust to a new environment, situation? Sensitive to changes in environment? routine? discipline?

How does the child react to discipline? How do you, in general, discipline? (Stress need for information and that you are not going to discipline them for their discipline procedures.)

Does he/she do what you ask? complete chores, and so forth?

Does he/she do anything that particularly annoys you or anyone else?

Why does it annoy you? How have you attempted to resolve this problem?

Wrap Up

If you could wish for three things for your child (the sky is the limit), what would you wish for?

APPENDIX B
ONSET OF STUTTERING: A CASE STUDY

INTRODUCTION

Many factors influence the detail and dependability of information gathered regarding the nature of events surrounding the onset of stuttering. One important factor is the interval of time from the onset of stuttering to the first interview between the parents of a stuttering child and a speech clinician. In most cases the speech therapist has to rely on the memory of parents about their reactions to and events concomitant with the beginnings of the stuttering problem. Any factor(s) that might dull parental memories, such as the length of time between the onset of stuttering and the parents' recollections about this, would, of course, interfere with the clearest possible understanding of the onset and development of stuttering.

The importance of the time interval between the onset of stuttering and the first interview was stressed by Johnson and others (1959). In these studies on the onset of stuttering, it seems that attempts were made to study "stuttering cases . . . in whom stuttering was of recent origin."[1] These researchers

[1]W. Johnson and others, *The Onset of Stuttering* (Minneapolis, MN: University of Minnesota Press, 1959), p. 15. Reprinted by permission.

apparently felt that the shorter the time period between onset and interview, the more detailed and dependable the information concerning the onset of stuttering would be. Even so, the median interval between date of onset of stuttering and date of initial interview (in the earliest study) was 5 months and 18 days. In a later study, the median interval was 17 to 17 ½ months (the exact median interval being dependent upon whether one uses the mother's or the father's report of the date of onset). The shortest interval for the first study was four days; for the later study, the shortest interval was less than one month. Therefore, even though Johnson and his co-workers interviewed a few cases within a short interval after onset, that is, one month or less, the bulk of the cases were seen several months to a year after onset of stuttering. The fact that parents, in general, wait a while before bringing their stuttering child to a speech therapist may say something in and of itself about the nature of the onset and development of stuttering. Whatever the case, our understanding of the onset of stuttering would be enhanced if we could interview parents and their children as soon as possible after the reported beginnings of stuttering.

In general, we are seeking to provide further information about the nature of the onset of stuttering. Specifically, we present a detailed account of a mother's and father's description of their son's incipient stuttering problem. This account appears uniquely capable of at least partially achieving the previously stated purpose for two main reasons: (1) The time interval between the reported onset and the initial interview was only eight days, and (2) the parents had discussed between themselves and written down the events surrounding the beginnings of their son's speech problem.

PROCEDURE

The parents, Mr. and Mrs. F. (the father was 52 years of age and the mother was 37), were interviewed both separately and together. Their son, age three years, eight months (he will be called Sammy here) was separated from his parents during the majority of this interview. It was not possible to do an extensive hearing evaluation or intelligence testing because of the limits on the parents' time. Therefore, it was felt that the available time would be most profitably spent in questioning the parents (especially the mother, who had apparently first diagnosed her son's speech as being stuttered) about the onset of the stuttering problem and about their son's speech and language development in general. Informal evaluation of the child's articulatory, phonatory, and language usage did not suggest the presence of any problem(s). (Formal testing of these areas was impractical since the child was uncooperative and also cried during much of the time he was separated from his mother.) One whole-word repetition was noticed, but this was not considered unusual for a child of his age. In short, Sammy appeared to be well within normal limits for a child his age in the areas of motor, intellectual, and speech-language development. (Once again, it should be noted that such statements were made on the basis of informal evaluation and not from formal testing.) At the end of the interview, the parents were counseled regarding 1) the findings of the diagnostic and 2) their future management of their son's speech problem.

THE INTERVIEW

The mother, who did the majority of the talking for both parents, was asked to describe from the beginning, the events surrounding the onset of the stuttering problem. Mrs. F. said that she had first noticed something wrong with Sammy's speech on the night of Monday, 1/31/72 (the date of the first interview was Tuesday, 2/8/72). At that time the family was watching the television program "Laugh-in," when a person on the program began mocking a stuttering person. Shortly thereafter, the mother said she noticed Sammy stuttering in apparent imitation[2] of the television character. The mother reported that neither she nor her husband said anything to the child about his speech behavior, but Mrs. F. said that she did look very shocked, an expression that she was sure her son had noticed. The mother then recalled that she had remarked to her husband, in the presence of their son, "Did you hear that?" in reference to Sammy's speech behavior. The father then replied to the mother, still in Sammy's presence, that the boy had done the same thing just a minute ago. However, both parents reported that neither of them had, at any time, mentioned anything directly to their son about his speech behavior. Neither parent could say for sure whether, when Sammy's stuttering was first noticed, he was using force or more effort than usual to produce speech. The mother did report that for the next two days she noticed the child producing several disfluencies, but she still did not mention these disfluencies to her son.

During these next two days, Tuesday, 2/1, and Wednesday, 2/2, Mrs. F. said that she noticed the child several times repeating the word *mother* or prolonging the initial /m/ of the word *mother*. On the third day, Thursday, 2/3, the mother reported that she got frustrated with her son's speech. She reported that on this day, if her son began to repeat a syllable or word, she yelled at him to "shut up and start over again." Mrs. F. also reported that on that day she told Sammy to "stop talking that way" when she noticed him repeating a sound or a word. The mother's frustration with her son's speech

---

[2]Even after intensive questioning, neither mother nor father could clearly describe the nature of this imitation; the only thing the mother could say was that she was so shocked at Sammy's stuttering that she could not remember the exact nature of the stuttering.

behavior is probably what led her to call me on the phone that day, Thursday, 2/3. In our telephone conversation, she expressed her concern about her son's speech and referred to his problem alternately as stuttering or double talk. All of these scoldings and reprimands, the mother reported, resulted in Sammy's crying. (However, the mother commented that he would start to cry whenever she would even "look cross-eyed at him.")

Both parents described their son's speech problem as being cyclical in nature, that is, some days he stuttered more than other days. The mother felt that most of her son's trouble developed at the beginning of a sentence he was formulating about something that was new or unclear to him. At these times, Mrs. F. said that he would repeat the first syllable of the first word or two of the sentence until he "got his train of thought." When questioned about the cyclical nature of their son's stuttering, the parents gave the following examples: Saturday 2/5, the mother was home alone with the child and only one stuttering was noticed; however, on Sunday, 2/6, when the father was home alone with the child, Mr. F. reported that Sammy stuttered all day.

When the parents were asked for their opinion as to why their son had a speech problem, the mother responded that Sammy stuttered primarily because he imitated the television performer. However, Mrs. F. stated that the imitation might have "brought to the surface some quirk or defect in his brain" that maintained the stuttering response well after the initial imitative response. The mother felt that some *quirk* or *defect* would have to be present to explain why her son had remained disfluent as long as he had.

The mother described Sammy as being in need of constant attention from her (she called him her "constant shadow"). She also felt that Sammy was very aggressive since he was constantly hitting his older siblings or pestering the cat. The mother, reportedly, attempted to deal with her son's misconduct by yelling or screaming at him. (Mrs. F. stated that she never hit any of her children. Sammy was the last for her four children, and only the three younger children still lived with the parents.) Sammy reacted to this yelling, according to the mother by crying, getting upset, or by telling his mother, "Don't yell at me." Both parents described their son's motor, social (for example, toilet training), and speech development as being essentially normal.

In general, the father's responses to most questions about his son's development suggested that he was not too concerned with any facet of Sammy's maturational progress and, in fact, seemed to believe that his son was essentially normal for his age. However, the mother felt that Sammy was somewhat slow in his overall development, and she also felt he could behave better. On the other hand, Mrs. F. commented that she was unable to see how her son's speech could be defective when the rest of him was "perfect." In fact, the mother indicated considerable concern over the fact that Sammy might be less than perfect in something, since everyone in his family always "tried to be perfect in everything they did."

When questioned with regard to whether they had any relatives with speech problems, the father said that his 30-year-old son (by another marriage) began to stutter when he was 14 years old. Mrs. F. said that she thought that her husband's son, even as an adult, was "hesitant when he talks." The mother went on to report that her sister's daughter had a speech problem when she was young, that is, her speech was very unclear and difficult to understand. Neither parent reported any major trauma or accident, either psychological or physical, that Sammy had ever been involved in.

DISCUSSION

From the information gathered during this interview, it could be stated that nothing seemed to be grossly wrong with Sammy, either psychologically or physiologically. Furthermore, there were no apparent speech or language problems; that is, the child appeared to be articulating speech and receiving and expressing linguistic mesages adequatley for a child of his age. What, then, was the problem? I believe that it was just such normalcy of development that led the parents to react to their son's speech. That is, as Johnson (1961) points out, "parents are most likely to decide their children are stuttering when they are hesitating and repeating for no reason that the parents can detect."[3]

This hypothesis seems to have even more merit when it is remembered that the mother did not become really concerned with her son's speech until the third day after the initial imitative response. At first, both parents were relatively tolerant of the child's speech problem becuase they felt he was simply imitating the television performer, but when the child persisted into the third and fourth days, the parents (the mother primarily) both started to worry over and react to the child's speech behavior. (Further support for this idea comes from the fact that the mother reported that she at first described the child's speech behavior as double talk and that it was not until the third day that she realized he was stuttering!)

Of course, the parental admonitions to "shut up and start over again" fit into the Johnsonian *diagnosogenic model* (Johnson, and others, 1967) in that the parents were then reacting to their own diagnostic label of stuttering. And, of course, as the model would predict, Sammy might

> learn to doubt that he can talk smoothly enough to please the people he talks to, mainly his parents. . . . What this amounts to is that he learns to be afraid that

[3]W. Johnson, *Stuttering and What You Can Do About It* (Minneapolis, MN: University of Minnesota Press, 1961), p. 126. Reprinted by permission.

"he will stutter" and that if he does he, along with "the stuttering," will be disapproved.[4]

However, in the present situation, the child hopefully, will never get to the point where he has learned to react to his parents' reactions to his speech by attempting to avoid stuttering. This may be the case since the parents were given the following:

1. Information regarding the normal development of speech and language, especially the period during which children are normally disfluent
2. Advice to listen to the *content* of the child's expressions instead of to *how* the child expresses himself
3. Advice to reduce the psychological tension and stress placed on the child when he does not do exactly what is expected of him
4. Advice to allow the child to talk as much as possible without any attempt to change the content or manner of his verbalizations

Furthermore, in attempts to clarify the proceeding points, the parents were given a copy of W. Johnson's (1949) "An Open Letter to the Mother of a Stuttering Child." [Currently we might also use Ainsworth and Fraser's 1988 or Cooper's (1979) pamphlets.] It was felt that the parents' level of understanding was such that, following the informal counseling they received, they would be able to derive benefit from Johnson's "Letter." The parents were instructed to check back in six months, no matter what the status of their son's speech and language development.

In conclusion, even within the limits of the interview procedure, it would appear that the short time interval between the date of onset of stuttering and the first interview in this case probably enhanced the detail and dependability of the information derived concerning the onset and development of Sammy's stuttering. Of course, such factors as low intelligence or hearing loss cannot be ruled out as contributing factors, but as already mentioned, the probability that such factors are contributory appears to be slight. Furthermore, the information procedure would appear to strongly support the diagnosogenic model of the onset of stuttering. This does not imply that some other model might not adequately explain the findings with regard to the child's onset of stuttering. However, it does suggest the viability of the hypothesis that stuttering finds its beginnings or onset in parental reactions to the child's normal developmental disfluencies.

It must be emphasized that before we are ever to get a clearer understanding of the origins of the stuttering problem, we must procure more and more cases like Sammy's in which effects of time have not had a chance to erase the necessary details. For as long as we are to deal with human memory and human biases, as it appears we must when we attempt to understand the

[4]Ibid., p. 68.

onset of stuttering through interview techniques, we must attempt to eliminate all factors that tend to cloud and distort human recollections about past events and perceptions.

APPENDIX C
NOTE TO
A BEGINNING
SPEECH-LANGUAGE
PATHOLOGIST

CLINICIANS AS PEOPLE

Before we became speech and language clinicians, we were people, and we will be people after we stop being clinicians. We need to know as much about ourselves as people as we do about communicative disorders if we really want to become effective clinicians. This is not a plea for encounter sessions, T-groups, psychoanalysis, and the like (even though some of us, from time to time, may need and seek such experiences). Rather it is a plea for the need to consider ourselves as people, people with frailties, people with strengths, people who are constantly learning how to facilitate learning in other people and hopefully, ourselves.

Many of the problems that parents bring to us are problems we still wrestle with within ourselves. Many of our young clients' concerns we had as children ourselves or are concerns we have with our own youngsters. We should not feel helpless knowing these things. Instead, we may feel some relief that our clients share in the same human condition that we are experiencing.

Starting from a base where we recognize our humanness and all that it entails, we have a lot less farther to fall when we come up against the difficulties of changing certain aspects of the human condition. Let us then consider some aspects about ourselves that will be factors in our dealings with clients with communicative disorders.

A CLINICIAN'S NEED TO BE SELF-ANALYTICAL

Somewhere between total oblivion to our mistakes and complete paralysis if a mistake is made is the area that clinicians should strive for. Happy-go-lucky clinicians who bumble through diagnosis and management are constantly amazed that their performances are not always the best. Conversely, clinicians who are paralyzed with fear that they will make a mistake are constantly amazed that they ever do anything right.

The ability to be appropriately self-analytical is a skill that is not easily acquired, but it is a skill well worth the acquisition. Clinicians who are continually growing, in the professional sense, are the clinicians who are capable of turning the errors they produce back into the system. Many clinicians resist the development of self-appraisal skills for a variety of reasons, none the least of which is the real threat to self that such personal scrutiny represents. Such clinicians are often confused between their *self* (personality) and their *behavior*. These clinicians can advise Mrs. Jones to tell Tommy, "I do not like having orange peels thrown on the rug," instead of the usual, "Tommy, why are you such a bad boy?" However, these same clinicians cannot apply this logic to their own self-analysis.

Knowing when you are going in the right or wrong direction is fundamental to your continued improvement as a clinician. Surely, other professionals and personnel will tell you how you are doing and if they like or dislike your work, but if you are *totally* dependent upon them for your feedback and monitoring of performance, it is going to be a long, long time before you start to see substantial improvement in your performance. You really have to work at developing an objective appraisal system for your *own* performance. It will not come overnight. You will have to develop sensitivity for other people's *unspoken* feelings, ideas, and so forth, and change your performance accordingly. You will have to be a better reader of clinical situations and adapt yourself appropriately.

Obviously, self-analysis will, from time to time, indicate to you that you are in error. Knowing you are in error will require you to modify your performance. Your ability to modify and entertain the notion that you are in error will take maturity and compromise on your part. The temptation to negate your errors and assign the blame to your client, the parents, your supervisor, your professors, the system, and so forth, will be great. However, such passing of the buck will not allow you to fully develop to the greatest extent possible. You will have to shoulder the responsibility for your errors and performance and attempt to modify them appropriately.

The monitoring of your clinical performance requires diligence but not necessarily paranoid caution. You can be relatively flexible in clinical situations as long as you realize that you are capable of changing your inappropriate clinical procedures. Your ability to monitor and change is as much an assumption for you as for your client if you cannot monitor and modify your own behavior, how do you expect your client to do so?

A PERSONALITY "SUITABLE" FOR BECOMING A CLINICIAN

Interpersonal relations are obviously of importance to the speech-language pathologist. The personality of the clinician does enter into the clinical equation that equals effective diagnosis and management. But what personalities are best? What are the necessary interpersonal relations that go into effective clinical operations? To begin, we must distinguish between the personality we *are* and the personality we *become* in the clinical setting. It has been said somewhere that we wear many masks for the different people we interact with. That is, we modify, to some degree, our interpersonal relations depending upon the person(s) we deal with. Consequently, different people may get different ideas or perceptions about our personalities.

We must realize that our *basic personality* may not be the reason we have clinical difficulties; however, our ability to play a role (personality) appropriate for the therapy setting may be less than adequate. We may not be putting on a wardrobe suitable to wear into the therapy room. And I am not talking about jeans versus a skirt or a T-shirt versus a shirt and tie. I am talking about the type of person you come across to your client as being while you are interacting with him or her in the clinical environment.

Now, it is also obvious that the larger the discrepancy between your basic personality and your *clinical personality*, the more uncomfortable your clinical duties will become. However, who ever said that you should feel comfortable all the time? Aren't you entitled to your moments of unease and uncertainty? We said that certain clinical roles will facilitate therapeutic endeavors, but we did not say it would always be easy or comfortable for you to enact those roles.

Your clinical personality should be as nonjudgmental as possible. You must become as sensitive a listener as possible, as objectively critical and at the same time appropriately reinforcing as you can be. You must convey belief that the person can and will change. You must convey an interest in the person as a person, and not just as a stutterer or as a set of interesting behaviors. Rogers' clinical tenet of *unconditional positive regard* is a good facet to add to your clinical personality. You must be able to open yourself up to a client's questions, about who and what you are, but at the same time realize when you need to take charge and shift the focus of the therapy interaction. Above all, your personality must convey to the client a sincere interest in his or her welfare, without becoming emotionally involved to the point where your objectivity vanishes and your ability to assist the person diminishes.

Do you have to be outgoing to be a good clinician, or can you be the shy, retiring type and still be effective? This question is inappropriate. Let us see what you do in the clinical setting. If you are continually cracking jokes to maintain attention, running off at the mouth, and being in general a hail-fellow-well-met, but giving clients no indication that you care about them or their problems, your clinical personality is inappropriate. Clients are apt to say of such clinicians, "Well, he's a nice person, but I don't think he understands me and my problem." On the other hand, if you religiously run through your clinical exercises, give minimal exposure to your personal frailties, and are basically standoffish, then you have problems. Of these clinicians clients usually say, "They seem to know about my problems, but they really don't care about me, the person." In essence, your clinical personality, whatever its form (and this form may have to be changed depending upon the client or clinical setting), must convey and reflect

1. Interest in the client as a person
2. Knowledge about the problem(s) at hand
3. Ability to assist the client in making change and belief that such change is possible
4. Objective assessment of behaviors, situations, and personal variables and minimal judgmental statements
5. Sensitivity towards the client's and your involvement in the human condition first and his or her problem(s) second

THE DEVELOPMENT OF A CLINICIAN: FROM CLASSROOM TO CLINIC

We take courses (short and long), sit through endless lectures, participate in seminars, and involve ourselves in independent studies. Our education is long and demanding. And then, one day, we step into the clinic for our first diagnostic or therapy session.

Suddenly, it seems, we are in another realm. We face a different world of real people with real problems who want our help and guidance and comfort. Gone are the books discussing hypothesis A versus hypothesis B. No more do we engage in the fascinating seminar discussions on whether a particular problem is learned or inate. We are on the line with a client, and time must be spent in a professional way. The way we spend this time, however, is the crux of our professional abilities.

Not all information we achieve in our education is readily applicable to the clinical process. This does not mean the information is useless, but sometimes clinicians express this opinion. What they appear to fail to realize is that education develops particular thought processes as well as it provides specific course content. Instead of accepting black or white approaches to the world, education tells us that many events are situated along a continuum. Such a relativistic notion does not excuse clinicians from making decisions; however, it should influence the type of decisions they make. Similarly, education instructs that problem solving, which asks answerable questions, tests them, and rejects and/or accepts hypotheses on the basis of findings is more appropriate than waiting for the answer from the expert(s).

Education expands horizons and our abilities to deal with change; it does not simply fill empty vessels. Surely, you cannot think in a vacuum. No one expects you to deal with communicative disorders without certain basic facts, figures, information, and concepts, but somewhere along the way, it is up to you to bridge the gap between classroom and clinic.

We often hear the claim, by clinicians in trouble. "If I'd only had so and so in such and such course then I'd be all right." The truth is, however, that these clinicians are not applying even the limited amount of information they do have. They appear to see no relation between what they learned and what they must do in the clinic. They seem to expect the clinical process to take care of itself ("All I need is experience"). Experience, in and of itself, will lead them nowhere if the experience does not involve their active participation. Practice does not make perfect. Perfect practice makes perfect.

Student-clinicians having trouble in the clinic do not seem able to transfer from academic to clinical setting. This lack of transference may result from a number of things: They did not really learn the content of their courses, (classroom excellence is often reflected in clinical excellence) or they did not really change their thought processes as a result of their education (they are still waiting around to be shown how to do it).

Many times such clinicians seem unable to compartmentalize their personal from their professional lives. Problems at home creep into and interfere with their clinical performance ("I couldn't concentrate on therapy because I'm worried about getting my car fixed").

Problem student-clinicians avoid evaluations by their supervisors and professors with the claim, "I tried to reach you but you weren't in." Interestingly, student-clinicians *without* clinical concerns always seem to find their supervisors and professors in their offices. The less than adequate student-clinician claims, "No one told me I was doing poorly." Perhaps, this is so, but often they were told and they did not hear or listen. Short of being told, "We are flunking you out," problem student-clinicians do not seem to understand their supervisors when they say there are concerns or problems with the student's performance. Such students appear to lack the ability to self-analyze and to receive and act upon objective criticism they receive from their supervisors and professors.

A really unfortunate situation arises when student-clinicians, who have received negative objective evaluations of their clinical performance, begin to rely too much on supervisor-professor input for their clinical endeavors.

They seem to be looking to some big person for help because they have received negative evaluation, and they become tremendously unsure of how to proceed. This fosters a vicious cycle where supervisors begin to see clinicians as overly dependent on feedback for clinical performance. Student-clinicians, in turn, come to rely too much on this feedback and do not develop their ability to problem solve and perform independently. Such cycles are difficult to break once started; we need to be aware of their potential for development so that we can head off their very existence.

Looking to others for assistance and suggestions is reasonable and appropriate, but when it becomes routine and habitual, it has the real potential for thwarting personal growth and independence. Self-responsibility for our lives, while never easy, is an absolute must for the development of an independent clinician. We all lapse back into stages of dependence, but hopefully we pick ourselves up off the floor and try to regain self-responsibility for our acts. It is our responsibility to apply course content to clinical endeavor. We must be the person to employ the necessary problem-solving orientation to the clinical situation. An active role is needed on the part of the clinician; passivity will result in little change and growth. Although it may be a comfort to blame external factors for our inabilities, in the long run it is we ourselves who must come to grips with the demands of the clinical interaction and try to rise to the challenge.

Self-analysis, problem solving, dedication to the task at hand, independence of thought and action, creative reactions to new situations, and the ability to transfer information from class to clinic are some of the more important hallmarks of a good student-clinician. Although very few people achieve all these hallmarks to the ideal degree, many people are working to achieve such goals. They are at least aware of the presence of these goals and believe them to be of importance. We can become all the clinician we can become as long as we realize that we are the ones who have to do the becoming.

HOW MUCH TRAINING YOU HAVE HAD

There is a great temptation to become defensive when a patient or client asks you how much training you have had. There are times when we do not like people poking around into our professional credentials. How we handle such questions, however, reflects as much on our training as it does on our maturity, experience, and so forth.

First, if at all possible, find out why you are being questioned. Maybe you say to the person, "I understand your interest, but why do you ask?" In any case, try to find out why you are being questioned about your credentials. Sometimes clients are shopping around for the best (in their opinion) clinician, and other times they are simply testing you. It is important to distinguish between the two motivations.

Second, look to yourself. What signals are you giving that elicit such a question? Is it your apparent uncertainty, or is it your lack of ease with a client, or what? Remember to keep in mind the difference between your uncertainty as a clinician-person and your uncertainty regarding the handling of a particularly unique, difficult, or unclear case. If you are young (especially your physical appearance and manner of expression), you can just expect more queries about your credentials or experiences. There is no need to become defensive. Remember, experience comes from going through the experiences you are going through.

Finally, have your past successes (or lack thereof) with a particular age client, parent, or communicative disorder finally caught up with you? Perhaps, if time or money permit, a course in the area of concern (no matter if you have had a course with the same title or not) may be a wise investment. We are never, thank goodness, too old to learn or relearn. If nothing else, start picking up books and journals and read.

"MY CHILD'S BEEN WITH YOU FOR THREE MONTHS AND I DON'T SEE ANY CHANGE"

Lack of progress, or no apparent new behavior, is often the beginning of the end of a therapy program. Parents who do not see any progress become less likely to chauffeur little Johnny in for his twice-a-week therapy. Johnny, likewise, is apt to become frustrated, less willing to work, and less motivated if he detects lack of progress, and the clinician, poor person, becomes depressed at the living testimony to his or her ineptness.

Surely, one does not want to whitewash incompetent methods that have resulted in minimal clinical progress. Likewise, one does not want to excuse the reluctant client and his or her parents who will not or cannot cooperate in the therapy process to bring about a change. We must, however, realize when lack of progress is really telling us something about the problem(s) we are dealing with.

First, have we evaluated and diagnosed the situation correctly and completely? Are we ignoring some important variable, for example, a limited attention span, because we believe the client can rise above such trivia and exert enough will power to improve? Therapy, it has been said, is a continual diagnostic experience; however, many times we forget this in the rush to fill the therapy hour with methods to effect the cure.

Second, does lack of progress really indicate that perhaps we are expecting change prior to change being possible? Are we becoming unnecessarily anxious with the slowness of the behavioral change process? Parents, particularly, are susceptible to wanting to speed up the pace of their child's development. Parents give us important clues to this when t ey tell us that Billy's stuttering "is holding him back and if he can lick this thing he'll be able to do much . . . he has so much potential . . . he's got to change it now before it's too late." They become impatient with our procedures, especially when those procedures do not work on his speech. Clearly, it is our role to tell parents, from the beginning, approximately how long therapy will take and what steps it will involve. Children must crawl before they walk, and parents must be made to understand this. No matter how much they love their child and desire for their child's well-being, the learning process cannot be sped up. There are no free lunches.

Third, clients may become depressed at the rate of progress because they envisioned you as the guru who was going to lift the stuttering burden off their shoulders without any sweat, pain, work, and travail on their part. It comes as a surprise to them when they learn that behavioral changes require them to work and practice every day at changing their speech. What is wrong, they think; it is not supposed to be this hard. I thought this speech doctor was supposed to cure me. Some doctor!

The client, like the impatient parent, must realize that change takes time, work, and patience. The longest journey begins with a single step. We, as clinicians, must clearly articulate to the clients our goals and subgoals and the time frame within which such goals will be realized. We must set our clients up for the inevitable wall of inertia they will meet when they begin to try to change their old, well-learned, but inappropriate, behavior. If we expect more stuttering before less stuttering, we should tell the client and the parents. We might explain that for change to occur, the client must diminish his or her circumlocutions and avoidances and acutally stutter. Likewise, we should tell the client and parents what they might look for in terms of signs of early improvement, for example, decreased duration of stutterings.

Even the most seemingly depressing situation like that of a no progress client is an opportunity for developing our clinical skills and assisting our client. Asking questions about the whys of the no progress evaluation will provide the opportunity. Looking for answers from the experts and books will provide us some assistance, but we may maximize the potential of the opportunity. Our progress as clinicians, like that of our clients, has a certain price, but fortunately all of us have the potential to pay this price.

APPENDIX D
CHILDREN WHO STUTTER: SUGGESTIONS FOR THE CLASSROOM TEACHER

From time to time, classroom teachers will have children who stutter in their class. What follows is information as well as suggestions that should better help teachers understand and deal with these children.

(1) *Children who stutter should be treated similarly to their peers.* Teachers should try to deal with children who stutter as they would any other "normally" developing child. While all children have special needs, "special" classroom activities do not need to be created to deal *routinely* with children who stutter. Neither should these children be *routinely* excluded from specific classroom activities. Treat the child who stutters, as much as possible, like the other children in the classroom.

(2) *Some "kinda help" is the "kinda help" these kids can do without.* Teachers should make every attempt to cease and desist any and all direct corrections of the young stutterer's pronunciation of speech sounds, expressive language usage, or speech disfluencies (that is, stutterings) *while* the child is routinely coversing with the teacher or other children. These corrections seem to make intuitive sense—they are frequently used by parents and other listeners—but if they really helped there would be little reason for therapy with stutterers.

Of course, a teacher should feel free to help young stutterers who misspell a word while writing, mispronounce a word while reading aloud during reading class, or who, during a grammar lesson, use incorrect syntax. These corrections are the type that the teacher uses with *all* children in class. However, teachers should try to avoid any and all corrections that, although well intended, call undue or inappropriate attention to the child's speech and language problem. Sometimes these corrections can wind up becoming part of the problem rather than part of the solution.

(3) *Accentuate the positive, eliminate the negative.* As much as possible, on days when the child who stutters seems particularly fluent (that is, doesn't stutter), the teacher should try to draw the child out and encourage him to talk and read. Conversely, on days when he or she is particularly disfluent (that is stuttering a lot), the teacher should call less frequently on the child to talk, recite, or read aloud in class. Encouraging the child to talk is best done on good days, while encouraging quiet or nontalking activities is best done on bad days.

(4) *Once children begin to speak, they should be allowed to finish.* Teachers should try—just as they do when normally fluent children speak—to let the young stutterer complete or finish his or her words, phrases, or sentences. Interrupting and filling in words for the child, correcting the child's vocabulary or grammar usage, and so forth *while* the child is talking may seem as if it helps, but it does not. These interruptions convey a less than positive message to the child about both his or her speaking abilities as well as the teacher's evaluation of them. Teachers and other adult listeners can't expect the young stutterer's peers to listen and not interrupt if they, as adults, continue to do the opposite.

(5) *Group speaking, singing, or reading.* Where and whenever possible, teachers should try to incorporate choral or group reading aloud, speaking, or singing in the classroom. These should not be special activities, but appropriate for and consistent with classroom activities and objectives. These acts maximize the young stutterers' chances for producing speech just like that produced by his or her normally fluent peers and should contribute to positive feelings about self and speaking abilities.

(6) *If you can't master the subject, master the other kids.* Some children tease or mock other children for a variety of reasons; for example, (1) they themselves are having trouble mastering subject material, so they try to "master" other children by ridiculing and/or putting them down; (2) they may feel that any attention is better than no attention at all and, to them, other people's negative reactions to their teasing are worth it if they get increased attention; and (3) they are uncomfortable with differences and really don't understand

that their mocking, teasing, or ridiculing hurts the other child. Whatever the case, if the situation arises where another member of the class *frequently* or *routinely* teases the child who stutters about his or her speech or related matters, the teacher should intervene.

First, when the child who stutters is out of the room, the teacher should give a short lecture to the class discussing how different people develop in different ways when learning different skills, for example, riding a bike, learning to talk, read, write, and the like. This talk may need to be given a few times, each time while the young child is out of the room, and the teacher should observe the lectures' influence on the child doing the teasing. Second, if, after such lectures, the teasing continues, the teacher should take aside the child doing the teasing and have an "information-sharing" conversation with the child. This conversation should describe the various ways in which children differ in their development and how teasing and ridicule do not help children who are different; it just makes them feel bad. The teacher should try to deliver this message in a firm but polite manner and minimize the teasing child's sense that he or she is being punished. This conversation may have to take place more than once. Any improvement in the ways in which the child who teases interacts with the young stutterer should be subtly but clearly reinforced by the teacher.

APPENDIX E
STUTTERING
DIAGNOSTIC REPORT

A SAMPLE OF A SYRACUSE UNIVERSITY
DEPARTMENT OF COMMUNICATION SCIENCES AND DISORDERS
GEBBIE SPEECH AND HEARING CLINICS

Speech and Language Diagnostic Report

I. Background Information

Name: Charles Baker

Address: 0000 North Road
Anywhere, N.Y.
Zip Code

Telephone: (315) 888-9999

Parents: Ann Baker
Ronald Baker

Siblings: Susie, 6

Faculty Supervisor:
Edward G. Conture, Ph.D.

Date of This Evaluation: 4/5/88

Date of Birth: 6/22/79

Age at This Evaluation: 8;9

Referral: Ms. Jane Doe
Speech-Language
Pathologist
Anywhere Elem. School

Tentative Diagnosis: Mild Stutterer*

---

*Rating a 3 on the 0 (no stuttering) to 7 (very severe stuttering) Iowa Scale for Rating the Severity of Stuttering (Johnnson, Darley, and Spriesterback, 1964).

II. Summary Statement

On April 5, 1988, Charles, accompanied by his mother, Mrs. Baker, was seen at the Syracuse University Gebbie Speech and Hearing Clinics for a speech and language evaluation. During the evaluation, Charles produced an average of 6 speech disfluencies per 100 words of conversational speech (range: from 3 to 13 speech disfluencies per 100 words), which included the following disfluency types (listed from *most* to *least* frequently occurring): sound/syllable repetitions, inaudible prolongations, audible prolongations, interjections, whole-word repetitions, and revisions. The mean duration of Charle's speech disfluencies was 0.6 seconds (range: from examiner's reaction time to 2.2 seconds).

Examination of Charles's oral-peripheral speech mechanism during (non) speech activities revealed no gross structural/functional abnormalities of his lips, teeth, tongue, mandible, or hard and soft palates. Charles's vocal quality and vocal pitch variability were judged to be within normal limits. Charles's speech sound production was inconsistently (53% occurrence) characterized by lateralized sound productions of the phonemes /s/, /z/, and /ʃ/ in all word positions at both single-word and conversational speech levels. Charles' receptive and expressive English language abilities were judged to be well above what would be expected for a child of Charles's chronological age (8 years; 9 months).

During a one-hour interview, Mrs. Baker provided information regarding Charles's speech and language development, and his medical, social, and familial history. Reportedly, the Baker family speaks both English and non-English languages. According to Mrs. Baker, Charles produced his first word, in English, at the approximate age of 8 months. Mrs. Baker expressed that her primary concern regarding Charles's speech is his production of speech disfluencies, which reportedly began occurring "approximately two years ago."

Based upon the results of the parent interview and present evaluation, it was recommended to Mrs. Baker that indirect speech therapy for Charles's fluency concerns is presently (4/5/88) *indicated*. It was further suggested to Mrs. Baker that she and Charles attend the Gebbie Speech and Hearing Clinic to participate in this Clinic's Parent-Child Fluency Group (beginning Thursday 5/25 at 4:15 p.m.). Detailed suggestions (see Recommendations) were provided to Mrs. Baker for facilitating Charles's speech fluency at home.

III. General History

During a one-hour interview, Mrs. Baker provided information regarding

Charles's speech and language development, as well as his medical, social and familial history. Mrs. Baker reported that her pregnancy with Charles was approximately "four weeks premature," and that his delivery was Caesarian. Mrs. Baker reported that Charles was born with a bump on his head as a result of "his head hitting the cervix" prenatally. Reportedly, the bump disappeared "within a few days" and Charles was "fine."

Mrs. Baker stated that Charles achieved developmental milestones within normal age expectations. Medical history was reportedly unremarkable, and Charles's current health is good. However, Mrs. Baker reported that Charles has suffered six or seven ear infections, with the most recent infection occurring in the winter of 1987. According to Mrs. Baker, in each instance Charles's ear infection was unilateral, no fluid discharge was noted, and the infection "only lasted for a couple of days." Mrs. Baker reported that Charles had an audiological (hearing) evaluation in September, 1987 and no hearing loss was evident.

In terms of Charles's speech and language development, Mrs. Baker reported that Charles babbled at approximately 2 or 3 months of age, and he produced his first word, which was in English, at about 8 months of age. She further reported that when Charles was 12 months old, he began to produce simple two- and three-word phrases.

With regard to the onset of Charles's stuttering, Mrs. Baker reported that she and her husband were the first to notice Charles's speech disfluencies "about two years ago." Mrs. Baker demonstrated the type of speech disfluencies, namely inaudible sound prolongations, that she and her husband initially noticed in Charles's speech.

According to Mrs. Baker, she and her husband observed that Charles's stutterings have become more frequent "in the past six months." She further reported that Charles's third grade teacher at the Anytown Elementary School concurrently noticed that Charles's speech disfluencies had increased. Consequently, Ms. Jane Doe, speech-language pathologist at Anytown Elementary, recently (3/10) contacted the Gebbie Speech Clinic, referring Charles for the present evaluation (4/5).

Mrs. Baker described that in the past six months Charles has continued to inaudibly prolong the first sounds and syllables of his words. She reported that Charles has recently demonstrated physical behaviors which occur during his stuttering. These behaviors include "eye movement" and tension in his facial muscles. Mrs. Baker described Charles's current speech by stating that "he hesitates on the first sound of the word."

According to Mrs. Baker, Charles currently has specific difficulty producing /k/, /h/, and /g/ in the initial position of words. Mrs. Baker stated that when Charles attempts to produce a word beginning with /k/, /h/, or /g/, that word "just won't come out." In addition, she explained that Charles is likely to stutter initially when "he answers the telephone." Mrs. Baker stated that she believes Charles avoids certain situations in school such as reading aloud and "show and tell time" in an attempt to avoid stuttering.

Mrs. Baker further stated that Charles "gets frustrated" when he is not able to produce a word. She reported that he has said to her, "It just doesn't come out; I try." Mrs. Baker stated that she and her husband try to help Charles stop stuttering by telling him to "slow down and say it again." Reportedly, Charles's younger sister, Susie, is not aware of Charles's speech disfluencies, and often "fills in the word" that Charles is stuttering on.

With regard to familial history of stuttering, Mrs. Baker reported that her own first cousin, who currently resides outside the United States, stutters. She reported that, in accord with her family's non-United States culture, it is not considered appropriate for family members to talk about a stuttering problem. Thus, Mrs. Baker was unable to provide any further information regarding her cousin's speech disfluencies. She reported that no other family members stutter; however, she was not certain about some of these relatives since a number of them reside outside the USA.

Mrs. Baker reported that Charles is an "intelligent boy," and that he is in the "top five percent" of his third grade class. Reportedly, Charles "enjoys school" and gets along well with his peers. Mrs. Baker further reported that Charles "used to be quite sensitive" and would cry when he was disciplined. She stated that she feels Charles's participation in "wrestling has helped him to be stronger." Reportedly, Charles enjoys sports and also plays the violin.

Mrs. Baker expressed the hope that the present evaluation (4/5) would provide Charles with ways to "stop stuttering."

IV. Speech and Language

During the present evaluation (4/5) Charles's conversational speech ranged from 3% to 13% disfluent, and averaged 6% disfluent (6 speech disfluencies per 100 words spoken). Disfluency types (listed from *most* to *least* frequently occurring) included:

1. sound/syllable repetitions (e.g.: "b-b-b-ball").....................................49%**
2. inaudible sound prolongations (e.g.: "——get") 26%

**Percentages (%) refer to the percent of the total number of speech disfluencies produced in a sample of 100 words spoken.

3. sound prolongations (e.g.: "ssssister") 13%
4. interjections (e.g.: "um") 7%
5. whole word repetitions (e.g.: "the-the") 4%
6. revisions (e.g.: I went, I came") 1%

The mean duration of Charles's speech disfluencies was 0.6 seconds (range: from the examiner's reaction time to 2.2 seconds).

The consistency effect, that is, the extent to which speech disfluencies occur on the same words during successive repetitions of the same material, could not be computed due to the fact that Charles only produced one speech disfluency during this imitative task.

Administration of the *Stocker Probe Technique,* which associates the level of communicative responsibility with the frequency of speech disfluencies, resulted in Charles producing a *total* of 14 speech disfluencies in response to 50 questions asked in reference to common objects. Charles's typical level of breakdown (the level at which speech disfluencies were *most* frequent) was level V (7 speech disfluencies per 10 questions asked at this level). His typical levels of recovery (the levels at which speech disfluencies were *least* frequent) were levels I and II (0 speech disfluencies per 10 questions asked at each level).

The *Stuttering Severity Instrument* (SSI) (Riley, 1980) was administered to assess the severity of Charles's stuttering behavior. Charles received a frequency task score of *10,* a duration score of *2,* and a physical concomitant score of *1,* for a *Total* score of *13,* which is equivalent to a severity rating of "mild" on the SSI.

The *Stuttering Prediction Instrument* (SPI) (Riley, 1981) was administered to predict the chronicity of Charles's stuttering behaviors from his history of, reaction to, and demonstration of speech disfluencies. Charles received a reaction score of *5,* a part-word repetition score of *3,* a prolongations score of *0,* and a frequency score of *13,* for a *Total* score of *21,* which is equivalent to a chronicity rating at the upper limit of "mild" on the SPI.

The *Peabody Picture Vocabulary Test Revised* (Form L) was administered to assess Charles's receptive vocabulary recognition abilities. Charles achieved a vocabulary recognition age equivalency score of 14 years, 4 months (14;4) which is well above what would be expected for his chronological age (8;9).

The *Expressive One-Word Picture Vocabulary Test* was administered to assess Charles's expressive vocabulary skills. Charles achieved a Language

Age (age equivalency) score of 14 years (14;0), which is well above that which would be expected for his chronological age (8;9).

The *Khan-Lewis Phonological Analysis* was administered to assess the phonological processes (systematic sound changes that affect entire classes of sounds) that occurred in Charles's use of English at the single word level (see Addendum A). Charles produced single words using one nondevelopmental phonological process, Lateralization, in which the fricatives /s/, /z/, and / ʃ /are produced with lateral air emissions in all word positions (e.g., "scissors" [ṣɪɚz̧]).

Examination of Charles's oral-peripheral speech mechanism revealed *no* gross structural abnormalities of the lips, teeth, tongue, mandible, or hard and soft palates. Function of Charles's oral-peripheral speech mechanism was assessed during the following non-speech activities:

> Tongue Mobility was examined. Depression of the tongue tip toward the chin, lateralization of the tongue tip, elevation and extension of the tongue tip, and rapid lateral movements were judged to be adequate for the purposes of speech production.

> Palatal Mobility was examined. Velar elevation was judged to be adequate on sustained and repetitive productions of /a/.

> Vocal Pitch Variability, Quality, and Related Behaviors were examined. Charles was able to raise and lower his vocal pitch from low to high (and vice-versa) both continuously and in discrete steps following the examiner's model. Vocal pitch variability was judged to be within normal limits during each task and in conversational speech. To obtain an approximate indication of the efficiency with which Charles's vocal folds function during phonation, Charles was asked to sustain the phonemes /s/ and /z/ three times in succession, and the ratio between average /s/ and /z/ duration was computed. Charles's average s/z ratio was 0.95 (average duration of sustained /s/ and /z/ was 16.08 and 17.01 respectively), which suggests that the efficiency of his vocal fold approximation is adequate during phonation ("normal" voice s/z ratio is 0.99).

Subtests of *The Quick Neurological Screening Test-Revised* were administered to assess Charles's fine and gross body movement, balance, and coordination. Charles exhibited *adequate* balance and/or rate, range, force, and coordination of movement during the following neuromuscular activities:

1. Fine hand movement during writing
2. Tactile recognizing of figures
3. Tracking the movement of an object with his eyes
4. Vocally and motorically reproducing sound patterns
5. Touching index finger to nose then to the examiner's hand held in midline
6. Rapid sequential touching of thumb to each finger, with both left and right hands

7. Rapid pronation/supination of hands on thighs
8. Identification of simultaneous two-point touch of hands and/or cheeks by examiner with eyes closed
9. Walking forward and backward heel-to-toe in a straight line with eyes closed
10. Standing on one leg with eyes closed
11. Skipping

V. Recommendations

Based on the results of the present evaluation (4/5) and parent interview, the following findings and recommendations were presented to Mrs. Baker:

1. Indirect speech therapy for Charles's fluency concerns is presently *indicated*. Mrs. Baker was informed of this clinic's Parent-Child (P/C) Fluency group, which meets on Thursdays from 4:15 to 5:15 p.m. (for older children). It was recommended to Mrs. Baker that she and/or her husband and Charles attend the P/C Fluency group, initially with the possibility of becoming enrolled in the group for the summer and fall semesters (Summer: May 25 to June 29; Fall: September 7 to December 7). Questions regarding the P/C Fluency group can be directed to Dr. Edward Conture at 443-4485. Depending upon the results of P/C group therapy, Charles may be advised to begin individual therapy late Fall/early Winter.

2. It was recommended to Mrs. Baker that she and her husband make the following communicative changes:

a. *Parents cease and desist corrections.*

Mrs. Baker (and other listeners in Charles's environment) should avoid as much as possible any *direct* corrections, criticisms, or instructions to Charles to change, modify or in any way modify his speaking behavior (e.g.: "slow down. . . , take a deep breath. . . , think about what you are saying. . . , relax. . ."").

b. *Parent model and use a slower speech rate.*

Speak at a slower rate of utterance when talking to or in the presence of Charles. (Mrs. Baker's current average rate of speech is 269 words per minute (wpm) with a range of 129 to 424 wpm. Similarly, Charles's present average rate of speech is 266 wpm, with a range of 123 to 451 wpm. Conversely, an "ideal" speaking rate is 160 to 180 words per minute). It was explained to Mrs. Baker that by using a slower rate of speech, she and her husband can provide a communication model for Charles that will facilitate Charles's development of a slower speaking rate and more fluent speech production.

c. *Parents increase their "pause time."*

Increase (to approximately 1 to 2 seconds) the "pause time" between the termination of Charles's speech and the initiation of the parent's own speech. By increasing their own pause time, the parents can attempt to decrease Charles's apparent communicative time urgency, that is, his feeling of being "rushed" to verbally communicate.

d. *Parents minimize interruptions/talking for child.*

Avoid, as much as possible, verbally interrupting Charles while he is speaking. It was suggested to Mrs. Baker that she and her husband provide a good communicative model in which they do NOT finish utterances or supply words for Charles. By decreasing the amount of interruptions of Charles's speech, the parents can help to further decrease Charles's apparent time urgency.

e. *Parents use shorter, simpler sentences.*

Reduce the length and complexity of the utterances directed at Charles. For example, say, "I see the dog." rather than "The big dog, who is actually a mongrel, is the one I see.") By speaking in shorter, less complex sentences, particularly when Charles is stuttering the parents can provide Charles with a model that is "easier," or more attainable for Charles, given that his speech production mechanism is still developing.

It was suggested to Mrs. Baker that observation of Fred Rogers (of "Mr. Roger's Neighborhood," a PBS children's show) could provide herself and her husband with insights into adult communications with children in which appropriate *speaking rate, pause time, and sentence length and complexity* are used.

3. It was recommended to Mrs. Baker that the parents consider making some "lifestyle" changes with regard to the following issues:

a. *Lifestyle Time Pressures:* Mrs. Baker was encouraged to observe her family's own time pressures and attempt to minimize any rigid, inflexible, or arbitrary schedules for the times when Charles or the rest of family must get up, eat breakfast, lunch, and dinner, take out the trash, do other chores, go to bed, and so forth.

b. *Perfectionism and Sensitivity:* It was explained to Mrs. Baker that Charles's apparent sensitivity towards his own behavior and its correctness makes it difficult for him to forgive, forget, and disregard any speech errors he does produce. It was suggested to Mrs. Baker that she and/or her husband occasionally model some imperfections in their own behavior, that is, when showing Charles how to do something, they can show him that leaving something slightly out-of-line is "okay." Mrs. Baker was encouraged to occasionally model behavior that is non-perfect, rather than continually feeling or assessing her own behavior and that of others as being either "all right or all wrong."

4. Mrs. Baker was given a copy of *If Your Child Stutters: A Guide for Parents* (third edition, Speech Foundation of America, Ainsworth and Fraser, 1988).

Approved by: Submitted by:

_____   _____
LRL, M.Ed.   E.H., B.S.
Graduate Assistant   Graduate Clinician

_____
Edward G. Conture, Ph.D.
Faculty Supervisor

cc: Ronald and Ann Baker
0000 North Road
Anywhere, NY Zipcode

Addendum A

Administration of the *Khan-Lewis Phonological Analysis* revealed the following sound production errors at the single-word level.

Phonological Processes

1. *Lateralization:* (53% occurrence) In all positions of words, /s/, /z/, and /ʃ/ are lateralized, meaning that the air escapes over the sides of the tongue.

    s - z; e.g.: santa claus /sæntə klɔz/—→ [ṣæntə klɔẓ]
    z - z; e.g.: scissors / sizɚz /—→ [ṣizɚẓ]
    ʃ - ʃ; e.g.: shovel / ʃʌvəl /—→ [ʃʌvəl]

The following sound production error was observed for one instance in the following single word item:

    1. Stopping: In the initial position of the following word, the glide, /j/ is replaced by the voiced stop, /d/:
    e.g.: yellow / jɛlo/—→ [dɛlo]

REFERENCES

ADAMS, M., 1974. "A Physiologic and Aerodynamic Interpretation of Fluent and Stuttered Speech," *Journal of Fluency Disorders*, 4: 78–89.

_____, 1977. "A Clinical Strategy for Differentiating the Normally Nonfluent Child and the Incipient Stutterer," *Journal of Fluency Disorders*, 2: 141–148.

_____, 1980. "The Young Stutterer: Diagnosis, Treatment and Assessment of Progress," *Seminars in Speech, Language and Hearing*, 1: 289–299.

_____, 1987. "Voice Onsets and Segment Durations of Normal Speakers and Beginning Stutterers," *Journal of Fluency Disorders*, 12: 1333–40.

ADAMS, M., B. GUITAR, and E. CONTURE, 1979. "A review of biofeedback procedures for school-age stutterers" *Journal of Childhood Communication Disorders*, 3: 8–12.

ADAMS, M., F. FREEMAN, and E. CONTURE, 1984. "Laryngeal Dynamics of Stutterers" in *Nature and Treatment of Stuttering: New Directions*, eds. R. Curlee and W. Perkins (Wien/New York: Springer-Verlag).

ADAMS, M. and P. HAYDEN, 1976. "The Ability of Stutterers and Nonstutterers to Initiate and Terminate Phonation During Production of an Isolated Vowel," *Journal of Speech and Hearing Research,*, 19: 290–296.

ADAMS, M. and P. RAMIG, 1980. "Vocal Characteristics of Normal Speakers and Stutterers During Choral Reading," *Journal of Speech and Hearing Research*, 23: 457–469.

AGNELLO, J., 1975. "Voice Onset and Voice Termination Features of Stuttering," in *Vocal Tract Dynamics and Stuttering*, eds. L.M. Webster and L.C. Furst (New York: Speech and Hearing Institute).

AINSWORTH, S. and J. FRASER (eds.), 1988. *If Your Child Stutters: A Guide for Parents*, 3rd ed. (Memphis, TN.: Speech Foundation of America).

AMMONS, R. and R. AMMONS, 1962. "The Quick Test (QT): Provisional Manual," *Psychological Reports*, 11: 111–161 Monogr. Suppl. I–VII.

Andrews, A. and J. Cutler, 1974. "Stuttering Therapy: The Relationship Between Changes in Sympton Level and Attitudes," *Journal of Speech and Hearing Disorders*, 39: 312–319.

ANDREWS, G. and A. CRAIG, 1988. "Prediction of outcome after treatment for stuttering," *British Journal of Psychiatry*.

ANDREWS, G., A. CRAIG, A. FEYER, A. HODDINOTT, P. HOWIE, and M. NIELSON, 1983. "Stuttering: A Review of Research Findings and Theories circa 1982," *Journal of Speech and Hearing Disorders*, 48: 226–246.

ANDREWS G. and M. HARRIS, 1964. *The Syndrome of Stuttering* (London: Heinemann Medical Books).

ANDREWS, G., P. HOWIE, M. DOZSA, and B. GUITAR, 1982. "Stuttering: Speech Pattern Characteristics Under Fluency-inducing Conditions," *Journal of Speech and Hearing Research*, 25: 208–216.

ANDREWS, G. and R. INGHAM, 1971. "Stuttering: Considerations in the Evaluation of Treatment," *British Journal of Disorders of Communication*, 6: 427–429.

ANDREWS, G. and M. NEILSON, 1981. "Stuttering: A State of the Art Seminar," Paper presented to Annual Conference of Speech Hearing Language Association, Los Angeles, California.

ATAL, B., J. CHANG, M. MATTHEWS, and J. TUKEY, 1978. "Inversions of Articulatory-to-Acoustic Transformation in the Vocal Tract by Computer-sorting Technique," *Journal of Acoustical Society of America*, 63: 1535–1555.

ATKINS, C., 1988. "Perceptions of Speakers with Minimal Eye Contact: Implications for Stutterers," *Journal of Fluency Disorders*, 13: 429–436.

AXLINE, V. M., 1947. *Play Therapy* (Boston: Houghton Mifflin).

BAILEY, A. and W. BAILEY, 1982. "Managing the Environment of the Stutterer," *Journal of Childhood Communication Disorders*, 6: 26–39.

BAKEN, R., 1987. *Clinical Measurement of Speech and Voice* (Boston: Little, Brown and Co).

BARR, H., 1940. "A Quantitative Study of the Specific Phenomena Observed in Stuttering," *Journal of Speech Disorders*, 5: 277–280.

BARSKY, A., 1988. *Worried Sick* (Boston: Little Brown and Co.).

BATES, E., 1976. "Pragmatics and Sociolinguistics in Child Language," in *Normal and Deficient Child Language*, eds. D. Morehead and A. Morehead (Baltimore, MD: University Park Press).

BAUMAN, L. with R. RICHE, 1986. *The Nine Most Troublesome Teenage Problems and How to Solve Them* (Secaucus, NJ: Lyle Stuart Inc.).

BEATTIE, G., 1983. *Talk* (Milton Keynes, England: Open University Press).

BEATTIE, M., 1987. *Codependent No More* (New York: Harper/Hazelton).

BEECH, H. and F. FRANSELLA, 1968. *Research and Experiment in Stuttering* (Oxford England: Pergamon Press).

BEECHER, H. K., 1955. "The Powerful Placebo," *Journal American Medical Association*, 159: 1602–1606.

BEITCHMAN, J. R. NAIR, M. CLEGG and P. PATEL, 1986. "Prevalence of Speech and Language Disorders in 5-Year-Old Kindergarten Children in the Ottawa-Carleton Region," *Journal of Speech and Hearing Disorders*, 51: 98–110.

BENSON, H., 1976. *The Relaxation Response* (New York: Avon Books).

BENSON, H. and M. D. EPSTEIN, 1975. "The Placebo Effect: A Neglected Asset in the Care of Patients," *Journal American Medical Association*, 232: 1225–1227.

BENSON, H. and D. McCALLIE, 1979. "Angina Pectoris and the Placebo Effect," *New England Journal of Medicine*, 300: 1424–1429.

BETTLEHEIM, B., 1985. "Punishment versus Discipline: A Child Can Be Expected to Behave Well Only If His Parents Live by the Values they Teach." *Atlantic*, 256 (November): 51–56.

BINGHAM, J., 1961. *Courage to Change: An Introduction to the Life and Thought of Reinhold Niebuhr* (Boston: Little, Brown and Co.).

BLOOD, G. and R. SEIDER, 1981. "The Concomitant Problems of Stutterers," *Journal of Speech and Hearing Disorders*, 46: 31–33.

BLOOD, G. and I. BLOOD, 1984. "Central Auditory Function in Young Stutterers," *Perceptual and Motor Skills*, 59: 699–705.

BLOODSTEIN, O., 1949. Conditions Under Which Stuttering is Reduced or Absent: A Review of Literature, *Journal of Speech and Hearing Disorders*, 14: 295–302.

BLOODSTEIN, O. Hypothetical Conditions Under Which Stuttering Is Reduced or Absent, *Journal of Speech and Hearing Disorders*, 15: 142–153.

———, 1960a. "The Development of Stuttering: I. Changes in Nine Basic Features," *Journal of Speech and Hearing Disorders*, 25: 219–237.

———, 1960b. "The Development of Stuttering: II. Developmental Phases," *Journal of Speech and Hearing Disorders*, 25: 366–376.

———, 1961. "The Development of Stuttering: III. Theoretical and Clinical Implications," *Journal of Speech and Hearing Disorders*, 26: 67–82.

———, 1975. "Stuttering as Tension and Fragmentation," in *Stuttering: A Second Symposium* ed. J. Eisenson (New York: Harper & Row, Pub.).

———, 1987. *A Handbook on Stuttering.* 4th ed. (Chicago: National Easter Seal Society for Crippled Children and Adults).

———, 1988. "Science in Communication Disorders: Letter to the Editor," *Journal of Speech and Hearing Research*, 53: 3347–48.

BOBERG, E., ed., 1981. *Maintenance of Fluency* (New York: Elsevier).

BOEHMLER, R., 1958. "Listener Responses to Non-Fluencies," *Journal of Speech and Hearing Research*, 1: 132–141.

BOONE, O., 1977. *The Voice and Voice Therapy*, 2nd ed. (Englewood Cliffs, NJ: Prentice-Hall, Inc.).

BORDEN, G., T. BAER, and M. KENNEY, 1985. "Onset of Voicing in Stuttered Fluent Utterance," *Journal of Speech and Hearing Research*, 28: 363–372.

BORDEN, G., D. KIM, and K. SPIEGLER, 1987. "Acoustics of Stop Consonant-Vowel Relationships During Fluent and Stuttered Utterances," *Journal of Fluency Disorders*, 12: 175–184.

BRADY, W. and D. HALL, 1976. "The Prevalence of Stuttering among School-age Children," *Language, Speech, and Hearing Services in Schools*, VII: 75–81.

BRAYTON, E. and E. CONTURE, 1978. "Effects of Noise and Rhythmic Stimulation on the Speech of Stutterers," *Journal of Speech and Hearing Research*, 21: 285–294.

BRAZELTON, T. B., 1974. *Toddlers & Parents* (New York: Dell).

BRAZELTON, T. B., 1983. *Infants & Parents* (New York: Bantam/Delcorte).

BROWN, R., 1973. *A First Langauge/The Early Stages* (Cambridge, MA: Harvard University Press).

BRUTTEN, G., 1982. "The Speech Situation Checklist for Children: A Discriminant Analysis." Paper presented to THE Annual Meeting of American Speech, Language, and Hearing Association, Toronto, Canada.

BRUTTEN, G., K. BAKKER, P. JANSSEN, and S. VAN DER MEULEN, 1984. "Eye Movements of Stuttering and Nonstuttering Children During Silent Reading," *Journal of Speech and Hearing Research*, 27: 562–566.

BRUTTEN, G. and D. SHOEMAKER, 1967. *The Modification of Stuttering* (Englewood Cliffs, NJ: Prentice-Hall, Inc.).

CAMPBELL, J., 1986. *Winston Churchill's Afternoon Nap* (New York: Simon and Schuster).

CANTWELL, D. and L. BAKER, 1985. "Psychiatric and Learning Disorders in Children with Speech and Language Disorders: A Descriptive Analysis," *Advances in Learning and Behavioral Disabilities*, 4: 29–47.

CARKHUFF, R. R., 1973. *The Art of Problem-Solving* (Amherst, MA: Human Resource Development Press).

CARUSO, A., J. ABBS, and V. GRACCO, 1988. "Kinematic Analysis of Multiple Movement During Speech in Stutterers," *Brain*, 111: 439–455.

CARUSO, A. and E. BURTON, 1987. "Temporal Acoustic Measures of Dysarthria Associated with Amgotrophic Lateral Sclerosis," *Journal of Speech and Hearing Research*, 30: 80–87.

CARUSO, A., E. CONTURE, and R. COLTON, 1988. "Selected Temporal Parameters of Coordination Associated with Stuttering in Children," *Journal of Fluency Disorders*, 12: 57–82.

CHILDERS, D. and A. KRISHNAMURTHY, 1984. "A Critical Review of Electroglottography," *CRC Critical Reviews in Biomedical Engineering*, 12: 131–161.

CHILDERS, D., J. NAIK, J. LARAR, A. KRISHNAMURTHY, and G. MOORE, 1983. "Electroglottography, Speech and Ultra-high Speed Cinematography," in *Vocal Fold Psysiology: Biomechanics, Acoustics and Phonatory Control*, eds. I. Titze and R. Scherer (Denver: Denver Center for the Performing Arts), pp. 202–220.

COLTON, R. and E. CONTURE, in press. "Problems and pitfalls of electroglottography." *Journal of Voice.*

CONTURE, E., 1974. "Some Effects of Noise on the Speaking Behavior of Stutterers," *Journal of Speech and Hearing Research*, 17: 714–723.

———, 1982. *Stuttering* (Englewood Cliffs, NJ: Prentice-Hall, Inc.).

———, 1982a. "Stuttering in Young Children," *Journal of Developmental and Behavioral Pediatrics*, 3: 163–169.

———, 1983. "The General Problem of Change," in *Stuttering Therapy: Transfer and Maintenance*, eds. J. Fraser and H. Gregory (Memphis, TN: Speech Foundation of America).

———, 1987a. "Facts and Myths," in *To the Stutterer: A Guide for Teens* (Memphis, TN: Speech Foundation of America), pp. 16–27

———, 1987b. "Studying Young Stutterers' Speech Production: A Procedural Challenge," in *Speech Motor Dynamics in Stuttering*, eds. H. Peters and W. Hulstijn (Wein/New York: Springer Press), pp. 117–139.

———, 1987c. "Fluency and Beyond: Self-help Mutual-aid," *SPEAK EASY Newsletter*, y: 6–7.

———, 1989. "Childhood Stuttering: What Is It and Who Does It?" Unpublished manuscript.

CONTURE, E. and E. BRAYTON, 1975. "The Influence of Noise on Stutterers' Different Disfluency Types," *Journal of Speech and Hearing Research*, 18: 381–384.

CONTURE, E. and A. CARUSO, 1978. "Book Review: The Stocker Probe Technique for Diagnosis and Treatment of Stuttering in Young Children (a test developed by Beatrice Stocker)," *Journal of Fluency Disorders*, 3: 297–298.

CONTURE, E. and A. CARUSO, 1987. "Assessment and Diagnosis of Childhood Disfluency," in *Progress in the Treatment of Fluency Disorders*, eds. L. Rustin, D. Rowley, and H. Purser (London, England: Taylor and Francis), pp. 57–82.

CONTURE, E., R. COLTON, and J. GLEASON, 1988. "Selected Temporal Aspects of Coordination During Fluent Speech of Young Stutterers," *Journal of Speech and Hearing Research*, 31: 640–653.

CONTURE, E. and E. KELLY, 1988a. "Nonverbal Behavior of Young Stutterers and Their Mothers." Paper presented to annual conference of American Speech, Hearing, and Language Association, Boston, MA.

CONTURE, E. and E. KELLY, 1988b. "Remediation of Stuttering in Young Children: A Parent/Child Fluency Group Approach." An unpublished paper presented to the Second Oxford Dysfluency Conference, Oxford, England.

CONTURE, E., G. McCALL, and D. BREWER, 1977. "Laryngeal Behavior during Stuttering," *Journal of Speech and Hearing Research*, 20: 661–668.

CONTURE, E. and D. METZ, 1974. "The Influence of Rhythmic Stimulation on Certain Vocal Characteristics of Stutterers." Paper presented to the fourteenth annual convention of the New York State Speech and Hearing Association, Kiamesha Lake, NY.

CONTURE E., M. ROTHENBERG, and R. MOLITOR, 1986. "Electroglottographic Observations of Young Stutterers' Fluency," *Journal of Speech and Hearing Research*, 29: 384–393.

CONTURE, E. and H. SCHWARTZ, 1984. "Children Who Stutter: Diagnosis and Remediation," *Communication Disorders*, 9: 1–18.

CONTURE, E., H. SCHWARTZ, and D. BREWER, 1985. "A Further Study of Laryngeal Behavior During Stuttering," *Journal of Speech and Hearing Research*, 28: 233–240.

CONTURE E. and E. VAN NAERSSEN, 1977. "Reading Abilities of School-Age Stutterers," *Journal of Fluency Disorders*, 2: 195–300.

COOPER, E., 1978. "Intervention Procedures for the Young Stutterer," in *Controversies About Stuttering Therapy*, ed. H. Gregory (Baltimore, MD: University Park Press).

———, 1979. *Understanding Stuttering: Information for Parents* (Chicago: National Easter Seal Society for Crippled Children and Adults).

———, 1980. "Stiology and Treatment of Stuttering," *Ear, Nose and Throat Journal*, 59: 60–76.

———, 1986. "Treatment of Disfluency: Future Trends," *Journal of Fluency Disorders*, 11: 317–327.

———, 1987. "The Chronic Perserverative Stuttering Syndrome: Incurable Stuttering," *Journal of Fluency Disorders*, 12: 381–382.

COX, N., 1988. "Molecular Genetics: The Key to the Puzzle of Stuttering," *ASHA*, 30, 36–40.

CRAIG, A. and G. ANDREWS, 1985. "The Prediction and Prevention of Relapse in Stuttering," *Behavior Modification*, 9, 427–442.

CRAIG, A., J. FRANKLIN, and G. ANDREWS, 1984. "A Scale to Measure Loss of Controlled Behavior," *British Journal of Medical Psychology*, 57: 173–180.

CROSS, D. and H. LUPER, 1979. "Voice Reaction Time of Stuttering and Nonstuttering Children and Adults," *Journal of Fluency Disorders,* 4: 59–77.

CULLINAN, W., 1988. "Consistency Measures Revisited," *Journal of Fluency Disorders,* 13: 1–10.

DALTON, P. and W.J. HARDCASTLE, 1977. *Disorders of Fluency* (New York: Elsevier).

DALY, D., 1980. "Differentiation of Stuttering Subgroups with Van Riper's Developmental Tracks: A Preliminary Study," *Journal of the National Student Speech and Hearing Association,* 9: 89–101.

———, 1988. "A Practioner's View of Stuttering," *ASHA,* 30: 34–35.

DARLEY, F., A. ARONSON, and J. BROWN, 1975. *Motor Speech Disorders* (Philadelphia, PA: Saunders).

DARLEY, F. and D. SPRIESTERSBACH, 1978. *Diagnostic Methods in Speech Pathology,* 2nd ed. (New York: Harper & Row, Pub.).

DAVIS, D. M., 1939. "The Relation of Repetitions in the Speech of Young Children to Measures of Langauge Maturity and Situational Factors: Part I," *Journal of Speech and Hearing Disorders,* 4: 303–318.

———, 1940. "The Relation of Repetitions in the Speech of Young Children to Measures of Langauge Maturity and Situational Factors: Part II & III," *Journal of Speech and Hearing Disorders,* 5: 235–246.

DeJONG, R., 1979. *The Neurologic Examination,* 4th ed. (Philadelphia, PA: Harper & Row, Pub.).

DELL, C.W., 1980. *Treating the School Age Stutterer: A Guide for Clinicians* (Memphis, TN: Speech Foundation of America).

DOSSEY, L., 1982. *Space, Time and Medicine* (Boulder, CO: Shambhala Publications).

DODSON, F., 1970. *How to Parent* (New York: Signet).

DOUGLASS, E. and R. QUARRINGTON, 1952. "The Differentiation of Interiorized and Exteriorized Secondary Stuttering," *Journal of Speech and Hearing Disorders,* 17: 377–385.

DUNCAN, S., 1972. "Some Signals and Rules for Taking Speaking Turns in Conversations," *Journal of Personality and Social Psychology,* 23: 283–292.

DUNN, L. and L. DUNN, 1981. *The Peabody Picture Vocabulary Test-Revised* (Circle Pines, MN: American Guidance Service).

ECKEL, F. and D. BOONE, 1981. "The s/z Ratio as an Indication of Laryngeal Pathology," *Journal of Speech and Hearing Disorders,* 46: 147–149.

EDWARDS, M. and L. SHRIBERG, 1983. *Phonology: Application in Communication Disorders* (San Diego,. CA: College-Hill Press).

EGOLF, D. and S. CHESTER, 1973. "Nonverbal Communication and the Disorders of Speech and Language," *ASHA,* 15: 511–518.

EKMAN, P., 1982. "Methods for Measuring Facial Action," in *Handbook of Methods in Nonverbal Behaviors,* eds. K. Scherer and P. Ekman (Cambridge, England: Cambridge University Press).

ENGER, N., S. HOOD, and B. SHULMAN, 1988. "Language and Fluency Variables in the Conversational Speech of Linguistically Advanced Preschool and School-aged Children," *Journal of Fluency Disorders,* 13: 163–172.

ERICKSON, R., 1969. "Assessing Communication Attitudes Among Stutterers," *Journal of Speech and Hearing Research,* 12: 711–724.

FAIRCLOTH, S. and M. FAIRCLOTH, 1973. *Phonetic Science: A Program of Instruction* (Englewood Cliffs, NJ: Prentice-Hall, Inc.).

FEINSTEIN, A., 1970. "The Pre-therapeutic Classification of Comorbidity in Chronic Disease," *Journal of Chronic Disease,* 23: 455–468.

FINCHER, J., 1984. "New Machines May Soon Replace the Doctor's Black Bag," *Smithsonian,* 64–71.

FINKENSTADT, S., 1988. Personal communication regarding treatment of stuttering in teenagers.

FLETCHER, S., 1972. "Time-by-count Measurement of Diadochokinetic Syllable Rate," *Journal of Speech and Hearing Research,* 15: 763–770.

FLYNN, P., 1978. "Effective Clinical Interviewing," *Language, Speech, and Hearing Services in Schools,* 9: 256–271.

FOLKINS, J. and D. KUEHN, 1982. "Speech Production," in *Speech, Language and Hearing,* vol. I, eds. N. Lass, L. McReynolds, J. Northern, and D. Yoder (Philadelphia, PA: Saunders).

FOURCIN, A., 1974. "Laryngograph Examination of the Vocal Fold Vibration," in *Ventilatory and Phonatory Control Mechanisms,* ed. B. Wyke (Oxford, England: Oxford University Press), pp. 315–333.

———, 1979. "Laryngograph Assessment of Phonatory Function," Proceedings of Conference on

Assessment of Vocal Fold Pathology, National Institute of Health, Bethesda, MD. To be published.

FRANKEN, M. C., 1987. "Perceptual and acoustic evaluation of stuttering," in *Speech Motor Dynamics in Stuttering*, ed. H. F. M. Peters and W. Hulstijn (Wien/New York: Springer-Verlag), pp. 285–294.

FRANKEN, M. C., L. BOVES, H. PETERS and R. WEBSTER, 1988. "Perceptual and acoustic evaluation of fluency shaping stuttering therapy." Paper presented at Annual Conference of American Speech-Language-Hearing Association, Boston, MA.

FRASER, J. and W. PERKINS, 1987. *Do You Stutter: A Guide for Teens* (Memphis, TN: Speech Foundation of America).

FREEMAN, F., 1979. "Phonation in Stuttering: A Review of Current Research," *Journal of Fluency Disorders*, 4: 79–89.

FREEMAN, F. and T. USHIJIMA, 1978. "Laryngeal Muscle Activity during Stuttering," *Journal of Speech and Hearing Research*, 21: 538–562.

FRIEDMAN, S., 1989 "A review of Speech Viewer," *ASHA*, 31: 45–46.

FRUNKEN, M., 1987. "Perceptual and Acoustic Evaluation of Stuttering Therapy," in *Speech Motor Dynamics in Stuttering*, eds. H.F.M. Peters and W. Hulstijn (New York, NY: Springer-Verlag).

FURSTER, J., 1985. "Temporal Organization of Behavior," *Human Neurobiology*, 4: 57–60.

GERMAN, D., 1986. *Test of Word Finding* (Allen, TX: DLM Teaching Resources).

GINOTT, H., 1969. *Between Parent and Teenager* (New York: Avon).

GOLDMAN, R. and M. FRISTOE, 1972. *Goldman-Fristoe Test of Articulation (GFTA)* (Circle Pines, MI: American Guidance Service, Inc.).

GOYER, R., S. READING, and J. RICKEY, 1968. *Interviewing Principles and Techniques* (Dubuque, IA: William C. Brown).

GREGORY, H., 1973. *Stuttering: Differential Evaluation and Therapy*. Indianapolis, IN: Bobbs-Merrill.

_____, ed., 1978. *Controversies about Stuttering Therapy* (Baltimore, MD: University Park Press).

GREGORY, H. and D. HILL, 1980. "Stuttering Therapy for Children" in *Stuttering Disorders*, ed. W. Perkins (New York: Thieme-Stratton).

GUITAR, B., 1975. "Reduction of Stuttering Frequency Using Analog Electro-Myographic Feedback," *Journal of Speech and Hearing Research*, 18: 672–685.

_____, 1988. "Is it Stuttering or Just Normal Language?," *Contemporary Pediatrics*, 5: 1–10.

GUITAR, B., M. ADAMS, and E. CONTURE, 1979. "Clinical Feedback," *Journal of Childhood Communication Disorders*, 3: 3–12.

GUITAR, B. and E. CONTURE, 1988. "If You Think Your Child is Stuttering. . .," (a pamphlet), (Memphis, TN: Speech Foundation of America).

GUITAR, B., C. GUITAR, P. NEILSON, T. O'DWYER and G. ANDREWS, 1988. "Onset Sequencing of Selected Lip Muscles in Stutterers and Nonstutterers," *Journal of Speech and Hearing Research*, 31: 28–35.

GUITAR, B., and T. PETERS, 1980. *Stuttering: An Integration of Contemporary Therapies* (Memphis, TN.: Speech Foundation of America).

GUYTON, A., 1971. *Textbook of Medical Physiology*, 4th ed. (Philadelphia, PA: Saunders).

HALL, E., 1984. *The Dance of Life* (Garden City, NY: Anchor Press).

HALL, H., 1966. Help Wanted?: *A Guidebook for Parents and Therapists Dealing with Young Nonfluent Children* (Evanston, IL: Junior League of Evanston, Inc.).

HAM, R., 1986. *Techniques of Stuttering Therapy* Englewood Cliffs, NJ: Prentice-Hall, Inc.).

HANSON, B., K. GRONHORD, and P. RICE, 1981. "A Shortened Version of the Southern Illinois University Speech Situation Checklist for the Identification of Speech Related Anxiety," *Journal of Fluency Disorders*, 6: 351–360.

HARDY, J., 1970. "Development of Neuromuscular Systems Underlying Speech Production," in *Speech and the Dentofacial Complex: The State of the Art*, (Rockville, MD: *ASHA Reports*), Number 5: 49–68.

_____, 1978. "Basic Concepts—Neural Processes of Speech and Language," in *Processes and Disorders of Human Communication*, ed. J. Curtis (New York: Harper & Row, Pub.).

HARRIS, T., 1967. *I'm OK—You're OK* (New York: Harper & Row, Pub.).

HAYHOW, R., 1983. "The Assessment of Stuttering and the Evaluation of Treatment," in *Approaches to the Treatment of Stuttering*, ed. P. Dalton (London: Croom Helm).

HEALEY, C., 1982. "Speaking Fundamental Frequency Characteristics of Stutterers and Non-stutterers," *Journal of Communication Disorders*, 15: 21–29.

HEALEY, E. C., F. GROSSMAN, and G. ELLIS November, 1988. "Behavioral Characteristics of Adult Stutterers: Implications for Determining Treatment Strategies." Poster presentation to annual conference of American Speech, Hearing, and Language Association.

HEALEY, E. C. and P. RAMIG, 1986. "Acoustic Measures of Stutterers' and Nonstutterers; Fluency in Two Speech Contexts," *Journal of Speech and Hearing Research*, 29: 325–331.

HILL, W. F., 1985. *Learning: A survey of Psychological Interpretations*, 4th ed. (New York: Harper & Row, Pub.).

HILLMAN, R. and H. GILBERT, 1977. "Voice Onset Time for Voiceless Stop Consonants in the Fluent Reading of Stutterers and Nonstutterers," *Journal of Acoustical Society of America*, 61: 610–611.

HOWELL, P., A. HAMILTON, and A. KRYIACOUPOULOS, 1984. "Automatic Detection of Repetitions and Prolongation in Stuttered Speech," *Journal of Acoustical Society of America*, 79: 1571–1579.

HOWELL, P. and L. VAUSE, 1986. "Acoustic Analysis and Perception of Vowels in Stuttered Speech," *Journal of Acoustical Society of America*, 79: 1571–1579.

HOWELL, P. M. WILLIAMS, and L. VAUSE, 1987. "Acoustic Analysis of Repetitions in Stutterers' Speech," in *Speech Motor Dynamics in Stuttering*, eds. H.F.M. Peters and W. Hulstijn (New York: Springer-Verlag).

HOWIE, P., 1981. "Concordance for Stuttering in Monozygotic and Dizygotic Twin Pairs," *Journal of Speech and Hearing Research*, 24: 317–321.

HRESKO, W., D. REID, and D. HAMILL, 1982. *Test of Early Language Development* (Austin, TX: PRO-ED).

HUFFMAN, E. and W. PERKINS, 1974. "Dysfluency Characteristics Identified by Listeners as 'Stuttering' and 'Stutterer,'" *Journal of Communicative Diseases*, 7: 89–96.

HULL, F., P. MIELKE, R. TIMMONS, and J. WILLEFORD, 1971. "The National Speech and Hearing Survey: Preliminary Results," *ASHA*, 13: 501–509.

HUTCHINSON, J., 1974. "Aerodynamic Patterns of Stuttered Speech," in *Vocal Tract Dynamics and Dysfluency*, eds. M. Webster and L. Furst (New York: Speech and Hearing Institute of New York), pp. 71–123.

ILG, F. and L. AMES, 1960. *Child Behavior* (New York: Dell Pub. Co., Inc.).

INGHAM, R., 1984. *Stuttering and Behavior Therapy: Current Status and Experimental Foundations* (San Diego, CA: College-Hill Press).

_____, 1985. "Assessment of Stuttering in Children," in *Stuttering Therapy: Prevention and Early Intervention*, ed. J. Gruss (Memphis, TN.: Speech Foundation of America).

_____, March, 1989. "Critical Issues in Treatment Efficacy Research: Theoretical, Methodological, Ethical." Paper presented to Conference on Treatment Efficacy, San Antonio, TX.

JAFFE, J. and S. FELDSTEIN, 1970. *Rhymes of Dialogue* (New York: Academic Press).

JANSSEN, P., F. KRAAIMAAT, and S. VAN DER MEULEN, 1983. "Reading Ability and Disfluency in Stuttering and Nonstuttering Elementary School Children," *Journal of Fluency Disorders*, 8: 39–55.

JOHNSON, W., 1946. *People in Quandries* (New York: Harper & Row, Pub.).

_____, 1949. "An Open Letter to the Mother of a Stuttering Child," *Journal of Speech and Hearing Disorders*, 14: 3–8.

_____, 1961. *Stuttering and What You Can Do About It* (Minneapolis, MN: University of Minnesota Press).

JOHNSON, W., F. DARLEY, and D. SPRIESTERSBACH, 1963. *Diagnostic Methods in Speech Pathology* (New York: Harper & Row, Pub.).

JOHNSON, W. et al., 1959. *The Onset of Stuttering* (Minneapolis, MN: University of Minnesota Press).

JOHNSON, W. et al., 1967. *Speech-Handicapped School Children*, 3rd ed. (New York: Harper & Row, Pub.).

JOHNSON, W. and L. ROSEN, 1937. "Studies in the Psychology of Stuttering: VII. Effect of Certain Changes in Speech Pattern upon Frequency of Stuttering," *Journal of Speech and Hearing Disorders*, 2: 105–109.

JOHNSTON, J., and T. SCHERY, 1976. "The Use of Grammatical Morphemes by Children with

Communication Disorders," in *Normal and Deficient Child Language,* eds. E. Morehead and A. Morehead (Baltimore, MD: University Park Press).

KAIL, R. and L. LEONARD, 1986. "Word-finding Abilities in Language Impaired Children," *ASHA Monograph* 25.

KELLY, E. and E. CONTURE, 1988. "Acoustic and Perceptual Correlates of Adult Stutterers' Typical and Imitated Stutterings," *Journal of Fluency Disorders,* 13: 233–252.

KENNEDY, M., 1988. "Time & Time," *Sesame Street Parents Guide,* 14–17.

KENT, R., 1983. "Facts about Stuttering: Neuropsychologic Perspectives," *Journal of Speech and Hearing Disorders,* 48: 249–255.

KIDD, K., 1983. "Recent Progress on the Genetics of Stuttering," in *Genetic Aspects of Speech and Language,* eds. C. Ludlow and J. Cooper (New York: Academic Press).

KIDD, K., et al., 1977. "A Genetic Perspective on Stuttering," *Journal of Speech and Hearing Research,* 4: 259–270.

KIRITANI, S., 1977. "Articulatory Studies by the X-Ray Microbeam System," in *Dynamic Aspects of Speech,* eds. M. Sawashima and E. Cooper (Tokyo: University of Tokyo Press).

KLATT, D., 1975. "Voice Onset Time, Frication and Aspiration in Word-Initial Consonant Cluster," *Journal of Speech and Hearing Research,* 18: 686–706.

KLICH, R. and G. MAY, 1982. "Spectrographic Study of Vowels in Stutterers' Fluent Speech," *Journal of Speech and Hearing Disorders,* 25: 364–370.

KOSINSKI, J., 1966. *The Painted Bird* (New York: Pocket Cardinal/Houghton Mifflin Company).

KRAUSE, R., 1982. "A Social Psychological Aproach to the Study of Stuttering," in *Advances in the Social Psychology of Language,* eds. C. Fraser and K. Scherer (Cambridge, England: Cambridge University Press).

KRUPSKI, A., 1986. "Attention Problems in Youngsters with Learning Handicaps," in *Psychological and Educational Perspectives on Learning Disabilities,* eds. J.K. Torgesen and B.Y.L. Wond (New York: Academic Press), pp. 161–192.

LANGE, A. and P. JAKUBOWSKI, 1976. *Responsible Assertive Behavior (Champaign, IL: Research Press).*

LANGLOIS, A. and S. LONG, 1988. "A Model for Teaching Parents to Facilitate Fluent Speech," *Journal of Fluency Disorders,* 13: 163–172.

LEFRANCOIS, G., 1972. *Psychological Theories and Human Learning: Kongor's Report* (Monterey, CA: Brooks/Cole).

LE SHAN, E. 1963. *How to Survive Parenthood* (New York: Warner Paperback Library).

LOUKO, L., M. EDWARDS and E. CONTURE. November, 1988. "Phonological Characteristics of Young Stutterers and Their Normally Fluent Peers." Paper presented at Annual Conference of American Speech-Language-Hearing Association, Boston, MA.

LOVE, R. and W. WEBB, 1986. *Neurology for the Speech-Language Pathologist* (Stoneham, MA: Butterworth).

LUPER, H., 1982. "Intervention with the Young Stutterer," *Journal of Childhood Communication Disorders,* 6: 3–4.

LUPER, H. and R. MULDER, 1964. *Stuttering Therapy for Children* (Englewood Cliffs, NJ: Prentice-Hall, Inc.).

MALLARD, A. and W. WEBB, 1980. "The Effects of Auditory and Visual 'Distractors' on the Frequency of Stuttering," *Journal of Communication Disorders,* 13: 207–212.

MALLARD, A. and J. WESTBROOK, 1985. "Vowel Duration in Stutterers Participating in Precision Fluency Shaping," *Journal of Fluency Disorders,* 10: 221–228.

MANN, V., 1987. A software review of DSPS Realtime Signal Lab, *ASHA,* 29: 64–65.

MASTERS, W. and V. JOHNSON, 1970. *Human Sexual Inadequacy* (New York: Little, Brown and Co.).

MASTRUD, B., 1988. "The Oxfordshire Fluency Programme for Adolescent Stutterers." Paper presented to Second Oxford Dysfluency Conference, Oxford, England.

McDONALD, E., 1964. *Articulation Testing and Treatment: A Sensory-Motor Approach* (Pittsburgh, PA: Stanwix House, Inc.).

McMILLAN, M. and R. PINDZOLA, 1986. "Temporal disruptions in the 'accurate' Speech of Articulator and Defective Speakers and Stutterers," *Journal of Motor Behavior,* 18: 279–286.

McNIGHT, R. and W. CULLINAN, 1987. "Subgroups of Stuttering Children: Speech and Voice Reaction Times, Segmental Durations, and Naming Latencies," *Journal of Fluency Disorders,* 12: 217–233.

MERITS-PATTERSON, R. and C. REED, 1981. "Disfluencies in the Speech of Language Delayed Children," *Journal of Speech and Hearing Research*, 24: 55–58.

METZ, D., E. CONTURE, and A. CARUSO, 1979. "Voice Onset Time, Frication and Aspiration during Stutterers' Fluent Speech," *Journal of Speech and Hearing Research*, 22: 649–656.

METZ, D., J. ONUFRAK, and R.S. OGBURN, 1979. "An Acoustical Analysis of Stutterer's Speech Prior to and the Termination of Therapy," *Journal of Fluency Disorders*, 4: 249–254.

METZ, D., V. SAMAR and P. SACCO, 1983. "Acoustic Analysis of Stutterers' Fluent Speech Before and After Therapy," *Journal of Speech and Hearing Research*, 26: 531–536.

MEYERS, S. and F. FREEMAN, 1985a. "Are Mothers of Stutterers Different? An Investigation of Social-communicative Interaction," *Journal of Fluency Disorders*, 10: 193–210.

MEYERS, S. and F. FREEMAN, 1985b. Interruptions as a Variable in Stuttering and Disfluency," *Journal of Speech and Hearing Research*, 28: 428–435.

MEYERS, S. and F. FREEMAN, 1985c. "Mother and Child Speech Rates as a Variable in Stuttering and Disfluency," *Journal of Speech and Hearing Research*, 28: 436–443.

MILLER, N., 1944. "Experimental Studies of Conflict," in *Personality and the Behavior Disorders*, ed. J. Hunt (New York: Ronald Press).

MOORE, W. H., JR., 1984. "Central Nervous System Characteristics of Stutterers," in *Nature and Treatment of Stuttering: New Directions*, eds. R. Curlee & W. Perkins (San Diego, CA: College-Hill Press).

_____, 1986. "Hemispheric Alpha Asymmetries of Stutterers and Non-stutterers for the Recall and Recognition of Words and Connected Reading Passages: Some Relations to Severity of Stuttering," *Journal of Fluency Disorders*, 11: 71–89.

MOORE, W. and E. BOBERG, 1987. "Hemispheric Processing and Stuttering," in *Progress in the Treatment of Fluency Disorders*, eds. L. Rusting, H. Purser and D. Rowley (London: Taylor & Francis).

MORLEY, M., 1957. *The Development and Disorders of Speech in Childhood* (Edinburgh, Scotland: Livingstone).

MURPHY, A. and R. FITZSIMONS, 1960. *Stuttering and Personality Dynamics* (New York: Ronald Press).

MUTTI, M., H. STERLING, and N. SPAULDING, 1978. *Quick Neurological Screening Test, rev ed* (Novato, CA: Academic Therapy Publications).

NEELLEY, J. and R. TIMMONS, 1967. "Adaptation and Consistency in the Disfluent Speech Behavior of Young Stutterers and Stutterers," *Journal of Speech and Hearing Research*, 10: 250–256.

NEILL, A., 1960. *Summerhill: A Radical Approach to Child Rearing* (New York: Hart Associates).

NEILSON, M., 1980. "Stuttering and the Control of Speech: A System Analysis Approach," Ph.D. dissertation, University of New South Wales, Australia.

NEILSON, M. and P. NEILSON, 1987. "Speech Motor Control and Stuttering: A Computational Model of Adaptive Sensory-motor Processing," *Speech Communications* 6: 325–333.

NETSELL, R., 1973. "Speech Physiology," in *Normal Aspects of Speech, Hearing and Language*, eds. R. Minifie, T. Hixon, and F. Williams (Englewood Cliffs, NJ: Prentice-Hall, Inc.).

NIEBUHR, R., 1934. "Prayer," in *Bartlett's Familiar Quotations*, 14th ed., ed. E.M. Beck (Boston: Little, Brown and Co.).

ORNSTEIN, R., 1969. *On the Experience of Time* (Middlesex, England: Penguin Books).

ORTON, S., 1928. "A Physiological Theory of Reading Disability and Stuttering in Children," *New England Journal of Medicine, 199: 1045–1052.*

PADEN, E., M. NOVAK, and J. BEITER, 1987. "Predictors of Phonologic Inadequacy in Young Children Prone to Ofitis Media," *Journal of Speech and Hearing Disorders*, 52: 232–242.

PAVLOV, I., 1927. *Conditional Reflex* (Oxford, England: Oxford University Press).

PERKINS, W. H., 1970. "Physiological Studies," in *Stuttering: Research Therapy*, ed. J.G. Sheehan (New York: Harper & Row, Pub.).

_____, 1978. "From Psychoanalysis to Discoordination," in *Controversies About Stuttering Therapy*, ed. H.H. Gregory (Baltimore, MD: University Park Press).

_____, 1980. "Disorders of Speech Flow," in *Introduction to Communication Disorders*, eds. T. Hixon, L. Shriberg, and J. Saxman (Englewood Cliffs, NJ: Prentice-Hall, Inc.).

PERKINS, W., J. RUDAS, L. JOHNSON, and J. BELL, 1976. "Stuttering: Discoordination of Phonation with Articulation and Respiration," *Journal of Speech and Hearing Research*, 19: 509–522.

PETERS, J., J. ROMINE, and R. DYKMAN, 1975. "A Special Neurological Examination of Children with Learning Disabilites," *Developmental Medicine and Child Neurology*, 17: 63–78.

PINDZOLA, R., 1986a. "A Description of Some Selected Stuttering Instruments," *Journal of Childhood Communciation Disorders*, 9: 183–200.

PINDZOLA, R., 1986. "Acoustic Evidence of Aberrant Velocities in Stutterers' Fluent Speech," *Perceptual and Motor Skills*, 62: 399–405.

PINDZOLA, R., M. JENKINS, and K. LOKKEN, 1989. "Speaking Rates of Young Children," *Language, Speech and Hearing Services in Schools*, 20: 133–138.

POOL, K., F. FREEMAN and T. FINITZO, 1987. "Brain Electrical Activity Mapping: Applications to Vocal Motor Control Disorders," in *Speech Motor Dynamics in Stuttering*, eds. H. Peters and W. Hulstijn (New York: Springer-Verlag).

PREUS, A., 1981. *Attempts at Identifying Subgroups of Stutterers* (Oslo, Norway: University of Norway Press).

PRINS, D., 1974. "Motivation/Part One," in *Therapy for Stutterers*, ed. C. Starkweather (Memphis, TN: Speech Foundation of America).

PRINS, D., and C. HUBBARD, 1988. "Response Contingent Stimuli and Stuttering: Issues and Implications," *Journal of Speech and Hearing Research*, 31: 696–709.

PRINS, D., and F. LOHR, 1972. "Behavioral Dimensions of Stuttered Speech," *Journal of Speech and Hearing Research*, 15: 61–71.

PROSEK, R., A. MONTGOMERY, and B. WALDEN, 1988. "Constancy of Relative Timing for Stutterers and Nonstutterers," *Journal of Speech and Hearing Research*, 31: 654–658.

PROSEK, R. and C. RUNYAN, 1982. "Temporal Characteristics Related to the Discrimination of Stutterers and Nonstutterers; Speech Samples," *Journal of Speech and Hearing Research*, 25: 29–33.

PURSER, H., 1987. "The Psychology of Treatment Evaluation," in *Progress in the Treatment of Fluency Disorders*, eds. L. Rustin, H. Purser, and H. Rowley (London: Taylor and Francis).

REES, N., 1980. "Learning to Talk and Understand," in *Introduction to Communication Disorders*, eds. T. Hixon, L. Shriberg, and J. Saxman (Englewood Cliffs, NJ: Prentice-Hall, Inc.).

REYNOLDS, G., 1968. *A Primer of Operant Conditioning* (Glenview, IL: Scott, Foresman).

RIEBER, R. W., ed., 1977. *The Problem of Stuttering: Theory and Therapy* (New York: Elsevier).

RILEY. G., 1980. *Stuttering Severity Instrument for Young Children.*, rev. ed. (Tigard, OR: C.C. Publications).

RILEY G., 1981. *Stuttering Prediction Instrument for Young Children* (Tigard, OR: C.C. Publications).

RILEY, G. and J. RILEY, 1979. "A Component Model for Diagnosing and Treating Children Who Stutter," *Journal of Fluency Disorders*, 4: 279–293.

RILEY, G. and J. RILEY, 1982. Evaluating Stuttering Problems in Children, *Journal of Childhood Communication Disorders*, 6: 15–25.

RILEY, G. and J. RILEY, 1986. *Oral Motor Assessment and Treatment* (Tigard, OR: C.C. Publications).

RILEY, G. and J. RILEY, 1988. "Looking at a Vulnerable System," *ASHA*, 30: 32–34.

ROBB, M., J. LYBOLT, and H. PRICE, 1985. "Acoustic Measures of Stutterers' Speech Following an Intensive Therapy Program," *Journal of Fluency Disorders*, 10: 269–279.

ROBINSON, F., 1964. *Introduction to Stuttering* (Englewood Cliffs, NJ: Prentice-Hall, Inc.).

ROSENBEK, J. et al, 1978. "*Stuttering Following Brain Damage*," *Brain and Language*, 6: 82–96.

ROTHENBERG, M., 1981. "Some Relations between Glottal Airflow and Vocal Fold Contact Area." *Proceedings of the Conference on the Assessment of Vocal Pathology* (ASHA, Reports #11), eds. C.L. Ludlow and M.O. Hart (Rockville, MD: American Speech Language Hearing Association).

ROTHENBERG, M. and J. MAHSHIE, 1980. "Monitoring Vocal Fold Abduction through Vocal Fold Contact Area," *Journal of Speech and Hearing Research*, 31: 338–351.

RUNYAN, C., and M. ADAMS, 1978. "Perceptual Study of 'Successfully Therapeuterized' Stutterers," *Journal of Fluency Disorders*, 3: 25–29.

RUSTIN, L., 1987. "The Treatment of Childhood Dysfluency through Active Parental Involvement," in *Progress in the Treatment of Fluency Disorders*, eds. L. Rustin, H. Purser and H. Rowley (London: Taylor and Francis).

RUSTIN, L. and F. COOK, 1983. "Intervention Procedures for the Disfluent Child," in *Approaches to the Treatment of Stuttering*, ed. P. Dalton (London: Croom Helm Ltd.).

RYAN, B., 1980. *Programmed Therapy for Stuttering Children and Adults.*, 3rd ed. (Springfield, IL: Charles C. Thomas).

RYAN, B., 1978. "Stuttering Therapy in a Framework of Operant Conditioning and Programmed Learning," in *Controversies About Stuttering Therapy*, ed. H. Gregory (Baltimore, MD: University Park Press).

SACCO, P. and D. METZ, 1987. "Changes in Stutterers' Fundamental Frequency Contours Following Therapy," *Journal of Fluency Disorders*, 12: 1–8.

SACCO, P. and D. METZ, in press. "Comparison of Period by Period Fundamental Frequency of Stutterers and Non-stutterers over Repeated Utterances," *Journal of Speech and Hearing Research*.

ST. LOUIS, K., and A. HINZMAN, 1988. "A Descriptive Study of Speech, Language and Hearing Characteristics of School-aged Stutterers," *Journal of Fluency Disorders*, 13: 357–373.

SAMAR, V., D. METZ, and P. SACCO, 1986. "Changes in Aerodynamic Characteristics of Stutterer' Fluent Speech Associated with Therapy," *Journal of Speech and Hearing Research*, 29: 106–113.

SCHIAVETTI, N., 1975. "Judgments of Stuttering Severity as a Function of Type and Focus of Disfluency," *Folia Phoniatrica*, 27: 26–37.

SCHIAVETTI, N., P. SACCO, D. METZ, and R. SITLER, 1983. "Direct Magnitude Estimation and Interval Scaling of Stuttering Severity," *Journal of Speech and Hearing Research*, 12, 568–573.

SCHINDLER, M., 1955. "A Study of Educational Adjustments of Stuttering and Nonstuttering Children," in *Stuttering in Children and Adults*, eds. W. Johnson and R. Leutenegger (Minneapolis, MN: University of Minnesota Press).

SCHUM, R., 1986. *Counseling in Speech and Hearing Practice* (Rockville, MD: National Student Speech Language Hearing Association) Clin. Series No. 9.

SCHWARTZ, H. and E. CONTURE, 1988. "Subgrouping Young Stutterers: Preliminary Behavioral Perspectives," *Journal of Speech and Hearing Research*, 31: 62–71.

SCHWARTZ, H., 1987. "Subgrouping Young Stutterers: A Physiological Perspective," in *Speech Motor Dynamics in Stuttering*, eds. H. Peters and W. Hulstijn (Wien/New York: Springer-Verlag).

SCHWARTZ, M.F., 1976. *Stuttering Solved* (Philadelphia, PA: Lippincott).

SHAEFER, C.E., 1978. "Raising Children by Old-Fashioned Parent Sense," *Children Today*, November-December. A publication of the Children's Bureau, ACUF, DHEW.

SHAMES, G., and D. EGOLF, 1976. *Operant Conditioning and the Management of Stuttering* (Englewood Cliffs, NJ: Prentice-Hall, Inc.).

SHAMES, G., and C. FLORANCE, 1980. *Stutter-Free Speech: A Goal for Therapy* (Columbus, OH: Chas. E. Merrill).

SHAMES, G. and C. SHERRICK, 1963. "A Discussion of Nonfluency and Stuttering as Operant Behavior," *Journal Speech and Hearing Disorders*, 28: 3–18.

SHAPIRO, A., 1964. "Factors Contributing to the Placebo Effect: Their Implications for Psychotherapy," *American Journal of Psychotherapy*, Suppl. 1 18: 73–88.

SHAPIRO, A., 1980. "An Electromyographic Analysis of the Fluent and Dysfluent Utterances of Several Types of Stutterers," *Journal of Fluency Disorders*, 5: 203–231.

SHAYWITZ, S. and B. SHAYWITZ, 1985. "Attention Deficit Disorders," in *Psychiatry*, Vol. 2, eds. J.O. Cavenar et al., pp. 1–15.

SHAYWITZ, B., S. SHAYWITZ, and T. BYRNE, 1983. "Quantitative Analysis of Computed Tomographic Brain Scans in Children with Attention Deficit Disorder," *Neurology*, 33: 1500–1503.

SHEEHAN, J., 1958. "Conflict Theory of Stuttering," in *Stuttering: A Symposium*, ed. J. Eisenson (New York: Harper & Row, Pub.).

———, 1970a. "Reflections on the Behavioral Modification of Stuttering," in *Conditioning in Stuttering Therapy*, ed. C. Starkweather (Memphis, TN.: Speech Foundation of America).

———, 1970b. "Personality Approaches," in *Stuttering: Research and Therapy*, ed. J.G. Sheehan (New York: Harper & Row, Pub.).

———, 1975. "Conflict Theory and Avoidance-Reduction Therapy," in *Stuttering: A Second Symposium*, ed. J. Eisenson (New York: Harper & Row, Pub.).

———, 1978. "Current Issues on Stuttering and Recovery," in *Controversies About Stuttering Therapy*, ed. H. Gregory (Baltimore, MD: University Park Press).

SHEEHAN, J. and M. MARTYN, 1970. "Stuttering and Its Disappearance," *Journal of Speech and Hearing Research*, 13: 279–289.

SHRIBERG, L., and J. KWIATKOWSKI, 1980. *National Process Analysis (NPA): A Procedure for Phonological Analyses of Continuous Speech Samples* (Baltimore, MD: University Park Press).

SHRIBERG, L, et al., 1975. "The Wisconsin Procedure for Appraisal of Clinical Competence (WPACC): Model and Data," *ASHA*, 17: 158–165.

SIEGEL, G., 1970. "Punishment, Stuttering and Disfluency," *Journal of Speech and Hearing Disorders*, 13: 677–714.

――――, 1988. "Science and Communication Disorders: A Reply to Bloodstein," *Journal of Speech and Hearing Disorders*, 53: 348–349.

SKINNER, B.F., 1953. *Science and Human Behavior* (New York: Macmillan).

SKOLNICK, M.L. and G.N. McCALL, 1972. "Velopharyngeal Competence and Incompetence Following Pharyngeal Flap Surgery; A Video-Fluroscopic Study in Multiple Projections," *Cleft Palate Journal*, 9 1–10.

SMITH, A. and C. WEBER, 1988. "The Need for an Integrated Perspective on Stuttering," *ASHA*, 30: 30–31.

SOCHUREK, H., 1987. "Medicine's New Vision," *National Geographic*, 171: 2–41.

SPOCK, B. and M. ROTHENBERG, 1985. *Dr. Spock's Baby & Child Care: Fortieth Anniversary Edition* (New York: Dutton).

ST. LOUIS, K. and A. HINZMAN, 1988. "A Descriptive Study of Speech, Language and Hearing Characteristics of School-age Stutterers," *Journal of Fluency Disorders*, 13: 331–356.

STARBUCK, H., 1974. "Motivation/Part Two," in *Therapy for Stutterers*, ed. C. Starkweather (Memphis, TN.: Speech Foundation of America).

STARKWEATHER, C. ed., 1974. *Therapy for Stutterers* (Memphis, TN.: Speech Foundation of America).

STARKWEATHER, C. W., 1982. *Stuttering and Laryngeal Behavior*, (Rockville, MD: *ASHA, Monographs*), 21.

STARKWEATHER, C. W., 1987. *Fluency and Stuttering* (Englewood Cliffs, NJ: Prentice-Hall, Inc.).

STERN, J., L. WALRATH, and R. GOLDSTEIN, 1984. "The Endogenous Eyeblink," *Psychophysiology*, 21: 22–33.

STEVENS, K., D. KALIKOW, and T. WILLEMAIN, 1979. "Research Note: A Miniature Accelerometer for Detecting Glottal Waveforms and Nasalization," *Journal of Speech and Hearing Research*, 18: 594–599.

STOCKER, B., 1976. *Stocker Probe Technique for Diagnosis and Treatment of Stuttering in Young Children* (Tulsa, OK: Modern Education Corporation).

STROMSTA, C., 1986. *Elements of Stuttering* (Oshtemo, MI: Atmorts Publishing).

STROMSTA, C. and S. Fibiger, 1980. "Physiological Correlates of the Core Behavior of Stuttering." Paper presented to eighteenth *IALP Congress*, Washington, D.C.

TANNER, D. and N. CANNON, 1978. *Stuttering: Parental Diagnostic Questionnaire* (Tulsa, OK: Modern Education Corporation).

TATE, M. and W. CULLINAN, 1962. "Measurement of Consistency of Stuttering," *Journal of Speech and Hearing Research*, 5: 272–283.

THOMAS, M. et al., 1972. *Free to Be You and Me* (New York: Bell Records).

THOMPSON, A., 1985. "A Test of the Distraction Explanation of Disfluency Modification in Stuttering," *Journal of Fluency Disorders*, 10: 35–50.

THOMPSON, J., 1983. *Assessment of Fluency in School-Age Children*, Resource Guide (Danville, IL: Interstate Printers and Publishers).

THORNDIKE, E., 1913. *The Psychology of Learning*, Educational psychology, II (New York: Columbia University's Teacher College).

THORNER, R. and Q. REMEIN, 1982. "Principles and Procedures in the Evaluation of Screening for Disease," in *Hearing Measurement: A Book of Readings*, 4th ed., eds. J. Chaiklin, I. Ventry, and R. Dixon (Reading, MA: Addison-Wesley Publishing).

TRAVIS, L., 1931. *Speech Pathology* (New York: Appleton).

TURNER, P., 1969. *Clinical Aspects of Autonomic Pharmacology* (Philadelphia, PA: Lippincott).

VAILLANT, G., 1977. *Adaptation to Life* (Boston: Little, Brown and Co.).

VAN RIPER, C., 1970. "Historical Approaches," in *Stuttering: Research and Therapy*, ed. J. Sheehan (New York: Harper & Row, Pub.).

_____, 1971. *The Nature of Stuttering* (Englewood Cliffs, NJ: Prentice-Hall, Inc.).

_____, 1973. *The Treatment of Stuttering* (Englewood Cliffs, NJ: Prentice-Hall, Inc.).

_____, 1974. "Modification of Behavior," in *Therapy for Stutterers*, ed. C. Starkweather (Memphis, TN.: Speech Foundation of America).

_____, 1975. "The Stutterer's Clinician," in *Stuttering: A Second Symposium*, ed. J. Eisenson (New York: Harper & Row, Pub.).

VENTRY, I. and N. SCHIAVETTI, 1986. *Evaluating Research in Speech Pathology and Audiology*, 2nd ed. (New York: Macmillan).

WALL, M. and F. MYERS, 1984. *Clinical Management of Childhood Stuttering* (Baltimore, MD: University Park Press).

WATSON, B. and P. ALPHONSO, 1982. "A Comparison of LRT and VOT Values Between Stutterers and Nonstutterers," *Journal of Fluency Disorders*, 7: 219–242.

WEBSTER, R., 1975. *The Precision Fluency Shaping Program: Clinician's Program Guide* (Blacksburg, VA: University Publications).

_____, 1978. "Empirical Considerations Regarding Stuttering Therapy," in *Controversies About Stuttering Therapy*, ed. H. Gregory (Baltimore, MD: University Park Press).

WEBSTER, W., 1988. "Neural Mechanisms Underlying Stuttering: Evidence from Bimanual Handwriting Performance," *Brain and Language*, 33: 226–244.

WILLIAMS, D. E., 1957. "A Point of View About 'Stuttering,'" *Journal of Speech and Hearing Disorders*, 22: 390–397.

_____, 1968. "Stuttering Therapy: An Overview," in *Learning Theory and Stuttering Therapy*, ed. H. Gregory (Evanston, IL: Northwestern University Press).

_____, 1971. "Stuttering Therapy for Children," in *Handbook of Speech Pathology and Audiology*, ed. L.E. Travis (Englewood Cliffs, NJ: Prentice-Hall, Inc.).

_____, 1974. "Evaluation," in *Therapy for Stutterers*, ed. C. Starkweather (Memphis, TN.: Speech Foundation of America).

_____, 1978. "A Perspective on Approaches to Stuttering Therapy," in *Controversies About Stuttering Therapy*, ed. H. Gregory (Baltimore, MD: University Park Press).

WILLIAMS, D. and L. KENT, 1958. "Listener Evaluations of Speech Interruptions," *Journal of Speech and Hearing Research*, 1: 124–131.

WILLIAMS D. and F. SILVERMAN, 1968. "Note Concerning Articulation of School-age Stutterers," *Perceptual and Motor Skills*, 27: 713–714.

WILLIAMS, D., F. SILVERMAN, and J. KOOLS, 1969. "Disfluency Behavior of Elementary-School Age Stutterers and Nonstutterers: The Consistency Effects," *Journal of Speech and Hearing Research*, 12: 301–307.

WINGATE, M. E., 1964. "A Standard Definition of Stuttering," *Journal of Speech and Hearing Disorders*, 29: 484–489.

_____, 1969. "Sound and Pattern in 'Artificial' Fluency," *Journal of Speech and Hearing Research*, 12: 677–686.

_____, 1971. "The Fear of Stuttering," *ASHA*, 13: 3–5.

_____, 1976. *Stuttering Theory and Treatment* (New York: Irvington Publishers).

WINITZ, H., 1961. "Repetitions in the Vocalizations of Children in the First Two Years of Life," *Journal of Speech and Hearing Disorders*, Monogra Supplies 7: 55–62.

WINITZ, H., 1969. *Articulatory Acquisition and Behavior* (Englewood Cliffs, NJ: Prentice-Hall, Inc.).

WINN, M., 1977. *The Plug-In Drug* (New York: Viking).

WOODS, C. and D. WILLIAMS, 1976. "Traits Attributed to Stuttering and Normally Fluent Males," *Journal of Speech and Hearing Research*, 19: 267–278.

WOODS, C. L. and D.E. WILLIAMS, 1971. "Speech Clinicians' Conceptions of Boys and Men Who Stutter," *Journal of Speech and Hearing Disorders*, 36: 225–234.

YAIRI, E. and N. F. CLIFTON, JR., 1972. "Disfluent Speech Behavior of Preschool Children, High School Seniors, and Geriatric Persons," *Journal of Speech and Hearing Research*, 15: 714–719.

YAIRI, E., 1981. "Disfluencies of Normally Speaking Two-year-old Children," *Journal of Speech and Hearing Research*, 24: 490–495.

_____, 1982. "Longitudinal Studies of Disfluencies in Two-year-old Children," *Journal of Speech and Hearing Research*, 25: 155–160.

_____, 1983. "The Onset of Stuttering in Two- and Three-year-old Children: A Preliminary Report," *Journal of Speech and Hearing Disorders*, 48: 171–178.

YAIRI, E. and S. JENNINGS, 1974. ''Relationship Between the Disfluent Speech Behavior of Normal

Speaking Preschool Boys and Their Parents," *Journal of Speech and Hearing Research*, 17: 94–98.

YAIRI, E. and B. LEWIS, 1984. "Disfluencies at the Onset of Stuttering," *Journal of Speech and Hearing Research*, 27: 155–159.

YOUNG, M., 1984. "Identification of Stuttering and Stutterers," in *Nature and Treatment of Stuttering: New Directions*, eds. R. Curlee and W. Perkins (San Diego, CA: College-Hill Press).

ZEBROWSKI, P., E. CONTURE, and E. CUDAHY, 1985. "Acoustic Analysis of Young Stutterers' Fluency," *Journal of Fluency Disorders*, 10: 173–192.

ZEBROWSKI, P. and E. CONTURE, 1989. "Judgments of Disfluency by Mothers of Stuttering and Normally Fluent Children," *Journal of Speech and Hearing Research*, 32: 307–317.

ZILBERGELD, B., and M. EVANS, 1980. "The Inadequacy of Masters and Johnson," *Psychology Today*, 14: 28–43.

ZIMMERMAN, G., 1980a. "Articulatory Dynamics of Fluent Utterances of Stutterers and Nonstutterers," *Journal of Speech and Hearing Research*, 23: 95–107.

——, 1980b. "Articulatory Behaviors Associated with Stuttering: A Cinefluorographic Analysis," *Journal of Speech and Hearing Research*, 23: 108–121.

ZIMMERMAN, J., V. STEINER, and R. POND, 1979. *Preschool Language Scale*, rev ed. (Columbus, OH: Charles E. Merrill Co.).

ZWITMAN, D., 1978. *The Disfluent Child* (Baltimore, MD: University Park Press).

INDEX